THE NEARNESS OF OTHERS

Searching for Tact and Contact in the Age of HIV

David Caron

University of Minnesota Press
Minneapolis
London

Portions of "Tact" were previously published as "Tactful Encounters: AIDS, the Holocaust, and the Problematics of Bearing Witness," *Yale French Studies* 118–19 (2010): 155–73. Portions of "Disclosure" were previously published as "Adventures in Online Cruising," *Achieve: A Quarterly Journal on HIV Prevention, Treatment, and Politics* 5, nos. 1–2 (2012): 6–9.

Copyright 2014 by the Regents of the University of Minnesota

Published by the University of Minnesota Press
111 Third Avenue South, Suite 290
Minneapolis, MN 55401–2520
http://www.upress.umn.edu

Library of Congress Cataloging-in-Publication Data
Caron, David (David Henri), author.
The nearness of others : searching for tact and contact in the age of HIV / David Caron.
Includes bibliographical references and index.
ISBN 978-0-8166-9175-3 (hc)
ISBN 978-0-8166-9179-1 (pb)
1. HIV-positive gay men—Biography. 2. HIV-positive gay men—Psychology. I. Title.
RC606.55.C37 2014
362.19697'920086642—dc23
2013050941

Printed in the United States of America on acid-free paper

The University of Minnesota is an equal-opportunity educator and employer.

20 19 18 17 16 15 14   10 9 8 7 6 5 4 3 2 1

Our hands are often carried where we direct them not.

—Montaigne

CONTENTS

Others / 53

Diagnosis

I GOT SLIM

On Wednesday, May 24, 2006, at three o'clock in the afternoon and about two hours before I was supposed to fly to Montreal for a dissertation defense and a carefully orchestrated weekend of dirty fun, in a dreary medical examination room decorated (there's got to be a better word really . . .) with images of body parts and admonitions to quit smoking before something really bad happened to me, I learned that I was HIV positive, and, just like that, my body, which for the past few years I had kept casually entertained with liquor, cigarettes, and strangers while giving little thought to any of it, reentered my mind, becoming once again the companion, familiar and strange, of my attempts at making sense of a world that, in the aftermath of 9/11, had become sick with wars, torture, and rebranded hatreds, and felt more vicious and more brutal with each passing day.

My doctor delivered the "bad news," as he called it, so swiftly and efficiently that I'd swear my whole world flipped over before his backside even hit the chair. The man was, after all, used to removing bandages by trade, and I had the impression that he would also make a great executioner. After he assured me that HIV no longer meant an automatic death sentence, he admitted somewhat sheepishly that, although several of his patients were HIV positive, this was the first time he had to tell one of them. I guess this explained the flash card he wasn't even pretending not to read from. This was a big event for him too, and he seemed a bit distraught by the whole experience, as if it had been his own bandage he had ripped off, his own pain he could not face. And please, do not read more than a touch of irony into this. Our difficulties may not have been of the same nature, or even degree, but, as odd as this may sound, sharing them helped both of us.

"Did you know?" he asked me with a mysterious tone and a penetrating gaze, as though the virus had given me some sort of supernatural powers. "Er, no," I replied. "I . . . I had no fucking idea, to be honest with you, and this comes as a bit of a shock." A few minutes later, I paid my $15 co-pay to a smiling staff person who told me to have a nice day, and I was on my way—but not to Montreal. In fact, I also canceled my annual trip to France (although not, for a million years, a long-planned outing to see Rufus Wainwright do Judy Garland at Carnegie Hall, an event so hyped that a friend of mine who tried in vain to find a ticket to the long-sold-out show crowned me "the luckiest faggot in all of New York") and, with two wars raging somewhere far away on a globally warming planet, I spent the rest of my summer working out like a maniac and cultivating my garden. Thank goodness, this Candide phase of blissful oblivion was to be short-lived. A man can eat only so much rhubarb. And it wasn't long before I remembered that I actually hate gardening. Still, my body soon looked so fit and so trim that when school started in the fall my friends and colleagues, who hadn't seen me in months, inundated me with compliments and concerned inquiries about the state of my health. "I'm perfectly fine," I told them, thinking, "For fuck's sake, can't I just look fabulous without everyone wondering what they're going to wear at the funeral? Gardening is no longer an automatic death sentence, you know."

It all went downhill after that. I thought I was at my sexiest when I really looked unwell, as some friends finally told me once I had put a few pounds back on. To make matters worse, the stress was such that I simply couldn't stand the contact of anyone other than my inner circle of friends. Between my fear of other people and other people's fear of me, my new slimness wasn't exactly put to good use. I know, there are many ways for a man to feel like a homosexual. There's the sharing of all sorts of cultural codes and social spaces, virtual and otherwise; the worshipping of dead stars; the rarefied exercise of unusual tastes; the excessive consumption of cocktails with Campari in them; the experience of shame, insults, and discrimination; and many other such niceties, but it doesn't hurt to have sex with men every once in a while. Men, however, wouldn't come near me and I wouldn't go near them. Oddly, I felt a simultaneous waxing and waning of corporeality.

I used to be generous with my body, you see. People would frequent it as we once did that restaurant in the East Village, Kiev, on Second Avenue—not the classiest joint in town, to be sure, but a no-nonsense kind of place, affordable, open all night, welcoming to the sort of people your mother warned you never to welcome and to the ones she never imagined could possibly exist, and capable of hitting the spot when the spot needed to be hit. Now it felt more like Ground Zero, with sightseers hovering curiously over it, yet staying at an awed distance. (Could it be rebuilt? reopened for business?) And, like Ground Zero, it had become one of the symbolic epicenters of a larger catastrophe that has claimed many lives for no good reason at all. I suddenly had the feeling that my body was not so much in the world but, rather, that the world, with its endless procession of catastrophes, wars, and acts of brutality and humiliation, was now in my body. I had become a synecdoche.

This book represents my attempt to put this body, my new, strange body, back where it belongs—right there in the rhythm of it all, ebbing and flowing with the crowd, a body among bodies, on the beat. Of course, this should also be an opportunity to reflect not just on my own body but on yours and on the body in general—on its simultaneous strangeness and familiarity and on its power to bring people in closer contact if one would only put one's mind to it.

FOOTNOTES

Adam Mars-Jones was wondering what the literature of AIDS should look like: "Perhaps only a customized form of the novel could adequately represent both the reality of the virus and its irrelevance, its irrelevance even to those whose lives it threatens. Imagine for instance a story interrupted by a footnote that grows to book length, the text never resuming." Think of this book's form more or less in the same way—a series of footnotes and no story resuming ever.

RB ON TB

Roland Barthes once wrote this caption above a photograph of himself taken after his recovery from tuberculosis: "Sudden mutation of the body (after leaving the sanatorium): changing (or appearing to change) from slender to plump. Ever since, perpetual struggle with this body to return it to its essential slenderness (part of the intellectual's mythology: to become thin is the naïve act of the will-to-intelligence)."

As I developed a genuine intelligence of my body—I mean, when it became more intelligible to my mind—I regained some of the weight I'd lost in the aftermath of the diagnosis. Was my initial desire to slim down at such a breakneck pace nothing other than a quest for physical erasure? A mad attempt at getting rid of the virus, the unwanted guest that crashed the party, by withdrawing not only the invitation but the host himself?

ALL AIDS, ALL THE TIME!

I had the terrible misfortune of testing positive for HIV on the eve of the epidemic's silver jubilee. It was indeed in early summer 1981 that the first articles appeared, describing unusual clusters of rare diseases among gay men in New York and Los Angeles. A quarter of a century later, I found myself caught in the hoopla surrounding the anniversary. Every newspaper, TV news show, and Internet wire service, it seemed, was giving AIDS the royal treatment. The four-letter word kept jumping at me from all corners at once. AIDS! AIDS! AIDS! AIDS!!! And it felt as though it was all about me personally—which of course it was. Picking up the *New York Times* in front of my house every morning became an ordeal. So did turning on my computer or the TV. What were they all going to say about me today? I didn't feel bombarded so much as stoned.

IT IS TEMPTING TO FORGET

2006. Twenty-five years of AIDS.

It is tempting to forget the morning rituals, when you inspected your body for lesions that might have appeared during the night and signal that *it* had started.

It is tempting to forget that when you asked, "Does this spot look purple to you?" you didn't need to say anything else for everyone around you to know just what was on your mind, if not on your skin, and how fast your heart was racing as you uttered the words as casually as you could because sounding casual seemed to increase the chances of a reassuring response.

It is tempting to forget that there was a time when gay men were hoping *not* to lose weight, that plump meant healthy and healthy reassuring. And reassuring, in a turnabout so shocking for us then, meant sexy.

It is tempting to forget that people were dropping like flies, that many gay men in cities like New York or San Francisco were crossing out name after name from their address books, sometimes losing their entire circle of friends and sometimes being the next name to be crossed out of other people's address books, and it is tempting to forget that many gay men who had long left their families behind in favor of friendships were now left only with mere acquaintances, no one close still living.

It is tempting to forget how parents who had once expelled their faggot son now rushed to his bedside to keep the lovers and friends away, to contest the will, and to snatch the spoils of a life lived far from the tender bosom of the family.

It is tempting to forget that women never "got" AIDS but somehow died of it by the thousands.

It is tempting to forget that the truth could only be whispered or screamed but seldom simply told.

It is tempting to forget that kids were chased out of schools by their friends' parents and by their friends and that their houses were burned to the ground.

It is tempting to forget that Ryan White was once described as a "homophiliac" in a newspaper.

It is tempting to forget the frightened medics and undertakers and the cops' face masks and latex gloves, as they arrested dying young men and women fighting for their lives.

It is tempting to forget ACT UP's unforgettable chant, "They'll see you on the news; your gloves don't match your shoes!"

It is tempting to forget angry queers screaming bloody murder and spitting out hosts in St. Patrick's Cathedral in New York.

It is tempting to forget the pictures of Dorian Gray on TV and on the pages of magazines, the emaciated faces covered with lesions, the hollow stares, and the feeling that one might as well have been looking at a charred and contorted body hanging from a tree, like Billie Holiday's strange fruit, as the crowd cheered.

It is tempting to forget gay-related immune deficiency and the gay cancer and the 4-H club—homosexual, heroin addict, hemophiliac, Haitian—and all the conspiracy theories and miracle cures that we knew were bullshit yet couldn't help but consider just in case, because madness could make sense.

It is tempting to forget the promise of a vaccine in about five years and that it felt like such an eternity that researchers sounded almost apologetic when explaining that retroviruses are particularly treacherous foes.

It is tempting to forget the calls for quarantine camps and tattoos and mass expulsions, "solutions" whose pros and cons were discussed with the sort of equanimity now applied to the debate on torture.

It is tempting to forget that nobody gave a shit.

It is tempting to forget that all this is still happening far, far away from here.

It is tempting to forget and it is easy.

NIGHTS YOU CAN'T SLEEP

Food you can't eat
Diseases you can't catch
Skins you can't touch
Sex you can't have
Friends you can't tell
Lovers you can't shelter
Facts you can't withhold
Silence you can't keep
Countries you can't enter
Jobs you can't hold
Bills you can't pay
Facilities you can't use
People you can't marry
People you can't count on
People you can't drink with
Fountains you can't drink from
Pools you can't swim in
Bus seats you can't sit on
Votes you can't cast
Freedom you can't enjoy
Roundups you can't escape
Time you can't have
Lives you can't live
Deaths you can't die
Nights you can't sleep

DEPRESSION IS CRAZY

For an academic to admit to being clinically depressed can be tricky, because to disclose that your mind isn't functioning as it should is to disqualify yourself, to risk rendering irrelevant everything you do or say as a professional thinker. Depression, in fact, often feels like being raped by thoughts, monstrous, deformed thoughts. They force themselves on your mind and leave you shattered and ashamed. It's simpler, at times, to give in to your attackers than to resist them, but you know that once they're done, the respite will be short-lived, and they're going to come for you again. Your thoughts are smarter than you when you're depressed, and you can't fool them very long. Sometimes depression feels as though no thought were involved whatever—like an effect without a cause. *It* happens and you don't know why. There may be warnings or there may be no warnings. There are, at times, signs that, like a prophecy, you can decipher only in hindsight, but nothing you can act on in any case. Even though depression is a madness that you are aware of, you read its signs but can learn nothing from them. You may find the strength to run for cover or you may not. Some mornings, you wake up and the nightmares begin. You can tell right away that your entire day will be pure hell, and because you can't just skip a day you only wait for it to end. Evenings feel like torture, mornings like death. Even when feelings remain under control, that is to say, kept under wraps, you know that, every morning, you open your eyes to find that one more little chunk of you has come off during the night, one more shaving has fallen under the plane, until, one day, the end ceases to feel tragic to you and more like a simple matter of making the state of things official—as easy as blowing out the last candle when you leave the room, because there's no one left in it. Depression doesn't make you a different person exactly, it makes you disappear little by little until nothing of you remains. It is therefore misleading to lament the high suicide rate among sufferers because, in truth, they have died long before they kill themselves. What is odd, though, is that, as you feel yourself gradually cease to exist, the force of the madness—this complete lack of discernment—overcomes your body. First inside. For a second or two, your eyes just stare blankly at familiar surroundings but do not quite make out what they see. Your hands hold objects whose purpose momentarily escapes them. The destination of a pen or a glass of water, once obvious, now seems baffling or obscured by clouds and cannot be recollected without time and efforts. Your legs can no longer carry the rest of you, and they slowly give way under the crushing weight. This is what, as a kid, I imagined it felt like to walk on Jupiter. And then the madness begins to push through your skin, stretching it so it makes you want to holler in pain. You could tear at the gentlest touch and find yourself exposed to the humiliation of inappropriate leaking. But then *it* starts oozing out. You're turning into some kind of werewolf. When that happens you're lucky to be home and alone. If not, as if drunk or high and desperate to appear sober, you can only hope that you will be able to walk undetected among the others, the living, the normal people, just long enough to pass the old, gray church, the first bridge, the second bridge, the Korean grocery store, the usual, the casual, the incomprehensibly banal, all these places you once barely saw but stand out as ominous landmarks today, one more block, almost there, a few more steps, just a few more steps until, finally, you can close the door behind you, lean against it, and stare at nothing, beaten, breathless, relieved at last to let the pain have its way with you because it's just easier that way and because, sometimes, the only relief you can expect to bring to your pain is pain of a different sort. It is astounding the amount of strength weakness requires, and the control and sharpness of thought that madness demands of the mad—and none of it recognized. Depression isn't sadness, it's madness, and trying to pass for sane feels excruciating for no other reason, perhaps, than it keeps reminding you of this inescapable truth: one is always depressed alone.

DEPRESSION AND LIFE

If Buddhism is correct and all life amounts to suffering, depression can become endemic only in cultures that do not have at their core a philosophy that takes this simple truth not only into account but as a foundation. What in lands far, far away from my house makes life so livable is the serene knowledge that it is unlivable. Depression, I believe, results from the tension between that knowledge and a stubborn resistance to it.

DEPRESSION AND METAPHOR

Given a choice, I'd pick HIV over depression any day. You can live with HIV. Depression, however, feels like such a complete denial of life that it becomes a challenge to even put it into words. Imagine chronic back pain so agonizing, so crippling that when it hits, you can no longer perform some of the most basic gestures required to function in the world around you. Even in moments of respite, you sense the pain's lurking presence, a constant companion, quiet at times but liable to strike without warning. Now imagine that pain not in your back but in your mind. That's depression.

The difficulty that one encounters when attempting to describe what depression feels like without resorting to corporeal metaphors testifies to the convenience of tropes with a strong evocative efficacy. But this also reminds us of our inability to think in purely abstract terms, of the deficiencies of pure reason. To relate, that is, to transmit and share our thoughts with others, we need the body. To put it metaphorically, as it were, corporeal metaphors are a bit like the body rushing back to reoccupy the space left vacant by its expulsion.

PASSING

I recognized early on that, in certain situations, it was better to keep the chaos in my mind safely hidden. In this I was helped by previous experiences of what you might call closetedness, or just discretion. Over the years, being gay, first, and now being HIV positive have given me the required skills with which to figure out when it is better to keep quiet and how to do it. With depression, things are a little different. When you are gay or poz, for example, discretion entails passing, whether explicitly or by omission, for someone or something you're not; in the case of depression you basically try to pass for you. In a sense, it is a bit like the opposite of the closet—yet still the closet. Unable to retrieve my old self buried too deep under the rubble of my past life, I sometimes find it more expedient to play him.

DEPRESSION AND INCONGRUITY

Depression kicked in when it occurred to me that not only was I HIV positive but I still had to do the laundry. Having entered the world of AIDS didn't mean that I'd abandoned the world I inhabited before—the world in which someone's got to do the dishes and light bulbs don't just change themselves.

There is something incongruous in the uneasy proximity of a world's crisis and your personal life, of a momentous disruption and the unruffled continuation of the mundane, of what's too big to grasp and what's too small to ignore, of the call to heroism and that of the everyday. Incongruous and productive. Two "events" as radically discontinuous in terms of magnitude and kind as AIDS and my laundry bled into each other when brought into contact. Household chores felt like an intolerably vulgar intrusion in the face of my seropositivity, yes, but the inescapable fact that menial tasks had to be performed also relegated HIV itself to secondary status, and this generalized dynamic of contamination cut the tremendous down to size and defamiliarized the quotidian.

The fact that from such disruption depression emerged signaled to me that HIV means disorder in many senses of the term but also that there may be something interesting in the opportunity it offered me to reassess everything. To look at a glass of water and wonder for a second or two what you're expected to do with it can have this sort of effect on a person.

DEPRESSED THINKING

Call it mulling, call it ruminating, it is a strange way to think, and a mind in darkness often convinces itself that it sees with clarity. But even though your thoughts seem to be going around and around without aim or point, they are thoughts, they are going somewhere—only they're not taking the straightest path to get there. Yet to think in circles and in excess, to ponder too much, too long, and too deeply—what French speakers call *ressasser*—is often perceived to be the opposite of thought because it doesn't go anywhere. Today, we largely see medicalization as progress because to think of depression as a pathological disorder cloaks it, as well as other mental disturbances, in the sort of objective discourse that is supposed to preclude moral judgment. It seems hardly necessary to show once more that this alleged objectivity of medical discourse is, in reality, shot through with ideology and moralism. Especially pernicious with this operation, however, is the way it isolates "the patient" by individualizing his or her suffering. To define depression as a disorder afflicting individuals allows order, by contrast, to remain the normal condition, and normalizing force, of the social. This is what I meant when I noted that one is always depressed alone: depression, understood as a disease of the mind, is too often denied its potential for relationality. Who in their right mind would want to partake in it? Pathologization isolates more powerfully than condemnation. Moral misery, however, loves company. In fact it thrives on it, which is why melancholia, unlike clinical depression, may represent an alternative way of thinking and being in the world as a kind of collective alienation. Depressed thinking, in other words, is thinking with and across difference, and it is a manner of sharing.

MAKING SENSE

The amount of attention I lavished on my body in the days, weeks, and months that followed the diagnosis looks, in hindsight, completely unreasonable. There was nothing I could do other than take my medications and update my vaccinations. Looking better or giving my days a semblance of order by filling them up to the brim with activities of all kinds—gardening? what was I thinking?—would have no bearing on my actual health, and I knew it. Of course, focusing on my looks didn't come out of nowhere. Since at least the nineteenth century, we have been trained to see beauty as a marker of health and to connect illness with disorder. The fact that I'd once written a book about these very matters didn't keep me from falling, ignorant, into their trap. I seemed to have lost my mind, and it all felt like complete clarity. You can go quite mad with worry, but you may not be aware of it. To worry is a uniquely temporal form of anxiety: it is time gone mad. To worry is to envision the future as completely unhinged from reason, that is to say, as the confirmation of radical disorder rather than as a source of meaning. Trying to look good after testing positive for HIV thus seemed to make sense.

When a while later, long after I, for one, had overcome that initial stage (I can't speak for others), I looked again at David Feinberg's AIDS novel *Eighty-Sixed* and couldn't repress a smile of recognition as I read this: *"After I was mugged three times in January of 1983, I started shaving every day."* The ostensible lack of logical connection between the two contiguous clauses of this sentence made total sense to me. Irrational as the narrator's behavior was, I could still *understand* it. I too had gone through seemingly crazy actions whose purpose was to restore order to a life that had found itself in utter disarray. Naturally, it wasn't the actions themselves that made sense but their normalcy and their power to anchor me to a world from which I felt myself drifting. The more these small actions blurred the boundaries between health, morality, and social conformity, the more they worked. Feinberg again:

> I used Q-tips on my ears. I flossed daily. I wore a tie to work. I
> ate three balanced meals. I started the day off with a handful of
> vitamins, milk, juice, toast, and bran cereal. I had a regular bowel
> movement at precisely ten o'clock. I slept for seven hours each night.
> I went to the gym every day. Each night I would apply moisturizer
> with care, making sure not to miss any spots.

Much later I realized that I went through these routines as if they had some mystical significance. On some superstitious level I believed that if I maintained the pattern, I would remain unharmed in the future.

But nothing guaranteed that the phone wouldn't ring in the middle of the night with bad news.

It's amazing how many of these same activities I, too, undertook with the same compulsion after I was mugged by my diagnosis. In these crazy months, being so systematic about such things felt just like reason. Except of course that behaving in a way that, if pathologized, would be called obsessive compulsive, is anything but, or rather, it is a simulacrum of reason. It is magical thinking masquerading as a system, a bit like religion.

If all these allegedly irrational behaviors made sense—and they did: they were not manifestations of denial but useful stages in a process of acceptance—it wasn't the sort of sense that one measures against an absolute, transcendent value but in relation to specific needs in a specific context. With the sudden irruption of senselessness in life, it seems wiser to resist the urge to restore sense and try, instead, to invent something new, thus acknowledging the incongruity—the absence of congruence—and work with it rather than against it. This may all have been madness passing as reason, but it did what it was supposed to. Call it need-based reason.

POLITICAL DISCOMFORT

As this book moves along, it will become clearer that my actual forays into the chaos of unreason provide opportunities to rethink the Enlightenment's concept of reason and the social order this concept has grounded. I am far from being the first scholar to do so, of course. My thinking owes much to Michel Foucault's early work, for example, and has found inspiration more recently in that of the Foucault scholar Lynne Huffer. And I do not mean to imply that the Enlightenment has ever constituted a homogeneous philosophy, that it was never uncontested from within, or that it wasn't altered by the material conditions that enable thought in the first place. The mind lives in the world, and the world is a mess. Precisely, the problems I raise have to do with the ways in which modes of thought have played out in people's actual lives, including my own.

Yet for someone like me, who was not only raised in France but trained as a scholar of French literature and culture, to criticize the Enlightenment may still raise political suspicions. True, before Jacques Derrida and the deconstruction of Cartesian thinking, a great deal of the political opposition to the Enlightenment came from a brand of extreme-right ideology rooted in its historical hostility to the French Revolution and the republican regime that emerged from it in fits and starts. Without getting lost in details, let's just say that the new right-wing nationalism that appeared in the 1890s argued against the influence of Kantian philosophy, against "Man" as an abstract, universal concept, and in favor of a kind of organic rather than contractual culture rooted in what Maurice Barrès called "the land and the dead" ("la terre et les morts"), a nation beyond the control of individual, rational subjects. The opposition between two incompatible ideas reached its first frenzied peak during the Dreyfus affair, which famously pitted Barrès against Emile Zola and laid out two camps that were to fight each other for supremacy in the twentieth century.

It would be shortsighted, however, to think that the demise of Nazi Germany has relegated irrational notions of culture to religious extremism and the political fringe. Case in point: the fascinating, if utterly depressing, controversy that is, as I am writing this, unfolding around the building of a so-called victory mosque at Ground Zero in Manhattan. Forget even that Park51, as the project is called, is neither a mosque (it's really a kind of Muslim YMCA with a prayer room) nor *at* Ground Zero (it's two blocks north of it). I'm not going to reargue the issue. What interests me here is how opponents of the project, whether cynical exploiters of popular anger or their gullible followers, are sometimes perfectly ready to admit that Muslims have a right to build the cultural center there but that it would be insensitive to do so. More forceful terms may include "affront," "offense" and "disrespect," and what all have in common is that they pertain to emotion rather than thought. So much so, in fact, that the conservative *New York Times* commentator Ross Douthat penned a column about the tension between "Islam and the Two Americas." This is what he writes:

> There's an America where it doesn't matter what language you speak, what god you worship, or how deep your New World roots run. An America where allegiance to the Constitution trumps ethnic differences, language barriers and religious divides. An America where the newest arrival to our shores is no less American than the ever-so-great granddaughter of the Pilgrims.
>
> But there's another America as well, one that understands itself as a distinctive culture, rather than a set of political propositions.

How "culture" is defined against (liberal-democratic) politics makes Douthat's column something Barrès could have endorsed. Needless to say, Douthat favors such a culture, the one populist conservatives have been calling "the real America," over the abstract principles on which the nation was founded. Of imam Feisal Abdul Rauf, the Sufi cleric who is "behind the mosque" (Muslim leaders and deciders, like the Jews of old, are always "behind," it seems, as if hiding something as well as themselves), Douthat says, "By global standards, Rauf may be the model of a 'moderate Muslim.' [Note the quotation marks.] But global standards and American standards are different."

This historical tension between a contractual kind of nation founded on universal principles and an organic, national one founded on inarguable emotions is indeed a reality in American society, just as it is in France and, I'm assuming, in every other country owing its dominant political culture to the Enlightenment's concept of reason. In the case of Park51, the rhetoric of sensitivity is intended to thwart all arguments based on law, logic, and principles, including ethical ones, in the name of an emotion supposedly so obvious and visceral that it need not and cannot be articulated, and so widely shared in the "culture" that not feeling it is a sure sign that one doesn't belong in it. Barack Obama's argument about constitutional rights is not just a sure loser, from this perspective; it is yet another indication that he is not really "one of us" and must therefore be foreign born and a Muslim, as so many Americans continue to believe in the face of indisputable evidence to the contrary.

This appeal to affect against reason as a basis for culture recalls a certain rhetoric that became popular in France and that Nicolas Sarkozy used often, first when he was interior minister and then as president. The term is *incivilités*, and it refers to a vague list of acts, such as vandalism, petty crimes, rudeness, and all sorts of improper social behaviors allegedly committed in public places by working-class kids who live in the projects and who are tacitly understood as being of immigrant origin. The word *incivilité* had become somewhat obsolete and literary until it was revived in recent years and popularized, one assumes, because it suggests that, thanks to their common etymology, civility and citizenship may also be organically connected and, it is implied, equally unavailable to people not born into it. The same logic allowed Sarkozy to order the deportation of thousands of Roma from France even though, as Romanian and Bulgarian nationals for the most part, they hold European Union citizenship. (This policy seems to be continuing under Sarkozy's successor.) This naked appeal to supporters of Jean-Marie Le Pen's Front National is explained by these angry voters' resistance to the sort of argumentative refutation and appeal to principles that have never had the slightest effect on the rise of the extreme Right in France since the mid-1980s.

Similarly, arguing in the name of legal rights and religious freedom against opponents of Park51 serves little purpose. Someone who agrees that Muslims have a right to build a cultural center near Ground Zero but should relinquish that right because it would be insensitive to claim it cares very little about the basic tenets of the constitution if a yet-to-be-defined sensitivity is enough to trump them in their eyes. When a point cannot be articulated, neither can a counterpoint. That's the trick: affect on one side, inaudibility or gibberish on the other (or jargon if the opponent's an academic). For Barrès, it mattered little that Dreyfus could be proved innocent of espionage; being Jewish was enough to make one a traitor. Ground Zero, as a site both real and symbolic, has become to some an American version of "the land and the dead," a milder version perhaps, but still a rich, nurturing soil for a sense of belonging that cannot be willed.

Obviously, the critique that animates this book is of a different kind. Universalism never liked me much, it's true, but I also find identity politics repulsive because, at their worst, they bear an unmistakable resemblance to fascism. Mandatory reason is causing me to suffer, but I do not expect nonthought or inarticulateness to bring any solace, as if by magic. I wouldn't be writing a book if it could—especially not a book about contact. What classical reason and fascist culture have in common, in the end, is the discriminating logic that propels them both. This doesn't entail an ethical or political equivalence between the two, only overlapping potentialities. But there exist in the world modes of thinking that don't fall in either of these two categories after all. So this book, then, is an attempt to bring together as many approaches to the elaboration of knowledge as I can without ever hoping to see them fuse into "the whole picture" or lead to a unifying conclusion. For one thing, I don't see knowledge that way, but, more crucially, who can see the "whole picture" of HIV, and what kind of conclusion would we be talking about exactly?

Through the different intellectual and thematic fragments that fill these pages, I don't simply intend to render the disjointedness of life with HIV. I do hope to convey some of that, of course, but this is also more than a formal experiment. One is not HIV positive in a cultural and political vacuum. In fact, there is no other experience of HIV than one that is saturated with politics and culture. That's why it's so messy and so slippery, so dynamic that it can never sit still long enough to constitute a stable object of knowledge. I am HIV positive in Ann Arbor, Michigan. I am an intellectual with a virus. I have access to excellent health care (I hope). I am HIV positive at a time when Islam is reviled by many. I am HIV positive after 9/11. I am HIV positive in a country engaged in a war on terror and on a planet warming like mad. I was HIV positive under George W. Bush and Dick Cheney, and now under the first African American president of the United States. I am HIV positive at a time when France rips headscarves off the faces of Muslim schoolgirls. I had an HIV-negative Chinese boyfriend for a while. I am an immigrant and the child of an immigrant. And if I am discussing HIV alongside torture or the forced unveiling of Muslim girls and women, it isn't simply because all involve certain bodies in problematic positions in relation to dominant cultures that feel disinclined to treat them fairly. All these events, these people, these bodies do not shed light on each other. They don't illuminate any larger, homogeneous truth but instead make their own contours blurrier through constant if ever-changing contact. They bleed into each other and contaminate thought itself.

THINKING OF BLEEDING

I'm doing the dishes. There's this really sharp knife. I don't know, perhaps I've had a bit too much to drink with dinner, perhaps I'm just too eager to show the friends who, as ever, have given me such loving and unquestioning hospitality that I'm trying to help out. Blood everywhere. All over the sink, the faucet, the dirty dishes—everywhere. I freak out, of course, but they seem to be OK with the whole gruesome incident. "Fuck, I'm so stupid," I say. "It's the knife that's stupid. I've always hated that knife," Nico replies. Blame the knife. The elegance of that man! I'm feeling ashamed and he's feeling guilty. Within two minutes, the place is cleaned up, and Guillaume has tightly dressed my hand. Of all the things that gay men inherit from their mothers, some are actually quite practical. Then we sit down at the kitchen table. The gushes of blood, it seems, have triggered a flow of words. I don't remember the details of what we talked about that night, only that we talked about *it*, and that although the big news was no longer so new and no longer so big by then, we had never really discussed it until the red, red blood on the white, white sink made it impossible to look away. Something had to come out and out it came. Gushing.

KIDS SAY THE DARNDEST THINGS

By and large, people were very nice to me when I was dead, but not everyone was so tactful.

One friend said to me: "So it *is* true, then. The more you sleep around the more likely you are to get it."

"Has this made you contemplate your own mortality?" asked a guy who obviously had issues I was wise to keep at bay. ("No, it hasn't," I should have replied, "but I'm beginning to contemplate yours right now.")

And there's the one who obviously had heard from someone else and, leaning over me, wrapped his arm around my shoulders, cocked his head ever so slightly and, in that . . . *tone*, inquired, "How *are* you?" I had the feeling that he actually cared very little how I was and that he only wanted me to know that he knew. Funny how a gay man's hand resting heavily on your shoulder used to say let's fuck but now means let's not. Funny how ostensible nearness really betrays distance sometimes. Funny how touchy (and probably unfair) this whole thing has made me.

And let's not forget those who saw the fact that I was dating an HIV-negative guy as an opportunity for me to rejoice: "You see? This shows that it's possible after all." Did they assume that only the HIV negative, such as themselves, may be the ultimate objects of my or anyone's desire?

Well, at least they said something.

NEGATIVE LOGIC AND A POSITIVE POINT OF VIEW

I once complained about this last point to a friend. He's HIV negative, and I didn't want to hurt his feelings, so I hastened to add, "Well, this may sound unreasonable of me, but I guess it's what you could call poz logic." "No," he retorted in the next breath, "it's not a logic, it's a point of view." Fair enough. The conversation took place in French, and I had used the phrase "une logique de séropo"—a poz person's logic—which didn't anchor what I called logic to an objective reality but to the subjectivity of someone drifting, rudderless, across rough seas, a far less stable proposition than the word *logic* alone would imply and perhaps even a contradiction in terms. So for the next couple of days, I mulled over this, wondering what the differences are between these two ways of thinking and whether each enjoys a particular relation to a specific serological (or sero-logical) status.

First of all, logic and point of view are not mutually exclusive. Because logic lays claim to the unspoiled, unsoiled objectivity that endows it with its legitimating power, it would be tempting to attach it to seronegativity, that is to say, to the status that represents the lack of contamination. In other words, logic is "clean." This could still account for the fact that HIV-negative people often behave illogically; they're only people, after all, material and imperfect vessels for abstract ideas. The inherent problem in the link between logic and purity is that the latter is not a permanent state. What defines the uncontaminated isn't its current status but the capacity to lose it, its susceptibility to infection. As an HIV-positive person, the fact of my contamination will never change. (Even in the unlikely event that someone discovered a cure that could rid my body of the virus, I don't think that I could ever again feel uncontaminated.) An HIV-negative person, however, cannot make a parallel claim to permanence, and if an HIV vaccine ever comes along, there are other viruses out there. To think of oneself as clean presupposes that one identifies in relation to dirt—a negative relation, to be sure, but a relation nonetheless. The notion of logic in relation to HIV status thus appears problematic from the get-go. Logic is logic much like reason is reason—thanks to the expulsion of what it isn't yet still is.

A point of view, then, represents a sort of ill logic, and it does so in two possible ways (at least) that make this mode of thinking especially pertinent in the context of HIV and AIDS. The illness of logic may be caused by some external entity that came into contact with it and entered it—a contingency in the full etymological sense of the term. Another way for logic to become ill would be for it to suffer from internal dysfunction, that is, a self-generated inability to put things, such as life, the world, and so on, in order. The first model would pertain to virology, the second to immunology.

But if logic isn't strictly objective, a point of view isn't strictly subjective either. Instead, we may think of a point of view as situational in that it indicates a certain localization in the world. It constitutes the thinking mode of the self-in-context. But situations, not to mention the world in which they take place, are both complex and ephemeral, unstable in terms of time and space. A point of view never reflects a person's organic relationship to a point that would guarantee the stability and clarity of a view. It always comprises a multiplicity of points, referenced or indexed, and thus a mode of viewing that doesn't imply objectification. It neither unifies the viewing subject nor reifies the viewed object. It is in that sense that a point of view cannot be strictly subjective (meaning, internal). Not only does it involve elements located in the world outside the subject, it also disrupts the very possibility of an enclosed, autonomous subject.

A point of view can therefore ground no claim to normativity. It emerges from a relational engagement with a variety of contexts—historical, social, scientific, moral, political, and so on—that are widely available for the sharing. It is contingent, but not in the way that ideology is the outcome of social relations. A point of view comes out of contacts and invents new ones with the help of whatever is at hand. It isn't simply that, say, Islamophobia affects my experience of being HIV positive because both are taking place in the same immediate environment; thinking about anti-Islamic sentiments, how they work, what they do, can help me make sense of my personal experience, and vice versa.

A point of view, then, constitutes a kind of bricolage applied to thought. A poz point of view in this case is not, structurally speaking, all that different from a queer one. It represents a convergence of multiple forces, many of them hostile, most of them external, that produce within a person's experience a divergent perspective that one may then redirect toward the world outside for various purposes. Just as "queer work," academically speaking, doesn't have to have homosexuality as its object, what we may call "poz work" may very well handle objects that, on the surface, have little in common with HIV and AIDS—except that these seemingly unrelated objects of examination contribute to the shaping of a poz experience. Such a point of view is both refracting and refractory; it breaks down the forces at play, laying out a web of connections but resisting the urge to synthesize them. Understood as bricolage, the point of view exposes the various components that brought it about, simultaneously altering and indexing their original intent.

"HOW CAN PLAIN CURIOSITY BE UNKIND?"

asks Hanif Kureishi in *My Ear at His Heart,* a book in which he dives into, and exposes, his family's archives, weaves his own text with those of others—chief among them his father's unpublished autobiographical novels—and wonders what right he has to do such things in the name of an exciting literary experimentation whose outcome remains by definition uncertain.

Questions, as such, are seldom indiscreet. No matter how personal they are, they do nothing more than come close to the edge. It is answers that may cross over to the other side and wreak havoc. We should be thankful that not all questions have answers, or else life would be unlivable.

TOWEL STORIES (1)

"Where's the towel you gave me the other day?"

"I threw it in the wash."

"But I hardly used it at all. It wasn't dirty."

"C'mon, it had blood on it, remember?"

His expression changed all of a sudden. He lowered his beautiful dark eyes almost imperceptibly, as if trying to avert what he thought would be my judging gaze.

"That was insensitive, wasn't it? I'm sorry."

It wasn't insensitive. It was, if not quite reasonable, at least understandable.

He was HIV negative.

He was a kind and touching lover.

And we kept our towels clean.

DIABETES? CHOLESTEROL? SOMETHING ELSE?

Hoping to reassure myself, early on, I told the nurse at the hospital that in the long run I'd rather be HIV positive than have diabetes. I tried very hard not to wonder too much what her perturbed expression actually meant, but it has left me with an uncomfortable, lingering doubt ever since. Other people, too, tried their best to sound reassuring, although it wasn't clear who it was they were trying to reassure sometimes, me or themselves. I'm guessing both. Let me be clear: the irritation I felt toward my friends now and then was the result of my own confusion, not of anything wrong they might have done. If they appeared collected and reasonable, I blamed them for dismissing the seriousness of what was happening to me; if they seemed distressed, they were at fault for freaking me out needlessly. The poor things just couldn't win. In truth, however, the shock wasn't mine alone, and my friends, too, had a lot to process in those early days. I expected (and received) support from them and didn't always realize that they needed some as well.

They often gave me something along the lines of "Some people have high cholesterol and they have to take a pill every day or they'll die. Today, it's the same thing with HIV." There's some truth to that, and if anything I appreciated the kindness. It stemmed from a desire to show that HIV is not something that marks you as radically different—even though the mere fact of implying as much confirms that it does, if not to my friends perhaps. Somehow these casual dismissals, affected or not and well intentioned as they were, seemed as inappropriate as unwarranted fears of my impending death. A friend of mine, who is also HIV positive, once told me in response to my frustration with such reactions, "To have HIV isn't a catastrophe but it isn't nothing either," an observation I take to be both comforting and perplexing; comforting because having to choose between nothingness and catastrophe feels a bit like deciding between chicken-feta sausage and baked brie with a mango-ginger reduction: you look down at the menu wondering how on earth your life could turn into such a pile of crap; perplexing because it still leaves a deafening silence halfway between two notions that stubbornly resist all easy attempts to put them into words. If it isn't a catastrophe and it isn't nothing, then *what the hell is it and how can I talk about it?* I don't know, really, but I don't think it's like cholesterol. No one feels nervous in your company because you have high cholesterol. Right?

(Update: My cholesterol level has now risen to such levels that, in light of new statistics indicating that otherwise healthy people living with HIV have a tendency to drop dead of heart attacks for no apparent reason, I now have to take another pill every day.)

THE AIDS CRISIS IS NOT OVER

If the AIDS crisis were over, people wouldn't still be dying of the disease in such high numbers.

If the AIDS crisis were over, people who have been on various combination therapies for years wouldn't be, as is increasingly the case, in such poor physical condition.

If the AIDS crisis were over, people with HIV wouldn't be in jail for failing to disclose their serostatus.

If the AIDS crisis were over, an HIV-positive status wouldn't be so problematic to disclose.

If the AIDS crisis were over, pozphobia wouldn't be so prevalent, so casual, so unconscious even.

If the AIDS crisis were over, my position as a patient wouldn't be a privileged one.

If the AIDS crisis were over, Detroit would be in better shape.

If the AIDS crisis were over, I wouldn't have written this book.

The AIDS crisis is not over.

SPEAKING OF HIV

I talk and talk about it, but I can't quite shake the feeling that I'm not really saying anything. I can tell people that I am HIV positive. I can do it in person, on the phone, through e-mail, anonymously or not. I can notify sexual partners and share the news with friends and sometimes they're the same people. I can tell how I think it happened and with whom, although I can never be sure. I can explain how I came to learn that I was HIV positive, why I got tested, how the results came, my doctor's slight unease, his exact words and body language, how I had to cancel a couple of trips. I can describe what it felt like that day and then the following days, weeks, and months. I can remember nearly every detail of my first appointment at the infectious diseases clinic. I can describe my subsequent hospital visits and my interactions with the personnel there. I can name my meds and say when I take them. I can tell you how stoned they made me feel in the beginning and how bizarre *A Star Is Born* looked that first evening. I can understand and explain how these meds work—or I could if I cared to read up on them. I can give exact figures and estimates: viral load, undetectable for now; CD4-cell count, not quite normal as of this writing but not terrible either. Should I call them T cells, like they do in the old novels and diaries? My life depends on these fucking cells, yet I'm never quite sure what they're supposed to be called. T4? CD4? I think they're the same thing. Does it matter that I know so little about HIV and AIDS? As a disease, I mean. Some people test positive and they embark on some kind of quest. They have to know everything about it, become experts. I haven't done that. For starters, I'm too impatient, and smoking (when I smoked) made it nearly impossible for me to stay in a library more than an hour at a time, so I never acquired the mind to undertake slow, painstaking research. If smoking cigarettes near priceless medieval manuscripts was allowed I might have written about the Black Death, who knows? But mainly, I don't want HIV to become my hobby, I don't want to "own it," as the kids say these days. I know why it was vital, in the early years, for activists to arm themselves with knowledge against an all-powerful, yet powerless, medical establishment. But now, I'm not so sure. When I want to feel equal to my doctor or, more exactly, when I want to remind him that we are, I draw him to *my* field. Rather than think like a doctor, I try to have him think like a critic. Anyway, I can consider myself lucky as well as unlucky. I can tell stories and I can describe facts. And I will. But that's it.

I don't know what it is to be HIV positive.

I am the object of other people's discourses.

I am:

a patient

an insurance company's customer

a regular yet unusual visitor to the local pharmacy

a statistic

a bit of a cliché

a potential criminal . . .

None of these identities are specifically pertinent to HIV. In fact I, and you, have endorsed some of them and will continue to endorse them for reasons unrelated to HIV.

I am NOT:

tragic

heroic

to be pitied

to be envied

interesting

special

strange

sick

dying

or an eighteen-year-old with no medical history, as the physician on duty put it to me as tactfully as she could one night at the ER. Whatever HIV makes me, or doesn't make me, stands only in relation to discourses, images, and narratives that have existed and will continue to exist outside me. My body just happens to be caught in them, alongside other people's bodies.

To be frank, I was surprised by all this. Not intellectually, I mean, but affectively. In the days following the diagnosis, I expected to be hyperaware of something going on inside my body. I thought I would feel infected, as if invaded by some alien life form. I sort of did at first. I know how silly this sounds, but it took almost two weeks before I could bring myself to shave again. I could cut myself, and I was afraid to see my own blood. But because my facial hair has turned mostly gray now, vanity soon reclaimed its rightful place in my life and that was that. So it was, and still is, about what—and who—is outside my body, a body that has never felt so singled out yet so devoid of autonomy. My body seems to be entirely caught up in a web of relations, and that's what makes it feel so real—not what's going on inside, which I cannot actually feel in any case, but its outer limits, its surface exposed to the touch or neglect of others, as it always was, of course, but nothing goes without saying now when it comes to my body.

It is in the eyes of others that, somehow, I first got the confirmation that my fears, triggered by a phone call from the doctor's office urging me to come over to "discuss" my test results—some discussion, really!—were justified. Anticipating that driving myself back was probably not going to be a good idea, I asked the friend who was supposed to give me a ride to the airport to take me instead to the doctor's right away. "Shit!" he said softly into the phone. Then he cried in the car on the way there. As soon I got there, walked to the window, and said my name, several pairs of eyes turned toward me, then down as if trying to take back what their small-town curiosity had already betrayed. "Go tell X that *he's* here." I could tell—or imagine, it really doesn't matter—that everybody knew what "he" had, and what they knew was this extraordinarily intimate thing about me that I didn't officially know myself yet and was still hoping wasn't true after all. As I walked out of the office with my friend, back toward the parking lot, all I remember saying is "I have no idea how it happened." There was no need to say what *it* was. He knew.

Is this, I now wonder, what Hervé Guibert meant when, a long, long time ago, he wrote:

> Long before my positive test results confirmed that I had the disease, I'd felt my blood suddenly stripped naked, laid bare, as though it had always been clothed or covered until then without my noticing this, since it was only natural, but now something—I didn't know what—had removed this protection. From that moment on, I would have to live with this exposed and denuded blood, like an unclothed body that must make its way through a nightmare. My blood, unmasked, everywhere and forever (except in the unlikely event of miracle-working transfusions), naked around the clock, when I'm walking in the street, taking public transportation, the constant target of an arrow aimed at me wherever I go. Does this show in my eyes?

Why does this sound so familiar? Remove the references to blood, or replace blood with the body, and you have a fairly accurate description of what it feels like to be a homosexual in a heterosexual world. Or perhaps a Muslim girl forced to remove her headscarf before entering a French public school. Unmasked or unveiled, the naked surface of the body reveals no truth; it simply exposes a person to public humiliation.

And one last thing: *A Star Is Born*—the version with Judy—*is* a bizarre movie, regardless of what you're on.

OLD FRIENDS, NEW FRIENDS

Is my HIV-positive body the same body I always had, only with HIV in it? Early on, I did feel invaded, inhabited, but no longer. Now the experience is more akin to a Kafkaesque metamorphosis. Do I have a different body, then—a body with HIV that is somehow not the same as a body without HIV? Or perhaps HIV is a supplement to my body, in the Derridean sense of the term, that is, an addition that also signals some foundational absence? This all depends on whether one considers the different stages of one's life to form a succession of events linked by an underlying narrative (whether revealed in hindsight or knowingly imitative) or, instead, revolutions that alter life's course in a radical and unpredictable way, forcing us to start all over again each time.

Truth is, it's both. If we see life as the relations that take place in it, then I can think, for example, of the old friends, the ones I made before anything out of the ordinary happened in my life, but also of the friends I made after I came out (as gay). Then there are the friends I made after I left for America and the friends I made after a very long relationship ended. Now there are the friends I made after HIV. Each set of friends feels somehow attached to a new self, unannounced and impossible for the earlier self to conceive because each is entirely made possible by and contained within a specific circle of friends. Yet my obsolete, discarded selves never really went away. They keep haunting the ones that have come after.

I wish I could be friends with my old selves, but they're like family, and I'm afraid we don't communicate very well.

FAMOUS LAST WORDS

No one ever did anger quite like Barbara Stanwyck. Whether young or old, she could reduce you to a quivering mess with her stare alone. And when she talked, she could make anyone who crossed her regret the day they were born. In one of her last appearances, in *The Thorn Birds*, she hurled this at poor Richard Chamberlain, who didn't want to fuck her for the stupid reason that he was a priest and made the even stupider mistake of reminding her of her age: "Let me tell you something, Cardinal de Bricassart, about old age and about that god of yours, that vengeful god who ruins our bodies and leaves us with only enough wit for regret. Inside this two-bit body, I am still young. I still feel. I still want. I still dream. And I still love you. Oh god, how much!"

How I idolize Barbara Stanwyck . . .

TOUGH AS NAIL POLISH

That I have turned to dead stars for solace and inspiration shouldn't come as a surprise, for, like the heavenly bodies after which they were named, they continue to shine down on us long after they have ceased to exist. I invoke camp, an outmoded, collective way of rereading obsolete forms, in order to reclaim, through the very act of mourning it, a gay sense of community that no longer seems so operational three decades into the epidemic. To put it more bluntly, it makes sense to turn to discarded cultural models of gayness at a time when gay culture has by and large shoved aside the HIV question and discarded the very people who embody it. To be specific, to rely on campy humor is still a way to face HIV by drawing on the resources of gayness itself, especially when it feels threatened. Today, just as it was in the early years, we are urged to step back from a certain "lifestyle" judged responsible by some for the epidemic. Early on, however, many AIDS activists understood that we had much more to gain by cultivating gayness than by toning it down. This so-called lifestyle could, in fact, provide us with the collective dynamic necessary to fight back, infusing our struggle with the power of collective self-creation—the very stuff of life, really—thanks to which we had always been able to invent and reinvent our sexual and social practices when looking for pleasure and strength in the face of danger. Camp emerged out of such needs, and even though it has repeatedly been given up for dead, I find it as resilient a force as Miss Stanwyck herself and, like her, just as vital now as it was then.

NO THERAPY

A friend to whom I'd shown an early draft of this book's first few pages believed that there ought to be something therapeutic in writing about all this. There isn't. Not that there couldn't be, I guess, but that's not what I'm after, that's all. I seek no relief, long for no well-being. This is not a comforting work of self-disclosure. It isn't about inner life but, rather, about outer surfaces. It is about skin given to other people's touch, however kind or unkind the touch turns out to be. (Can one—should one—ever control the afterlife of a gift?) It isn't about me; it is written to you. And I hope you appreciate it, because writing it has been hell.

Writing about HIV isn't in itself any easier or any more difficult than other kinds of scholarship, and the fact that there happens to be a personal dimension attached to it in this particular case doesn't really make a difference. Drawing pertinent and useful conclusions requires that I somehow extract myself from the objects of my analysis, which isn't so hard when you consider how diverse the experiences of HIV are. Furthermore, if I'm not looking for therapy here it's just because I don't think I need it—at least not in relation to being HIV positive. (I have my issues, like anyone else.) What has made this writing onerous, in its crisscrossing of the autobiographical and the scholarly, is the question of disclosure. Using the personal as an anecdotal springboard for theorizing, I could not dissociate my own disclosure from everything that's problematic about that act in general. Fear and vulnerability, humiliation and submission, but also control, anger, and defiance—I have spared myself none of this.

UNSPOKEN KNOWLEDGE

"For reasons that are well known to them." With the awesome swiftness of a falling ax, Joan Crawford famously cut her first two adopted children, Christina and Christopher, out of her will. What an interesting turn of phrase! How, I wonder, can something be simultaneously known and left unspoken? How does one *know* that one has been cast out? By what operation does the burden of knowledge—and it *is* a burden—fall on the shoulders of the excluded rather than on those of the very people who supposedly have "reasons" to exclude? Does it mean that knowledge and reason fall on different sides of the process of exclusion? Or is such knowledge shared? But if it is shared, shouldn't one expect it, by that very fact, to produce community rather than exclusion? This would imply, then, that exclusion is always a self-defeating proposition. I don't mean this in the now obvious sense, as it were, that one needs to produce an outside for the inside to exist, with the latter logically depending on the former, but, more subtly perhaps, in a way that may indicate something like affective intimacy. Furthermore, how can the contents of a sudden revelation be known before it is uttered? Can this be telling us something about why so many warnings fall on deaf ears until it is too late, making Cassandra's gift—the one she possessed and the one she offered—a curse? You know, as in "I should have known."

FROM HERVÉ GUIBERT'S HOSPITAL DIARY (I)

"I will ask and ask until they give it to me."

"Hospital is hell."

"You have to demand respect right away, it's exhausting."

"Allow me, Madam—or is it Miss?—to let you know that I think you behaved very badly with me the other night, be it humanly, ethically, and professionally."

"To turn psychological torture (the situation in which I'm in, for example) into an object of study, if not a work of art, makes torture a little more bearable."

"This morning I refused a pillowcase made of paper."

"You will have to wait for me to sink much lower than I am now before you can make me cross the hospital wearing that thing."

"I was martyred for peanuts: they were not even trying to make me confess the truth."

HOSPITAL VISITS

I was angry. It had taken me far too long to get the first appointment at the infectious diseases clinic. (Actually, HIV patients go to the internal medicine department, where, I was told beforehand, no one in the waiting area would know why I was there. "Internal medicine" is a bit like the black plastic wrapper in which *Poz* magazine comes in the mail. Anyway, after a while we all learn to recognize each other, and, as with homosexuality, a passing glance is all the confirmation we need.) My regular doctor had already told me that my blood had been tested against twenty-nine different combination therapies and that the virus offered no resistance to any of them. All I had to do was try to relax and wait for the call, which was supposed to come within a few days. Well, it didn't. Although I was better informed than many and I knew that I probably had little to worry about, I was still an emotional wreck. I had heard about the treatments' terrible side effects and how some patients had become sicker under the meds than they had been without them. In fact, that's exactly what happened to my friend Hervé. Like so many people, he actually became very sick when the meds started to work. The people at the hospital knew better, though, and they felt no need to see me right away. But I felt utterly neglected.

After two weeks that felt like two years, I got to see a nurse and a social worker. Both were fabulous. The nurse explained to me what I could expect the treatment to be like and that its main side effect could be kidney damage, which is entirely reversible in any case and, besides, affects primarily African American women. "I'd be very surprised if you died of HIV." "I know," I retorted. "I'll die of lung cancer." She smiled: "*That's* the spirit!" As for the social worker, she handed me a form and urged me to write my will. *That's* the spirit. And to contact and inform all the sexual partners I had during the previous three years. "Hmm . . . But it's, er . . . I . . . They . . ." "I know, I know, just do the best you can." This is how I learned that you may be tested anonymously but that your personal information has to be transmitted to the local health authorities once you are under treatment. Sure enough, a few days later I had to explain to the Washtenaw County official who called me at home that I had been very very bad and that there was no way in hell I could possibly contact people whose name I never even knew. She must have heard that sort of story before, because she didn't sound fazed at all. "Just do the best you can." Still, the kindly, understanding tone could not change the fact that twice in a row I found myself in the position of confessing to having been sexually promiscuous and contracting HIV. No one asked me to establish a causal relationship between the two, and that was the beauty of it: it was left to me to stitch the yarn together. And things didn't stop there either. As it turned out, in the state of Michigan, where this story takes place, I had also become legally obligated to divulge my HIV status to all future sexual partners before any penis entered any orifice, no matter whose or which and regardless of actual risk and whether protection is used. The question of disclosure had now taken center stage in my life, becoming inextricably linked to the disease itself and to its experience.

I finally got to see the doctor, a few more weeks later. It didn't go well at all. He entered the examination room with a young student in tow, and she was visibly freaking out. After a few minutes, and without a word of explanation, I was asked to pull down my pants and underwear and lie down on my side so that the two of them could take a close look at my rectum. Why? What the fuck were they expecting to see in there? A bunch of sweaty little viruses dancing bare chested to the beat of "It's Raining Men"? Is the rectum a cavernous disco? A back room? A crime scene to be dusted for fingerprints? What was the purpose of all this? To remind me that I was a diseased homo who had been fucked in the ass—you know, in case I had forgotten? To shame me? To force me once more to establish a narrative thread linking lovers' beds and hospital beds, gay sex and disease, pleasure and punishment, Eros and Thanatos? To assert power over my body? In all likelihood, they were looking for possible signs of other sexually transmitted infections, but why not say so, for heaven's sake? So I did what any self-respecting faggot would have done in similar circumstances—I bitched. I complained to the social worker that bringing a student to the first visit and making me feel like some sort of textbook was, at the very least, not quite tactful. From that day on, the doctor, who turned out to be a warm and charming man and who, in all likelihood, had no idea that he had upset me so and probably regretted it, always asked me for permission before inviting a student to the visit. Guibert would have been proud of this small victory, I think.

Yet bitching wasn't enough, believe it or not. I wanted to be respected and I wanted to be loved. I wanted to be a good patient. For example, I oh-so-casually informed everyone at the clinic that I, too, was an AIDS researcher in my own right, and one day I gave them a copy of my first book. Pretty pathetic, I know, but I found it important to establish the fact that I was a professor at the University of Michigan, just like my doctor. I have no idea whether anybody there ever read the book, because after the initial excitement this caused, nobody mentioned it again. Maybe they thought the book sucked and they didn't have the heart to tell me. (Later, one of the nurses wrote his own book on HIV. It sold rather well, he told me, and was soon picked up for a Kindle version. I was insanely envious.)

I also made them laugh every chance I got. Gene Kelly and Judy Garland said it best, with a little help from Cole Porter: "Be a clown, be a clown, all the world loves a clown." So a few months later, upon learning that I had to be tested for chlamydia and gonorrhea, I quipped, "Why bother? This is a bit like testing me for malaria. I haven't exactly been to Burundi lately, if you know what I mean." "I know exactly what you mean," my doctor (he was now *my* doctor like I was *his* patient) snapped back with a smirk. "But I hardly have to tell you, a Frenchman of all people, that sometimes the government exerts some control over doctors and their funding." Oh, the man could be funny too. Without my realizing it, we had moved from a Lon Chaney silent horror fest to the chatty final scene of *Casablanca*, when the crooked cop and the honest crook walk off together into the foggy night. A beautiful friendship.

FROM HERVÉ GUIBERT'S HOSPITAL DIARY (II)

"There arises, at the moment when the doctor exerts an intense suffering upon the patient, a curious feeling of love and respect that I believe to be mutual. There is something sacred to suffering. The doctor who made the patient suffer and the patient who suffered become friends of sorts, accomplices perhaps—but there's always modesty."

STAR ENTRANCE

The excruciating and tantalizing succession of stages—my primary care physician; then the nurse and social worker at the hospital; finally the AIDS doctor opening the door—evokes, to me, the narrative layering that precedes and sets up a star entrance, when, say, Lana Turner first appears all dressed in white, pausing at the door frame, as a pure image, in *The Postman Always Rings Twice*: a lethal and irresistible object of desire. The star.

I'm sorry, but shouldn't *I* get top billing here?

(I gotta get me a turban.)

The truth, though, is that Lana standing at the threshold tells me that she comes out of nowhere; that she didn't exist before I laid eyes on her; that it is also I who makes her a star and not just camera work or that famous *je ne sais quoi* known as "star quality."

As long as both our names appear above the title, I'll be willing to share top billing with my doctor. How's that?

STAR EXIT

Planning is everything. On my first visit to the AIDS clinic at the hospital, and right after I was told it would be extremely unlikely that I would ever die because of HIV, I was also urged to write my last will and testament, give a trusted person power of attorney over my affairs, register a living will, and so on. To expedite matters, I was handed a pile of forms and documents to attend to right away. They sat on my kitchen table for many weeks until, one day, they had entirely vanished under a pile of bills, recipes I had cut out from the *New York Times* but will never cook, articles I had promised myself to read without delay but never will, and other such stuff that just could not wait but did. Eventually I put all the documents pertaining to my death away on a shelf somewhere. I imagine they're still there.

If I should die in bed, I have several models to choose from. For a long time, I had a special fondness for Bette Davis's death in *Dark Victory*. Fore-warned of her imminent demise by the onset of blindness that strikes her as she is tending her garden with a friend, she walks slowly up the stairs to her bedroom, half clutching half caressing the banister (because she's blind, you see), lies down on her bed, and, looking fabulous, waits for death to take her. Other than for the Max Steiner score, the whole scene is rather moving in a simple sort of way. For a second, she thinks clouds are moving in, but not at all: it's that rare kind of brain tumor that is finally catching up with her. One of Bette Davis's finest moments, to be sure, and she simply looks ravishing in the entire movie. Yet I am tempted by something a little less understated (and which doesn't involve gardening), something more along the lines of the death of Juanita Moore at the end of *Imitation of Life* perhaps—as long as Lana Turner doesn't get all the best close-ups. A grandiose service in a monumental black church may be a bit much to ask, though, especially in Ann Arbor, but the horse-drawn carriage I find hard to resist. Especially in Ann Arbor.

In *Camille*, Garbo expires divinely from consumption in the arms of her lover, but that requires a lover. And consumption. Instead, I could walk sen-suously into the ocean like Joan Crawford in *Humoresque*. It's noble, highly cinematic, and easier on your friends, but I'm not sure Lake Huron would do the trick. I need waves. Of course, I could always go for Marlene Diet-rich's death in *Dishonored*. There's something rather appealing about dying all tarted up and dressed like a whore. But let's face it, my chances of getting my hands on a Prussian firing squad are rather slim.

I'll think of something.

THE DREAM SEQUENCE

The sticky residue of a night's dreams often clings to mornings and days. This phenomenon—strange, vivid dreams—is one of the best known and most curious side effects of the meds I'm on and must take at bedtime, and it can be so persistent that I have found it easier and more beneficial to my peace of mind to accept, once and for all, that the boundary between sleep and waking life has, if not entirely ceased to exist, at least become an object of serious dispute, and one that shows no sign of being settled anytime soon by the warring factions. I have, in other words, started to live two different but intermingling lives. Coming to terms with this has also been good for my plants, which kept dying, since I mostly watered them in dreams. (Just because my dreams are strange and vivid doesn't mean they were created by Salvador Dalí. Sometimes I just water plants, but in a strange and vivid way.)

So no, I did not actually pick up a cigarette yesterday, and it takes a disturbing amount of effort on the part of my rational self to convince my panicky self of that simple truth. Sure, these dreams are about failure and pertain to more than just quitting smoking, but it felt so good to smoke last night and, more important, it still feels so good long after it didn't happen. So why fight, really? Why not accept the true feelings generated by false realities and end this pointless tug-of-war between my competing selves? Isn't this precisely what grounds my love for fiction, for art, for old Hollywood, for all sorts of made-up stuff?

Overcoming their natural boundaries, a night's dreams never fail to infect the following day. They and their contents have now bled into my life for good and found their place alongside people and things. And as with people and things, I must face the fact that dreams I like and dreams I don't are now, not unlike HIV itself, the companions of my days. But they walk with me with such obstinacy that I have begun to wonder whether they are trying to claim their own spot in the sunshine or to drag me back with them into the darkness.

Let me be very clear: these reflections do not constitute some clever *mise en abyme* of one of this book's central arguments about the constant mingling of reason and unreason. What I describe here is a factual account of the phenomenon as I experience it almost daily. We all know the unsettling feeling of doubt that sometimes remains after an especially powerful dream. Was this really a dream? It must have been, right? Yes, yes, of course it was. Now imagine this feeling not with a single dream once in a while but several dreams at a time nearly every day of your life, and you may have an idea of how one experiences the nearness of two worlds that, incompatible as they may be, end up sharing certain features. Just as in my waking life I wonder whether a certain memory might not in fact have been dreamed, so in dreams do I sometimes suspect that what feels so real may well be a trick.

Two of the recurring characters in my dreams have been my father and my brother, both of them dead for years. The first time they appeared was not as if they had never died but as a return to life. "Denis's coming back!" someone yelled, and my mother, my sister, and I would feverishly prepare for the big arrival. Soon, father and brother were home for good, back in our lives and in theirs. Forget the fact that in real life both men had left home when I was a boy; the dreams were rather joyous at first, and I would wake up with the lingering warmth, slightly tinged with sadness, that follows the pleasure of having spent some time with people I loved. But it wasn't long before my friendly ghosts began to overstay their welcome. When, for example, my brother asked me to score some weed for him, I was suddenly reminded, inside my dream and out, that he and I were never that close to begin with, and it wasn't long before I wished that he would just go away again. Warmth gave way to guilt. In short, the vivid dreams, which had allowed my father and my brother to overcome their boundaries and creep into my waking life, have started to wear me out. These two men are, after all, dead, and having to remind myself of that fact every few mornings is far more onerous than remembering that I didn't start smoking again.

An obvious way to interpret these periodic visitations is to see them as signs that I may be the next to go. My father and my brother would not be back among the living for good, then, but rather would have made the trip to come get me. However, because I never have the "feeling" of being HIV positive in these dreams, I wonder to what extent the ghost that haunts them, and me, isn't in fact my old, dead self beckoning like the face of a missing person on a flyer. This feeling of being a lost child has recently found itself reinforced as my mother passed away, and she too joined the cast of nightly characters.

I DIED A THOUSAND DEATHS (ALL OF THEM GORGEOUS)

I died very well when I was a boy. Beautifully, in fact. Whether I was a Roman slave or an exiled oriental prince, a pirate or a Sioux—whichever allowed me to be half naked or wear feathers—my exits tended to be more drawn out and tantalizing than Ava Gardner's entrance in *The Barefoot Contessa*. I can never decide between a star entrance and a star exit which one is the more significant. If the first is always a form of unveiling, isn't the second the real moment of truth? And the truth is, I was not the sort of kid who lived happily ever after. Lying mortally wounded in the arms of a beloved comrade (or subordinate), I would make my men bear witness to my gorgeous agony, leaving them to wonder how they could possibly go on living without me. No point in trying; they couldn't. Should I urge them to keep up the fight no matter what, I made sure they understood that they needn't think about it too much because my demise would inevitably be followed by music swelling and the words "The End." I was an eight-year-old bossy bottom.

One of my signature deaths consisted in drawing my last breath in midsentence, halfway through a final revelation that would forever remain unuttered. Some moment of truth! What fabulous mystery, what buried treasure was I taking with me to the grave? Had we been a little older at the time, we would all have realized exactly what my deaths, which, in their over-the-top tragic beauty, evoked Garbo far more often than they did Robert Mitchum, were attempting to reveal and conceal at the same time— indeed to reveal *by* concealing. (Come to think of it, had we been a little older we might have been playing different games of unveiling, revealing, and concealing.) What *was* clear, however, was that I always died the victim of some sort of injustice and that, somehow, this made me impossibly desirable. Well, not in my friends' eyes maybe, but this was all taking place in a working-class neighborhood in Normandy, and I wasn't planning to stay there much longer—just long enough to have my desires forever shaped and frustrated by a childhood at once humdrum and uneasy.

To be alive is much more time-consuming than to be dead, and I had oceans to cross.

Others

THE NEW WORLD

I cannot date with any certainty the moment I became aware that I had entered another world. This new world exists in proximity to the old world, yours, where life continues to unfold as if nothing had happened. Mine isn't a subterranean world, however, nor is it in any way invisible if one cares to look. Rather, old and new world exist in a neighborly relationship of nearness, discordance, and discomfort. Within arm's reach or a stone's throw— the metaphor isn't mine to pick.

THREE THOUSAND DEATHS IN ONE DAY

It is easy to forget, given the torrent of stupid certainties and the idiotic fervor, unabated to this day, that have followed them, that the events of September 11, 2001, were very surprising. Her voice a mere mumble, the neighbor asked me for a cigarette as we were both standing on the sidewalk that sunny Tuesday morning, so clear and luminous—a reverse omen of the murkiness that was soon to envelop us like a treacherous fog. She didn't have any cigarettes herself, and I assumed that she must have quit but that if ever a situation demanded a smoke, this was it. We nodded, we raised our eyebrows, we didn't say anything. We just smoked. Soon Johnny walked by. He had just moved to the city to start grad school at NYU. Classes had been canceled, obviously, and he was on his way home. He didn't say much either. He shrugged and extended his arms a little, his palms turned upward in a universal gesture of baffled powerlessness. He smoked too. We didn't know what to say or what to think. We just stood there on an East Village sidewalk and smoked in near silence.

A few minutes later on Houston:

"Tower came down?"

"Yes."

"Man . . ."

Then Michael stopped by the apartment. "Well," he laughed, "I guess it's up to us to repopulate the earth!" This was funny because everyone in the room was gay. Well, you had to be there. And gay. At least we could still camp it up a little. It always seems to help, somehow. To think that, only two days before, we had had a passionate discussion on the respective (de)merits of *Earthquake* and *The Towering Inferno*. . . . Just two days. But camp always takes you back.

WAITING

So we waited. We waited for all the other planes still in the air to land and be accounted for. We waited for the second tower to fall. We waited for the president to come out of hiding and say something. We waited to know what the hell happened and whether a war had started. We waited for the moment when we wouldn't have to be waiting anymore.

We waited for Fourteenth Street to reopen so that traffic could flow again, so that grocery stores and, most importantly, bars could replenish their stocks. By Tompkins Square Park, the joint with the painted sign that said it never closed, closed. At Starlight, on Avenue A, the staff was passing around free booze. Every bar was full, and everyone there was drunk. No one wanted to stay home, it seemed. It was like a party, but sad.

Some waited for their friends or relatives to reappear and say, Look, I didn't die! Some waited to hear if they knew anyone who wouldn't reappear. And after a few days the wind turned and that smell flooded our neighborhood. We all decided to believe that it was coming from melted phones and computers and just leave it at that. But all the same, it was like breathing death, and we couldn't wait for the smell to go away.

It is always the case with waiting that something that hasn't happened yet or may never happen at all is shaping our present. Something unknowable, something that essentially doesn't exist, makes our lives what they are. In the end, today's material conditions and tomorrow's hypothetical ones become inseparable. We do not all wait for the same thing or things, of course. And we do not wait in the same way. There is no single way to wait. You may wait patiently or impatiently. You may hope or dread, be confident or doubtful. You can wish or pray for something to happen or not to happen. What we wait for and how we wait for it—what we do while we wait—says a lot about who we are. Or is it how we wait that shapes who we are? Does a desire for revenge emanate from a vengeful personality, or does it produce that personality? Is a person waiting for the second coming of Christ because he or she is a devout Christian or the other way round? What about Jews and the Messiah?

Does the very act of waiting together somehow bring us closer to one another? If so, could it be because whatever it is that we wait for and makes us different is in fact exterior to us and hasn't happened, doesn't exist? Was it when answers, revenge, and traffic finally came that the closeness some felt that day vanished into thin air?

I'm not one to believe in a nation miraculously unified in the wake of tragedy. I'm talking about a feeling more basic, vibrant, and real than that. I'm thinking of the guy, walking down endless flights of stairs inside the World Trade Center alongside a woman, a complete stranger, who was also trying to get out. Today I don't remember which tower and what floors, but at the time every detail of the story mattered. Both were in their late forties, I'd say, maybe older, frightfully normal, and now they were in that East Village bar, and the guy was regaling the crowd with the story of their narrow escape. He relished the attention and the free drinks. She was speechless, in a stupor almost, but he was from Brooklyn so there was no shutting him up, and he started wondering aloud about how complicated it would be for him to get home. And that's when I realized that the guy didn't want to go home at all! He was just putting the moves on the dame, see? (Sorry, but there was something very Jimmy Cagney about the whole scene.) In the middle of a cataclysm, someone was trying to grab a chance encounter and turn it into full-fledged contact. Look, the guy seemed to be saying, something terrible has happened that may very well change the world forever, and the subway's not working. Wanna get a room? How inappropriate yet completely fitting.

And why not? To move around in a city, to want to move around in a city, is a highly erotic affair. One takes to the streets in order to brush one's body against other people's bodies, preferably those of strangers. The city is full of them. In a city one seeks company. So I'm not sure what kind of imaginary national community was taking form on 9/12, and to be honest I'm not sure that I want to know, but on 9/11, in New York City, people were getting drunk and trying to sleep with strangers. Like on 9/10, really, only more so.

NEARNESS AND NEIGHBORLINESS

In her testimonial writings, Charlotte Delbo, a French Resistance fighter and Auschwitz survivor, repeatedly uses a specific rhetorical strategy that several critics, including myself, have commented on. Hoping to establish a relation of proximity with her readers in order to be able to transmit *something* of what she went through, Delbo must also try to frustrate our wish to know what we cannot possibly know, to deflect our desire for something like deep, subjective intimacy with someone whose experience will always remain partly beyond our grasp. The literary scholar Patricia Yeager, for one, has written beautifully about the need to resist the temptation of intimacy and proprietary knowledge when reading testimonies of trauma. Instead, Delbo's goal is to establish enough common ground for us to stand near her while maintaining the distance necessary to ensure that we will not be able to be in her place or appropriate what is not ours. Close, in other words, but not so close as to render her transparent to us and her experience fully knowable by others.

In the opening section of her trilogy, *Auschwitz and After*, Delbo describes what we immediately identify as a typical train station. Yes, we recognize this space, we've occupied it, or one just like it, we've used it, and, inevitably, we've shared it with throngs of other people, complete strangers for the most part. Soon, however, Delbo pulls the rug from under her readers' feet, and the description makes way for a very different train station—the arrival ramp of Auschwitz-Birkenau. The people exiting the trains here are not going home or to work or on vacation; they are Jews going to their deaths. In another passage, the narrator recalls the tales of colonial explorers nearly dying of thirst in the desert, stories whose orientalist local color once made them both exotic and familiar. And then, almost without warning, she depicts the far less heroic and far more disorienting experience of thirst that she went through in the swamps of Poland. Later in the book, a beloved childhood pet morphs into a bloodthirsty hound that tears a prisoner to pieces. There are other examples. These scenes dramatize just how far a reader may be able to go without, in essence, colonizing the witness by implanting into the testimony a kind of knowledge that is in fact the reader's own.

It isn't that Delbo is trying to trick us, of course. Anyone who picks up her books opens them with a certain set of expectations. Some readers, such as academics, for example, are also aware that the testimonial writing of trauma always raises questions of representation and that witnesses must rely on rhetorical tactics to ensure that something of the traumatic experience will be transmitted to others. Some authors use a degree of fictionalizing in telling their story, creating composite characters maybe, or imagining dialogues in order to verbalize for their readers' benefits what may have been only felt or thought at the time; others tactically inhabit familiar genres or registers that provide us with something resembling a roadmap into mostly uncharted territory. But all know that familiarity has its limits. Sharing an experience of the extreme involves negotiating these limits and problematizing the modalities of contact, since it is through contact between what they articulate that limits in general are established and felt to exist even though they have no tangibility of their own. Our eyes lie. Only when I touch you and you touch me do we know for certain where we begin and where we end.

If Delbo doesn't exactly lure unsuspecting readers into uneasy contact, she does beckon us, in a way; or rather, she makes an appeal for us to read her. The French phrase that comes to my mind here is *faire signe*. It means to signal or to wave at somebody, but literally "to make a sign." Indeed, if Delbo motions us to come near her, her mode of address foregrounds its status as sign. When we read the description of the train station in the opening pages, we know that it is meant to be typical, a series of signs that indicates not a train station but a "train station." In a similar way, we are asked to recognize stories of thirsty explorers as told in children's books whose purpose was to produce popular myths and a sense of national identity in colonial times. Readers are therefore keenly aware that the witness is relying on artifice but also that only through artifice—the substitution, for reality, of a representation flaunting its status as sign making—can we get near the truth.

Yet unlike the narrative device that Roland Barthes identified as a "reality effect," thanks to which we experience representation as if it provided us with a direct and unproblematic access to reality, nearness of the sort Delbo proposes can be experienced only at the same time as contiguity with and discontinuity from "true events." It is no accident that the events in question were also characterized by the same apparent contradiction. Without question, the Nazi enterprise was conceived and perpetrated by human beings and it occurred within human history, but it also drew the outer limits of humanity and history—contiguity and discontinuity. The tactical use of beckoning and nearness in *Auschwitz and After* mirrors, in a way, what appears to be the defining duality of its subject matter. This allows the witness to convey in form what could not be expressed in content without committing an injustice against the truth: the feeling for a limit that we can never really get at and return from alive. (Think of what Primo Levi wrote about the inevitable shortcomings of the survivors as witnesses.)

In her famous epigraph to her trilogy, Delbo tells us, "Today, I am not sure that what I wrote is true. I am certain it is truthful." It is in the nature of a sign to bring us close to the truth precisely by erecting a barrier between it and us. A sign connects and separates at the same time; it is liminal in essence, the threshold where a substitution may take place. *Faire signe* is thus about making contact. Because a sign can bring reality to us and us to reality only by standing in between, it all at once reveals and conceals, illuminates and obscures. In that sense, the avowed "signness" of Delbo's addresses to her readers may provide us with a way to rethink modalities of encounters away from the policing role of interpellation and in favor of the kind of relational dynamics, of contact, that I like to call neighborly. I ground it in the idea that no connection may seek to cancel the separateness of what it brings together without erasing itself as connection. Contact, in other words, may occur only on condition that it fall short of its own completion.

Needless to say, not all encounters are neighborly. Louis Althusser's cop hailing me, constituting me as a subject shot through with ideology, does not have friendly designs. The disciplinary discourses discussed by Michel Foucault do not either. In both cases, I find myself transparent and subjected to identification, knowability, and control by being called, if not always named. With discourses of power that get under my skin, I am assigned a place within a social structure, and simultaneously the social structure is assigned a place within me. But I am also made removable in an instant because my contours are so clearly outlined that my excision shall create no harm to the system. Interpellating in this manner doesn't beckon a person into a relationship of nearness, and it doesn't constitute a mute appeal either, for no contact has really taken place. Instead, the interpellation creates a sense of unbridgeable distance by making me feel my limits as if they had a tangible existence and as if I, as a subject, were not coextensive with others in the world outside. Instead of feeling our contours by touching each other, our contours keep us from touching.

Against this problematic notion of the autonomous subject, I find the idea of neighborliness conceptually useful. Neighborliness provides us with a spatial and social model that is simultaneously very concrete, in that many of us experience it in our daily lives, and rather difficult to define because it is more a matter of dynamics than space. As I have argued elsewhere, a neighborhood is a place both public and private, yet is neither exactly. It is, in fact, defined by the lived inability to distinguish the public from the private and by its power to undo the kind of social policing that the dichotomy was designed to enforce. A neighborhood functions a bit like a home— my neighborhood, your neighborhood—but it is not as ideologically determined as a home because, while familiar, it isn't familial. It is relational without being institutional. There, one doesn't feel *chez soi*, a proprietary feeling, but *comme chez soi*, a very different proposition that rests on the contiguity-discontinuity of a trope. Always connected to the city around it (there are no neighborhoods in villages and in certain kinds of suburbs), a neighborhood remains open for all to pass through, use, and change. Unlike "the home," and while it, too, is subject to rules of propriety or *convenance*, it cannot be so clearly endowed with a normalizing mission. It is too loosely delineated for that, its dynamics too ephemeral. But it is also a place of commonality so invested with affect that it cannot be structured coldly and efficiently either. In short, a neighborhood's communal dimension is enacted by the individuals who use it, but the people in it experience themselves as individuals only insofar as a community recognizes them as such, that is, in a collective, relational way. It is precisely this crisscrossing of seemingly incompatible forces and openness to change, errors, and misunderstandings that makes neighborliness such a productive, if elusive, concept. This requires us to envisage complex modes of relationality based on contact.

BECKONING AND APPEALING

We were walking in a group, laughing loudly about something or other, when, without warning, a fire station sneaked up on us near Washington Square Park. The flowers, notes, and portraits of the dead firefighters stunned us all at once into a heavy silence. The conversation picked up again after we'd left the station behind us, but the laughter sounded more forced somehow, until it died down altogether.

The way New York City reacted to 9/11, how the city mourned its dead, was distinctly urban. Unlike the suburbs, where life is largely centered on the family home, and villages, where everyone knows everyone, a city lives thanks to its streets and the constant crisscrossing of people, of selves passing others in public spaces where the known and the recognized (*le connu* and *le reconnu*) may not necessarily coincide or happen in the sequence that one would surmise from logic or morphology alone. The flyers with pictures of the missing and presumably dead—the disappeared, one would say in other contexts where bodies were not to be recovered—posted all over the city on pay phones, mailboxes, newspaper dispensers, and other such objects that we use or used to use daily without ever paying them much mind were even more moving to me than the portraits of the fallen firefighters outside the stations. The firefighters were brave, perhaps heroic. The civilians who died that day were people no different from the ones we pass on the streets every day, no different from us, who were now seeing the flyers—only those people were missing now. So we missed them. Even if we didn't know them. Their photographs were all over the streets for everyone to miss the dead, for the city to witness their disappearance and account for their absence. "Have you seen this person?" asked the flyers, or, more hauntingly, "Have you seen me?" I say "hauntingly" because it seems inappropriate to call those who authored the flyers authors; they were not authors, really, but more like vessels. The words are not etymologically related, but let's call this "proximity by proxy." Like witnesses of Auschwitz, friends and relatives lent their bodies to give shelter to the voices of the dead so that they might make their way to us. And being beckoned by the dead is quite different, ideologically speaking, from being interpellated by a cop.

On some of the flyers, the photograph, photocopied cheaply in black and white, was too dark for anyone to make out the missing person's features and recognize him or her. These images were all the more moving for that reason, as though they figured the very effacement of the disappeared and identified them not as Wall Street executives but as poor people. "Have you seen me?" asked the dead. But what could we answer? "No, I haven't seen you because you are no longer here. But yes, of course I have seen you, every day, or I have at least seen people just like you, like that Brooklyn fellow who was trying to bang another survivor, people who make this place a city because they are using its streets and sidewalks and newspaper dispensers and mailboxes. Every day, without thinking—until now."

Looking at a nineteenth-century photograph of a man about to be hanged, Roland Barthes was taken by the sudden confusion of time that ensued. The handsome young man who was going to die was, in reality, already dead. Linear time had collapsed. A photograph's *punctum*, as Barthes calls this unnamable "thing," this inconsequential detail that jumps out of the image and unexpectedly beckons to me and touches me, is also, in the end, time itself. If reason mandates that time come in succession, affect tells us otherwise. Reason separates; it splits the self from the nonself and categorizes each thing apart from the other. Affect pertains to simultaneity; it erases the gap between me and the world, the present and the past, giving me the impression that I am what I'm feeling. Reason is clean, affect murky. This isn't just a matter of Proustian musings, though, for I am convinced that there are ethical ramifications to all this. The portraits on the streets of New York after 9/11 may help us envisage a notion of time less brutal than that of History.

The affective dimension of 9/11 was not to be expressed in the studied, official pathos that followed the events and served to justify the takeover of two Muslim countries and the killing, torture, and humiliation of their "backward" people in the name of forward-looking modernity; rather, it was felt in the unspeakable sadness that greeted the sudden dissolution of boundaries once thought secure. The awareness that such undoing of safe categories could have radical consequences is, I believe, what the mainstream media (or whatever they stand for) were trying to nip in the bud when they kept telling us that America had, once again, lost its innocence. Time, though, is only what we think it is. Think of it as linear or reasonable, and war follows 9/11 the way an effect follows a cause; think of it as simultaneous and engorged with affect and what comes after loss, or rather continues it, isn't nostalgia but hauntedness—an absence less communicable perhaps than transmitted like an infection, or caught like an unexpected glimpse. Barthes's "first" *punctum*—the striking detail—"touches" in two ways, in that it is both a contact and an emotion. But so does the "second" *punctum*—time—when affective contact comes into play with the dissolution, or bleeding, of categories into one another, as, for example, when the photograph of a live person represents someone who has already died.

The awareness of such phenomena doesn't come effortlessly, however. Affect, as I define it here, may lead to a kind of nonrational knowledge, but it isn't a divine state of grace or a truth revealed, whole and im-mediate, as a blissful burst of oneness or fascist certainty. Even Proust's narrator ultimately has to *work* in order to make the past return at will and occupy its rightful place alongside the present. Accidents will happen, as will random encounters, but they will not do, and the labor of joy is no less demanding than the work of mourning. Yet I found myself angered at first by the people who had their pictures taken *purposefully* at the Union Square makeshift memorials and had their solemn faces posted in a way that seemed so disrespectful to the dead, whose own smiling portraits appeared all over town. "Look at me! Look how sad I am! I too have been affected by this trage-dy." The dead's question "Have you seen me?" signified lack and absence, whereas the implied interpellation "Look at me!" that I sensed from these more artistic portraits appeared to demand that we acknowledge the living's presence, our own presence. I know this was New York, but still, how narcissistic can a person be?

Hastily put together by friends and relatives and conveying grief by referencing a kind of happiness—through pictures of weddings, vacations, or birthday parties—that we know now to be a thing of the past, the flyers made up small works of witness rather than sentimental narratives. They paid no attention to aesthetic value, no mind to posterity. They were a kind of bricolage seeking to make contact, here and now, by relying on the ruins of the past—people and events and feelings no longer in existence. The sort of proximity enacted by witnessing is thus always an approximation. By beckoning us, the flyers foregrounded not their reality but their very signness, that is to say, their foundational absence. Indeed, every sign is an absence, since it works as a substitution, and in this case signness itself was the sign that allowed the "real" absence of the missing people to be "seen."

The Union Square portraits, however, felt so tasteful as to be tactless. They seemed too calculated, manipulative even. Worse, they gave a sense that they were self-serving rather than about any kind of collective dynamic, like people who engage in charity work just because it allows them to be acknowledged as good persons by their peers or to fool themselves into believing that they are. These artful portraits reeked of soulful depth and individual subjectivity. Their penetrating, self-important gazes were not beckoning me; they were shaming me. Fuck that. I was overcome by this icky mixture of anger and embarrassment, not knowing which of these two feelings was feeding off the other.

But perhaps I was wrong. Perhaps the pictures of the living didn't memorialize but sought, instead, to inscribe collective grief within the city-scape. In a sense, to bring the dead and the living into contact by establishing such a visual parallel made 9/11 no longer a spectacular historical event, to be watched over and over again on TV, but a matter of daily life writ small and sprouting from the ground up. A sign is a place of contact. It brings nearer who sends it and who receives it, whatever meanings the receiver intends for it to have and the meanings the receiver brings to it in the process. A sign first represents the space where interlocutors meet and try to negotiate the terms of their encounter. The "authors" of the flyers were not authors in the traditional sense. As their use of a borrowed first person indicates, they, like Holocaust witnesses for example, were merely being hospitable to the dead to whom they lent their bodies.

Eventually, the living beckoned by the dead on the flyers had themselves become vessels, relays of hauntedness without end, and beckoning had morphed into a more complex kind of appeal. Indeed, with the faces of the missing now everywhere, multiplied on objects of everyday usage and forming a kind of collective photo album without a single identifiable author, the city felt haunted. And with the author impossible to locate (or "dead" in Barthes's sense) authority, too, had fallen by the wayside and, with it, the unified and unifying source from which to produce knowledge and organize it in neatly delineated—clean, safe—categories.

If the faces of the living on the pictures at Union Square made them look as if they were dead, or at least touched by death, the portraits on the flyers were very often happy photographs that made the dead look as if they were still living. This uncanny sense of being in contact with the absent was enhanced by the direct address "Have you seen me?" and by the socially codified, and therefore sharable, expressions of intimacy depicted on photos exposed all over the streets. We kept running into them, in fact, so ubiquitous were the flyers below Fourteenth Street. "Have you seen me?" Here's that hunk on the beach again, and here's the beaming bride. "Have you seen me?"

Whenever and wherever they appealed, we answered. We looked at the proud graduate and at the Asian guy in a suit, every time they called out, until the dead were near us and we near them. Blurring the boundaries between the private and the public, the dead and the living, you and me, is what I called an urban way to mourn and a mode of sharing—being tactful to the dead.

INCOMPLETE STRANGERS

The feeling of slight discomfort that often greets a stranger's beckoning stems from a breach of boundaries, perhaps even of propriety. "Why are you calling me? I don't know you." But when a complete stranger beckons you, he or she ceases to be a complete stranger and becomes, if not exactly an acquaintance, at least an incomplete stranger. "You don't know me completely but you know the surface of me just as I know the surface of you."

It isn't hard to see why Romantics would have recoiled in horror at this. This sort of encounter turning into a contact is typically urban. It isn't premised on the oneness of a deep or transcendent self but on the contingent relationality of selves in transit. The incompleteness of the stranger to me mirrors my incompleteness to him or her. Our meeting doesn't remedy it (it is neither an illness nor a matter of unfinished business); it acknowledges incompleteness as our shared and permanent condition. But if this doesn't represent an affective meeting of souls, it isn't a meeting of minds either. So what kind of knowledge is the knowledge of the incomplete stranger?

Seeing the 9/11 flyers and recognizing the dead as our neighbors, or reading Delbo's rhetoric of nearness with the dead of Auschwitz, we are no longer complete strangers to other people's experiences of disaster. The sense of our own incompleteness is like the trace left in us, or on us, by a disaster we cannot "really" know. Like all traces, it is an absence that we can see. Lack obliges us toward the other, the alien, and makes us relate to him or her in a meaningful way, but in the mode of difference.

If I come to you who beckon me, the space I was occupying will now be empty. But if I was walking down a city street, or any other place defined not by individual ownership but by collective usage, every space that I occupy for a moment and then leave will be filled next by someone other than me yet like me. This interplay of difference and likeness defines the sign and all such substitutions and tropes. In this sense, beckoning understood as *faire signe* functions as a sort of trope, and this can explain why the portraits at Union Square worked. To beckon means to recognize that a distance exists and then to invite nearness. But nearness only, that is to say, proximity and distance at the same time. Intimation rather than intimacy.

GROUND ZERO

"The memory of friends is everywhere. It pervades the city. Buildings, skylines, corners, have holes in them—gaps; missing persons. And if the present is a cemetery, the future is a minefield."

These words were written about New York and appeared in Andrew Holleran's book of collected essays *Ground Zero* published in 1988. I extracted this from the piece of the same name, and, like the rest of the book, it's about AIDS. I don't read it now as eerily prophetic or anything. It could have been written about other collective traumas, such as the Holocaust or the Balkan wars of the 1990s. Hiroshima and Nagasaki may just as well come to mind, since, for a long time, the expression *ground zero* referred primarily to the point of impact of an atomic bomb. No, what strikes me about this passage's similarity to 9/11 is that its simultaneously narrow and diffuse focal point—the expansiveness of private loss, available for all to see—evokes the dual dimension of the urban catastrophe. If urban space is shared space, we must share it also with the missing.

"I'M GOING TO DIE, AREN'T I?"

Several years after September 11, 2001, some recordings of phone calls made to 911 by people trapped in the towers above the points of impact were made public. A woman told the operator, "I'm going to die, aren't I?" As I began to ask a friend of mine who was with me in New York that day if he had heard the tapes, he interrupted me with a brisk arm gesture and a mumble that meant yes, he'd heard them too but that he wasn't going to talk about it. I knew then that he had also been thrown back to that horrible day and to the inarticulable shock of it. These recordings could simply not, in any way, constitute a topic of conversation. I think it was the "aren't I?" that made this call resonate far beyond the 911 operator who received it.

HAPPY HOUR AT THE COX

There was Hervé, who said, "Ever since Mom left . . ." ("Depuis que Maman est partie . . ."). And there was this guy, a friend of Hervé's whom I had never met before, or since. He had recently arrived in Paris from Bordeaux. Gay life there had changed beyond recognition, he explained, and it was time for him to leave. He added, "And there were many passings" ("Et puis il y a eu beaucoup de décès"). *Décès* was such a strange word, I thought, so bland and legalistic, so disengaged (as if apolitical), so dispassionate (as if painless)—so not ACT UP. Inside me, a voice was screaming, "THEY'RE NOT 'DECEASED,' THEY'RE DEAD, OK? THEY'RE FUCKING DEAD!" And I was remembering how Hervé's gang of boys, back home in Caen, young, beautiful, fearless, had by then been entirely decimated, leaving him, as far as I knew, the sole survivor. But the friend from Bordeaux had paused and then lowered both his voice and his eyes ever so slightly when he uttered those words, in a way that embodied the contained, tactful withdrawal that the term *décès* so eerily and movingly conveyed.

Although I had known her since we were kids, I was never close to Hervé's mother and of course I didn't know the boys in Bordeaux, so I guess it was easy for me to call them dead. But Hervé and his friend were close to those they had lost, obviously. Their delicate, almost quaint words, which fell just short of expressing the magnitude of the loss they had suffered, nevertheless impressed it on me, transmitted it in the very distance left unclosed, like a door, between words and reality. They were euphemistic forms of tact that invited me to be equally restrained. Affect isn't located in words but in gaps, and this is especially true of grief and sorrow. What had sounded to me like a kind of avoidance—perhaps of denial—was in reality a mode of contact, whereas my inner protests, had I expressed them out loud (and especially so), would have betrayed denial: I was trying to deny that their words had touched me more than I'd cared to acknowledge at that moment. *I* was the one trying to keep death at bay, not them. How could they have?

And there was also the guy who had taken Hervé's bar stool after he went to the bathroom but who relinquished it on the spot and without a word when Hervé, still young and already so visibly frail then, looked at him, also without a word. The persistent reality of AIDS had seldom felt so palpable to me than in this brief, almost imperceptible exchange of silences.

A few years later, Hervé was still doing reasonably well. He was on the new protease inhibitors, and they held HIV disease in check. He was awfully tired, though, both physically and psychologically. And so very thin. He was suffering from terrible side effects that kept sending him to the hospital more often than he used to go before the treatment. He also had to deal with this new and unexpected situation. After having prepared himself for the inevitable, he now had to face the unsettling possibility that he may not die after all, not now, not of AIDS. In French circles at the time, this process was called "le deuil du deuil"—the loss of loss. Hervé explained to me how surprisingly difficult it had been for him. He was still trying to come to terms with it. He may have succeeded. And then he died.

NAKED ARAB BODIES

Is it because young Arab men caught America so nakedly unprepared, like an emperor with no clothes, its vulnerability exposed for the whole world to see and gawk at, that our leaders and a sizable portion of the people felt the need, in turn, to bare and humiliate Arab bodies? Is it as payback for its humiliating defeat in Algeria that the French Republic thinks it has the right to rip headscarves from the faces of Muslim girls who attend its public schools? Has reason always been barbaric and thus (etymologically) foreign to itself?

And has it always been so sexual? As Jean-Luc Nancy suggests, sensual desire and the desire for thought may not be so easily disentangled, and what takes the form of sex in the realm of the senses is a sort of openness to contact no different in nature from that of thought itself:

> If intelligible order escapes from the sensible [*le sensible*, what pertains to the senses] and exceeds it, it is in the sensible that the momentum for this escape and for this excess originates. Sensual ardor itself is already a desire for thought. There is thus no thought that isn't also sexual. Whether it manifests itself as a "homo" or a "hetero" sexuality, thought is in itself the opening of this difference to the incommensurable terms of which "sex" is both site and figure, form and force: difference, which isn't a relation to an object but, rather, touch and tension between beings.

What happens, though, when I need to deny this continuum between body and thought for fear of losing myself (my self) forever in an abyss of pure relationality and difference, of touch and tension? How can I resist my coming undone?

To expose someone else's body without his or her consent for the sole purpose of humiliation instantly and unwittingly transforms the reviled person into an object of desire—or perhaps reveals that person to have always been one. The quickest way to resolve this tension between the reviled and the desired, the hated and the loved, is rape—in particular anal rape, in that this specific mode of violent bodily penetration seeks to destroy the other person's personhood by undoing the very boundaries that are constitutive of it. Think, for example, of the NYPD officers who inserted a police truncheon into the rectum of Abner Louima, a Haitian man, or of the impalement by right-wing skinheads of a recently buried Jewish man in the old Carpentras cemetery in France. The link between anal rape and the humiliation of ethnic or cultural others is all too apparent. But the intimacy thus created (and as the historian Joshua Cole has shown in the context of the French-Algerian war, torture is a form of relational intimacy) has the immediate potential of ruining the entire project of subjugation and exclusion (a policing project); or, rather, intimacy reveals that the project is impossible to begin with because desire was always at work within. If torture enacts a form of intimate contact with that-with-which-there-must-be-no-contact, it does not, however, allow for a simple, unintended reversal—"really" exposing the torturer's inhumanity reasserting the humanity of the tortured.

In her take on Abu Ghraib, and specifically on the attention lavished on the torturers, the queer scholar Jasbir K. Puar makes a comment that I found so perplexing that I wonder whether it stemmed from a temporary lapse of judgment or careless reliance on ideological autopilot. She writes: "It is devastating, but hardly surprising, that the U.S. public's obsessive consumption of this story nevertheless did not result in any deep-seated or longer-term demand to know who the victims are, what they experienced and felt, and how their lives are today." Yes, there's got to be a way to make these guys talk.

What takes place when any contact occurs is always and necessarily reciprocal. This doesn't imply moral equivalence, especially in the sort of violent contact that we are discussing here, but it invites us to consider the situation in a more complex fashion. If you've seen Alex Gibney's *Taxi to the Dark Side*, a documentary film about Abu Ghraib, that showed interviews with American soldiers accused of committing acts of torture—the Bush administration's infamous "bad apples"—in parallel with actual footage of the acts they committed, you may have realized that what often emerges from these juxtapositions is the shared humanity of perpetrators and victims. After all, if making an ethical decision is by definition a sign of someone's humanity, does it change anything, in that respect, whether the decision is right or wrong? Isn't a "bad" person still a person? As a result, the film allows its viewers to shift their focus from the perversion of individuals, always easy to isolate and distance oneself from, to that of a system, our system, with which relations are not so comfortably severed because it also gives shape and meaning to our own existence.

In a story set during the Vietnam War, Anna Moï writes, "There is no such thing as mechanical torture. A man always intervenes to determine the right dose of suffering to be imparted on another man, or on a woman. Or on a young woman."

But a man never acts alone.

S-21

S-21 is the name at once innocuous and chilling in its efficient administrative brevity given to what used to be Phnom Penh's Tuol Svay Prey High School. The S stands for "Security prison." There, between 1975 and 1978, under the Khmer Rouge regime, more than seventeen thousand Cambodians were imprisoned and tortured, and those who didn't die were hauled on trucks for a short ride to be murdered just outside the city in a place we now call the killing fields of Choeung Ek. Bullets being in short supply, victims were often done in with the blow of a shovel to the backs of their heads. S-21 has now been transformed into the grandiosely named Tuol Sleng Museum of Genocidal Crimes. The place is terrifying, for obvious reasons—most of the rooms in the various buildings have been left essentially untouched and there is no obtrusive curating to soften the impact of the visit—but also for reasons more indirect, less immediately affective.

S-21 unmistakably recalls the school that it used to be. It looks more or less like all the other schools you see across Cambodia. The torture chambers were once classrooms. In some of them, instead of desks there is now a bare metal bed frame where prisoners were bound and tortured. On one wall sometimes hangs a large, very poor quality black-and-white photograph of a prisoner on that very bed, in that very room that was once a classroom, his body mangled and his face a bleeding mess; on the opposite wall, a blackboard. Between the two, on the floor, dark stains. Past horrors seldom feel that present. The cellblock consists of rows of tiny spaces separated by wooden partitions or bare brick walls, all of them appearing to have been put together in no time and at minimal cost by amateurs, which was of course the case. As a prison and as a museum, S-21 reeks of poverty and of making do. The unspeakable horror of the acts perpetrated there by poor people against poor people and the pompous name of what in wealthier countries would barely qualify as a museum at all seem shockingly out of proportion with the modesty of the place. As a result, it all works now as it worked then—eerily, brutally well.

Before going to Cambodia I traveled up and down Vietnam. In Hanoi, I made the obligatory visit to the infamous Hanoi Hilton, the old French Maison centrale where, during the American War, US prisoners were detained and some, like John McCain, tortured. With its dark corridors and dungeons and chains and, yes, its gruesome guillotine, the old prison looks today just like what you expect an old prison to look like. Perhaps because of its colonial origins, there is something very nineteenth century about it, like the French version of a Dickensian gaol maybe, and it seems to have been built to house the likes of Vautrin and Edmond Dantès. In reality, of course, many Vietnamese independence fighters were jailed, tortured, and killed there. But with time, and because unlike S-21 this prison was actually built as one, it has acquired a sort of literary patina that its Cambodian counterpart will never be able to claim.

What that visit to S-21 made clear to me, as I came to realize later in the persistent and disturbing aftermath of it, is that bricolage, for all its inventiveness, all its creative potential, has no *inherent* political value. Yes, bricolage may be an ingenious mode of resignification that allows the marginalized to inhabit and hijack social norms, not at the grand conceptual end of them, the way revolutionaries might, but at the small, practical end that directly polices their lives and that is therefore easier to handle and maneuver without much thought. But S-21 and 9/11 were forms of bricolage also. School buildings and planes were hijacked and repurposed, ordinary gardening tools and box cutters recycled to commit mass murder, and this transformation of everyday things we normally think of as good or just harmless if we think about them at all had much to do with the historical and cultural impact of S-21 and 9/11. Each may have started small, but their reverberations have been deafening.

THE MODERNITY OF TORTURE

Our modern, Western sense of self is a matter of abstraction. The universal Man has been severed from the materiality and contingencies of his body in order to make room for a new form of citizenship. Torture, however (and this is also true of rape or racism or pathologization), seeks to reassert the fundamental exteriority of others by defining them as and with their bodies, that is to say, as pre- or nonself entities. To reactivate an archaic form of punishment is intended to expel its victims from the realm of modern selfhood by transferring this archaism to them. As paradoxical as this may sound, the torturer's barbarity makes him civilized because it produces the victim as his binary other, the nonself whose expulsion is necessary for there to be a self. Like rape, like racism, like pathologization, torture represents an integral part of the modern project.

THE E.R. EPISODE

Disgust often gives a person a sense of impenetrable wholeness, hence its central role in the fear of HIV and AIDS. Years ago, something horrible happened to me at the emergency room of the University of Michigan hospital. Although what brought me there was no big deal, I realized that day that my skin wasn't as thick as I thought it was. The barely perceptible curl of a doctor's lip as she read my chart was all it took to break it. It was as if a bottomless abyss had suddenly opened, and everything—everything—had vanished into it in a never-ending fall. This episode became the recurring nightmare of my waking life: I know what it feels like to be judged less than a human being. Thankfully, other people live with that knowledge too, so we can get together and laugh about it.

TRUTH AND TORTURE

One of the most startling things to emerge from the debates on torture during the Bush era (other than the realization that torture was an object of debate) was that information obtained under so-called enhanced interrogation techniques is known to be unreliable, since prisoners will simply say anything to make their suffering stop. Of course, Montaigne argued that very point in the sixteenth century. Closer to us, Elaine Scarry showed that "the fact that something is asked *as if* the content of the answer matters does not mean that it matters." So why torture? If information extracted from prisoners in pain is far more likely to be false, the "truth" that torture seeks must be located elsewhere and its purpose other than the revelation of facts still unknown but whose possible existence is invoked to justify the unjustifiable.

As semantics and etymology imply, there exists a connection between unveiling and revealing and, as a logical and commonplace extension of this link into the realm of allegory, between nakedness and truth. What, then, is this truth that torture attempts to reveal through the forced disrobing of other people's bodies and their exposition to their tormentors' gaze? If "truth" made up under torture doesn't perforce precede its "revelation," it must follow it or come about with it, and it is the naked body that bears (and bares) it. In the specific case of Arab bodies, the search for truth inevitably draws from the long history of relations between Muslims and Christians and between "East" and "West" as entities said to be not just distinct and incompatible but also unequal. The truth that the Christian West has sought, from the Crusades to Abu Ghraib, is, as we have known at least since Edward Said's groundbreaking work on orientalism, its own sense of possessing a homogeneous cultural identity. And this sense of simultaneous oneness and rightness has been asserted by contrast and thanks to the humiliation of Muslims as religiously wrong and of Arabs as culturally duplicitous.

The French ethnologist François Bizot, a scholar of ancient Cambodian cultures, was captured by the Khmer Rouge guerrillas in 1971 and recently testified against his captor, the infamous Kang Kek Iew, better known as Duch, who came to oversee S-21. Reflecting on the purpose of the horrific acts of torture committed by the Khmer Rouge and the relation of such acts to truth, Bizot remarks:

Among the Khmer Rouge, this was a settled matter: no one was to reveal anything or recount his personal story otherwise than expected of him. In this context, proclamations of innocence and proclamations of guilt were made in the process, as each testimony anticipated the appropriate statement of what a given individual was entitled to display about himself. Hence, the systematic intervention of a torturer, whose investigating mission was not, as I naively believed, to obtain a genuine confession but, rather, compliance.

Compliance, that is, with a preestablished model of what we already know the victim to be and that I, on the other hand, am not. At a deeper level lies no truth other than the illusion that subject and object, self and other, I and you form distinct entities endowed with their own set of incompatible characteristics. Truth, therefore, is not *uncovered* by policing; it *is* policing—the revealed, or unveiled, truth of the police. Torture, it appears, has no other purpose than to invent a discourse of power that we may then call the truth. Or to put in a different way, torture, as a part of an apparatus of power and domination and, as such, discursive in nature, seeks, like all discourses, not to represent reality but to produce it—in this case, to produce a specific political reality.

Can nakedness, displayed, denied, or hinted at, be played with and affect modalities of power?

DINING WITH FRENCH PEOPLE

For an American academic—and I am one—to study the controversies that have taken place in France over Muslim headscarves before and after 9/11 feels a bit like landing on a distant and mysterious planet or falling down the rabbit hole into a world where everything seems to have been turned upside down and stopped making any kind of sense. I must confess my admiration for scholars such as the feminist historian Joan Scott, the anthropologist John Bowen, and others, who have so eloquently refuted every single argument ever put forth by proponents of the ban on religious symbols in French public schools. My own reaction, which I may very well explain by the fact that I am not just American but also French, has been far less sanguine and more along the lines of "Have you people completely lost your minds?"

Once, during a stay in Paris, I was invited to a (lovely) dinner at which I forgot once again to arrive twenty minutes late. (Immigration can be so disorienting, although not just to immigrants, I believe, which is one reason why it's so interesting.) At one point in the flow of the conversation, I expressed my exasperation with people who say "Ça m'agresse!" as a reaction to seeing women wearing a hijab on the streets. (Bowen's fine reading of this phrase, which describes something between feeling offended and assaulted, inspired me that night.) One of my friends, whose intelligence is not in doubt, replied, "I'm sorry but I do feel it is a form of aggression." In the republican culture of modern France, the term *public* traditionally refers, when used in a political sense, to entities run by the state or local government. A school can be public; so can a library, a museum, or a swimming pool. But a restaurant, for example, is not. As for the street, it is a dicey business. Is it an extension of the home, as so many people's behavior would suggest, and in this case private in nature? Or does it belong to the public sphere because it is maintained thanks to the citizens' taxes? The latter view explains why French people so often take their political grievances to the streets; the former why some find littering or kissing in public perfectly natural. Perhaps unfairly, I chose to ignore the fact that streets, by virtue of their spatial and cultural in-betweenness, inevitably get caught up in all sorts of friction, and I went on a rant about how slippery the definition of the "public" can become and how easily we go from public schools to government offices to the streets, which were supposed to belong to everyone and, if I'm not mistaken, to remain free from excessive state intervention. Case in point: the eventual banning of the niqab, the burka, and all full facial veils from the entire territory of the Republic. What I should have said was this: for a while now, young Arab men have been largely defined as delinquents (Nicolas Sarkozy used more controversial terms) who simply refuse to integrate into French society and whose alleged acts of so-called incivility are typically described as "aggressions." Now, it seems, time has come for the young women to be guilty of the same crime, and their hijabs are the telltale signs of their refusal to live in harmony with others. Thanks to a rhetorical trick, members of a minority subjected to racism and many forms of social exclusion find themselves redefined as the aggressors, while members of the majority become the victims. How clever. What a smart way to say, in essence, "I don't want to encounter these people in *my* neighborhood."

Another dinner, another story: I was once asked to participate in a graduate seminar at another university. I had agreed to talk about Guillaume Dustan, a gay, HIV-positive author who was rightly or wrongly made to embody a certain "ghettoized" gay lifestyle that once made a subject of controversy in France. During the dinner that followed, I found myself sitting next to one of the grad students, a young, white, French woman who soon started criticizing what she understood as my defense of *communautarisme*—the word often used in a variety of French discourses (political, philosophical, etc.) to mean, and denounce, something like identity-based separatism. Because the gay community hasn't occupied center stage in that debate since roughly the late 1990s, the discussion turned right away to Muslim girls and their attire. Of course, that's what the young French woman was trying to get at all along. She had no interest in homosexuals and wouldn't criticize them in front of me in any case.

I had recently finished Bowen's book, *Why the French Don't Like Headscarves*, so I was astonished to hear my dinner companion, who had been trained at the prestigious École Normale Supérieure, give me pretty much the entire roster of points that the American anthropologist had knocked down one after the other. *Communautarisme*, Islamist threats to France's secular culture and its strict division of the public and the private, attacks against women's rights and dignities . . . You name it, she said it. It is one thing to be convinced, as I was, by a scholar's analysis, but quite another to verify the accuracy of this analysis, so perfectly and in the flesh. Needless to say, having the book so vivid in my mind allowed me to be far quicker on the uptake than I usually am in similar situations. After listening to, and countering, a litany of complaints so robotic it verged on the creepy,

I finally told my interlocutor, "Do you honestly think that the best way to integrate young people into society, as you claim you want to do, is to expel them from school?" To which she replied, without missing a beat and in a tone of righteous indignation only the French can muster to perfection, "People don't get expelled from schools; *symbols* do!" An awkward silence fell around the table, interrupted, in more colorful versions of the anecdote, by the squishy sound of my lower jaw dropping into my plate of Moroccan couscous. The conversation kind of shifted to another topic after that.

Don't think me a braggart, however, for as French as I admit I remain sometimes, I claim no glory in having defeated my opponent in a verbal joust. I am well aware that from an intellectual standpoint, and perhaps even from an ethical one, the worst thing you can do with an argument is win it. Victory's a lousy teacher, its pleasures too fleeting and ordinary to constitute anything resembling a fruitful reward. And that last one required little effort in any case. Yet I recount these stories not only because they are absolutely true but because they illustrate with uncanny accuracy the strange phenomenon that has been taking place in France of late. Here's a country where the elites who produce, modulate, and impose dominant discourses have created a national identity based on reason, human rights, and intellectual sophistication, yet these same elites have embraced the exact opposites of these values without so much as a blink. The thing, of course, is that these sets of opposites cannot be disentangled, each term perpetually repelling and desiring its own negation, and it is a good thing to be periodically reminded of this fact. Still, how irritating.

Think of my second dinner companion. By blinding herself to an obvious reality—that actual human beings have in fact been expelled from public schools for wearing a hijab or legal equivalent (a "regular" scarf, a bandanna, etc.)—she made a statement that I could charitably describe as disingenuous. Yet the remark was also quite revealing, so to speak, and what it unwittingly uncovered by mentioning the centrality of symbols in this whole sorry affair was the aesthetic dimension of the political. I am not talking about an aestheticization of politics, as is the case with fascism, but, following the philosopher Jacques Rancière, of politics as inseparable from aesthetics to the extent that both are fraught with questions of visibility. If the body and the face have a long symbolic history, so, of course, does the veil that hides them from sight and signals their presence at the same time. The fact that the word *voile* (veil) has been, as Joan Scott and others rightly point out, so often used to refer to a headscarf that does not actually cover the woman's face, signals that we are indeed in the realm of symbols and, therefore, dealing with questions of aesthetics.

To expel symbols constitutes in itself a symbolic act, and so does forcing girls to remove their headscarves. In the first situation, actual headscarves, already metonyms for the Republic's latest inassimilable other, must be replaced in the public sphere with their symbolic, constitutive absence or privatization. In the latter situation, another symbol is created—the "unveiled" face that stands for the naked body. Indeed, in 2010 France finally made it unlawful to cover one's face in "public spaces" and did so in the name of individual freedom and gender equality. Politicians were fond of evoking "the whole territory of the Republic" in order to impart on people that nothing short of national integrity was at stake in the debate. But why would the visibility of one's face present a guarantee of equal treatment? France, after all, is also a country where it is customary to attach one's picture on a CV, thus opening the door to all sorts of discrimination. The following question arises now: How can this second mode of symbolization—unveiling—work to exclude Arab women from full citizenship as well as, or even better than, their physical expulsion from public schools would?

The answer to this question has to do with the place of the body in relation to the French model of universal citizenship. To aestheticize the body *as body* makes it that which must be the object of the gaze and, as such, cannot pertain to reason or have any access to it. And the operation also results in making the person thus defined by his or her body unable to escape membership in his or her "biological" group, such as sex or race. Religion inscribes itself within the same logic. Privatized by Western modernity, it finds itself "naturally" attached to women in a move that welds together reason's two opposites, irrationality and the body, and expels them both from the public sphere in one fell swoop. In other words, this form of corporeality underscores the person's inability to become an autonomous individual and to rise to the level of abstraction that is the necessary condition of citizenship in post-Enlightenment France. Scott shows very convincingly how, for a long time, this operation excluded women from citizenship and how French Muslims now find themselves facing a similar problem: "Muslims are now in a similar position. Of course, they do qualify for citizenship, but their membership in a religious community that does not conceive of individuals as able to recognize their beliefs in terms of public or private makes them not susceptible to abstraction, hence incapable of assimilation." And I would add all postcolonial and sexual others to the list. In fact, it is no surprise that colonial imagery was so sexualized, in one form or another, since most of the colonial expansion took place at roughly the same period as the invention of our modern categories of sex and sexuality and the development of ever-more effective virtual technologies of the gaze that sought to produce bodies impossible to abstract.

If reason has two opposites, does this entail that the political system that rests on it cannot hope to reach the sort of stability and oneness normally provided by the expulsion of a singular other? The desire to close what is a foundational loophole may explain the urge to pathologize madness and deviance during the century that followed the bourgeoisie's seizure of political power. If irrationality, in the form of madness, superstition, perverse desire, and whatnot, can be visible on the body, reason's two opposites would appear to be one and the same. The bourgeoisie, however, had always sought to define itself by occupying the middle ground, justifying its claim to power by representing the ideal of moderation against both lack and excess. What characterizes such a class is that it is surrounded by several others, hence its need of a more diffuse form of power that can allow it to deal with that multiplicity.

We have known at least since Foucault that visibility in itself provides no emancipation and that, in fact, it has served as a vector for the diffusion of liberal-democratic forms of power by multiplying and disseminating the points of contact—between power and bodies, for example. (Ask me what it feels like to be obligated by law to reveal/unveil the contents of my bone marrow in certain intimate circumstances. Then again, don't ask me; it's torture.) Visibility, therefore, possesses no intrinsic political value. Nothing does. Since politics pertains by definition to the relational, a thing's political value is thus always located in the interstices that simultaneously separate it from and connect it to other things, that is, where the relating takes place but nothing actually *is*. This is where the political plays itself out: in the distance without which no such thing called visibility can exist. In that sense, to aestheticize the other's body seeks to fill this distance with a very specific type of political relation, one in which the gazing subject dominates the objects of his gaze and produces the illusion that the gaze cannot be returned. As Scott points out, the fantasy of the veil, as opposed to the actual headscarves, finds its origin in the fear of being seen without seeing. The aestheticization and embodiment of young Muslim women thanks to their symbolic unveiling—their being made visible—is thus what allows the French Republic to use the discourse of integration to exclude people.

The diverse must be embraced the better to be denied, or: contacts must be established (a modern form of power dynamics) for there to be exclusion (the work of the police).

What matters politically, in the end, is what you do with visibility and invisibility (what, according to Rancière, frames what we call politics). So what is it, then, that some of these French Muslim women who wear a headscarf in public do? For one thing, wearing a headscarf inscribes Muslim women in public spaces—no small feat in a culture that mandates that religion and sex be privatized. But it does so in a way that doesn't make them the objects of a reifying gaze. Fighting symbol with symbol (what choice do they have if everyone understands the head as standing for the whole body?), they use the headscarf in a way that says, "I will not be aestheticized by the act of unveiling." The piece of cloth, which symbolically disrupts the hierarchization of a subject's gaze and an objectified body, also mediates between two power systems—a "progressive" West and a "regressive" Islam—that each have a long history of excluding women from full citizenship, either by exposing their bodies or by covering them. In that sense, wearing a hijab in France may be a tactical way for women to make an oppositional use of a small piece of fabric in order to expose and oppose the workings of power within two systems that may not have women's best interests in mind. Each woman wearing a hijab may not realize that this is going on, but the system seems to have sensed the danger somehow.

In the end, could this feeling of aggression some French people like to complain about be triggered not so much by the sight of hijabs in public places but instead by the visibility of Muslim women as citizens in the public sphere and therefore not out of place within the polis? Just as the "unveiling" of Muslim schoolgirls sought to cover up the oppressive agenda of the Republic's discourse of integration, the "veiling" of the same people may reveal the exclusion of Arabs by and from the French state. In a new twist on the old colonial paternalism—"This is for your own good and you'll thank us when you've grown up"—the republic forces women not to be coerced into wearing a hijab. This perverse form of enlightened coercion finds its justification in a liberal regime of the self. Such a regime refuses to acknowledge that the self does not represent a universal truth to be uncovered at last but a product of cultural mediations—in other words, a veil, a veil that veils the nothingness of pure difference. For some Muslim women, to reclaim public spaces with the headscarf points, perhaps not automatically but at least potentially, toward a different model of democratic, rather than republican, citizenship based on a relational concept of the self as an effect, rather than a precondition, of contact.

From such a democratic vantage point, we cannot consider the self the autonomous entity from which reason may arise and ground social contracts. Instead, the self results from contacts, always multiple and ever changing, between bodies. As Rosalyn Diprose puts it,

> If it cannot be said that the self remains unchanged through a series of actions, then promises cannot be made, contracts cannot be signed, no one could be taken at his or her word and, according to this view of things, social relations would have no basis. So to say that the self's identity is performed and reconstituted within the act is no trivial claim; it challenges the very foundation of the moral, social, and political relations of modernity.

To this I would add: if the self doesn't preexist the contract but is instead an effect of it, then selfhood is contracted, like a virus or other foreign body, thanks to unplanned encounters or because, for whatever reason, we let our guard down. This may create some degree of discomfort at the post office or the supermarket, but is it going to kill us?

ENCOUNTERING THE STRANGE

For non-Muslims, the very act of coming across people they can immediately identify as Muslim, right there on the streets or in some public administration, without expecting it, bursts with affect, often of the confusing kind. In other situations, perhaps other times, similar feelings of confusion have greeted encounters with people of color or gay men holding hands or Jews wearing a yellow star or the frail, wasting bodies the media once taught us to recognize as those of people dying of AIDS. So what do these anxious encounters with Muslimness tell us about encounters in general? (The French word *musulmanité* would contain an interesting possibility of wordplay with *humanité*, by the way.)

First of all, it is important to note how the categories of Arab and Muslim have bled into each other in public discourses and imagination. Roughly half the Arab population in the United States is in fact Christian, and we know that Iranians, Turks, Indonesians, or Malays, for example, while predominantly Muslim, are not Arabs. The same can be said of Berbers in North Africa. In France, several of the "affairs" that brought the question of the hijab to public attention concerned non-Arab converts. Yet because of the combined forces of France's colonial history and the immigration patterns that followed decolonization, "Muslim" has in effect become synonymous with "Arab," and a religious "problem" that had until recently raised few problems at all has served as a convenient excuse. Better, it seems, to cloak one's hostility to certain people in the grand principles of the nation than to admit that it boils down, in the end, to a matter of racism. With 9/11 and the invasion of Iraq in 2003, the fog of war has further clouded the issue, but, with the return of torture to the fore, it has also brought back the fact that, since the Algerian War, the relationship between French and Arabs has had a uniquely strong physical component. (Nothing quite like that has played such a role with other Muslims in France, such as people of West African origin.)

The historian Naomi Davidson asserts that current French hostility toward Islam, while claiming the mantle of secularism as a defining characteristic of the nation, has crystallized over Muslim embodied religious practices and that this has in fact been the case at least since the start of the colonial era. Arab Muslims have been caught in a double bind as a result. Asked to integrate within French secular culture, much as the Jews are said to have done, they have been simultaneously subjected to various discursive and institutional forces that made it impossible for them to do so. Jews, on the other hand, were provided after centuries of oppression with the necessary support that made their full citizenship possible. And from this I hypothesize that some people invoke the exemplarity of the Jews' integration mainly to produce Arabs as polar opposites while making Jews exceptional and thus undermining their alleged integration at the same time. The move, twinning Jews and Arabs as example and counterexample in a sort of intimacy that they themselves can experience only as conflict, is nothing short of brilliant, if diabolical.

To force the bodies of Muslims to play a central role in their othering betrays a founding tension in the Enlightenment's ideal of the contractual nation. Both practically and conceptually, cultural rejection cannot always be separated from racism—the likes of which, I would add, may not appear so nakedly in the wake of Auschwitz if the argument is to have an appeal beyond a small circle of unrepentant far-right activists. Indeed, dominant French culture forecloses all possibility of a discursive space from which to articulate a racist position that wouldn't simultaneously expel the speaker from the political mainstream. Every act of expulsion grounded in hostility toward other people's bodies must therefore assume a cultural form (battles over headscarves, rules of engagements in public places, women's rights, civic etiquette, etc.) while performing the irreducible corporeality of these others in order to expel them on this very basis. The controversies that, as I noted earlier, once greeted the development of a visible gay neighborhood in the Marais in the 1990s exemplify just such a move. Queers, then, were criticized for allegedly threatening the republican pact of universal citizenship.

With their focus on the corporeality of others in order to protect the integrity of one's own body, racism, like homophobia, thus forms a kind of embodied thinking, but one that can only piggyback on discourses of culture. The purpose is to give the impression that others are naturally (rather than discursively) embodied when said embodiment actually represents a projection and denial of the thinker's/speaker's own. Given the cultural framework in which this operation is taking place, the thinker/speaker must conceal his own embodiment for fear of disqualifying himself as a thinker/speaker. (And this position is indeed symbolically a male one, even though an actual woman may occupy it.) What emerges in the social realm is thus a principle of radical separation that has failed in thought—a foundational failure that must imperatively appear masked, or veiled.

Doubters could argue that the headscarf affairs are not racist at all, the irrefutable proof being that they often concerned French converts not of North African descent. But it is the converts themselves who embody precisely the fear of contact as contamination.

Feelings of aggression, with the strong physical undertones of the phrase *Ça m'agresse*, do signal what is essentially a refusal to make corporeal, as well as cultural, contact. It reveals that nearness, in such cases, is felt as out-of-placeness, a breach of boundaries—and of the social contract resting on them—that tends to produce anxiety about one's own sense of identity. People may interpret the signs of racialized Muslimness on the bodies of the people they see, but they do so in the strictest hermeneutic sense, that is, only to the extent that they uncover the meaning that these signs were already endowed with before a specific encounter has even taken place. People want to recognize their own projections, which they can do by denying the relational nature of meaning. For example, the condemnation of so-called radical Islam, a violent rejection of everything modern and Western that found its most shocking illustration in the collapse of the World Trade Center, is often nothing more than a veil thrown over the modern, Western form of radical rejection stemming from Cartesian thought: the expulsion of the other as radically distinct from and nonconstitutive of the self. The trick, once more, allows us to accuse of separatism the very people *we* have separated from us.

A more pleasurable kind of encounter, it seems to me, would occur in situations where the appeal of strange surfaces makes us aware that the in-betweenness that defines nearness brings together touch and separation, inside and outside, singular and plural, self and other, and so forth. We could call this the pleasure of difference.

TIMES SQUARE LOST

New York and its vanished landmarks have once again crept into my memory. Perhaps because of 9/11 or perhaps because of the idea of strange encounters, I'm thinking of the old, filthy Times Square as I discovered it in the summer of 1985, with its junkies and crazies and whores. "Want some company, honey?" asked the woman who came so close that her invitation sounded like a whisper in my ear over the cacophony of the city. Back then, you couldn't experience an evening on Broadway, a fun and glitzy night on the town, without at least a glimpse of the underbelly of it all. Pleasure, in other words, couldn't be dissociated from the discomfort of encounters with the strange, and New York would never let you forget what its fabulousness was built on and at whose expense. This was, after all, the Reagan years. People were dying of AIDS by the thousands in complete indifference, and homelessness was everywhere. Since then, Rudy Giuliani's Disneyfication of Times Square (a process Hanif Kureishi once had a narrator describe, in a Marxist way, as one in which "the real relations of production [are] concealed") has entailed hiding the unsightliness and pushing the sites where encounters and contact are possible all the way beyond even the margins. Celebration, U.S.A., Disney's new-urbanist community in Florida, is similarly surrounded by the poor and largely Latino population that works there but doesn't live there, as the cultural critic Andrew Ross has observed. In both cases, the purpose is to keep opposites neatly separated, aggression at bay, and order in the streets.

The first time I saw the new Times Square, it was very late on a warm summer night. 1999 I think it was. I encountered a nice white family, with young kids skipping around all happy and smiling and shit. Scary, scary stuff. There goes the neighborhood, I thought. Times Square? Definitely not the kind of place where you'd want to hang out after dark anymore. In this city I loved, I felt a little lonely and out of place.

"Want some company, honey?"

Yeah, as a matter of fact, I do.

IN THE CITY AND OUT

The notion of civility, like its near synonym urbanity, implies that a certain level of sophistication is to be found in cities. (A French equivalent of "civil" and "urbane" would be *policé*, a word with similar implications, this time from a Greek rather than Latin root.) If cities are defined partly by diversity and circulation, life together may be attained there thanks only to the careful management of differences and more or less tacit rules of etiquette. The alleged incivility of young French people "of immigrant origin" (*issus de l'immigration* says the capacious phrase of choice) may then be understood as a breach of etiquette that threatens the very possibility of *vivre-ensemble*. Men's "aggressions" and women's religiosity become signs that they do not belong in the city but outside it, in the *banlieues* with which they remain almost automatically associated in the minds of many.

But because civility is the mark of civilization, the refusal or inability to master etiquette doesn't entail only exteriority but also inferiority. The odious theory of the so-called clash of civilizations doesn't position the West and Islam side by side and equal. The incongruity of visible Muslims in a Western city signals at best their lack of sophistication and at worst their barbarity, that is, their outsider status as uncivilized foreigners. Islamic terrorism, in that sense, would thus constitute the ultimate act of incivility. It makes an awful mess in the city.

FROM PUBLIC SCHOOLS TO PUBLIC POOLS

Soon it wasn't just French schools anymore. If the management of some (privately owned) supermarket chain decides to sell halal products or, in neighborhoods with a large Muslim clientele, not to carry pork or alcohol at all, accusations of "Islamization" or "Talibanization" start flying and the blogosphere goes wild. There were outcries when some Muslim women asked for women-only hours at public swimming pools. Surely people had made such requests before, and even though I don't know for sure what happened locally, I suspect that the countrywide controversy erupted only after the headscarf had become a national *affaire*. And there were other "problems" at many government offices and administrations and other public venues, which gave the impression that some sort of cultural invasion was taking place that would soon result in a complete takeover of the country by foreign forces. As you can imagine, 9/11 and its aftermath didn't help.

The *Jewish Journal of Greater Los Angeles* once ran a cover story titled "The Rise of Muslim Europe." The front page featured a veiled Mona Lisa. Converted by choice or by coercion? In the spring of 2010, I took a trip to Toronto at a time when Quebec's own attempts at banning Muslim veils and headscarves in public places were making the Canadian news. A local daily featured on the top half of its front page, which made it visible in vending machines all over town, the photo of a woman whose face was covered by a black niqab leaving only her eyes visible—her pale green eyes that looked blue only three feet away. A friend of mine laughed when I showed her the picture: "Well, she could be Berber, I suppose . . ." The point both papers were trying to make was simple enough: if left unchecked, Muslims will not just seek the right to dress the way they want or to practice their religion freely but they will force the rest of us to adopt their backward ways. We fear contact as a kind of contagiousness. Forced unveiling, like mandatory disclosure, represents a symbolic attempt to make something like a virus visible to keep it at bay.

Not convinced? Consider this. In France, tensions also arose when young men and boys (of color) were turned away from pools because, out of modesty, they preferred to swim wearing longer and looser shorts rather than the mandatory small, tight swimming trunks that, for cultural reasons, they deemed too revealing. Again, from this side of the Atlantic, the controversy borders on the surreal. The stated reason to refuse the young men access to the pool was that they could possibly have worn their shorts on the streets and that swimming with them on would be unsanitary. The obvious solution—loaning clean shorts on the premises—seems to have crossed few people's minds. And what happened to chlorination? The rhetoric of hygiene in portrayals of foreigners, immigrants, and in this case people considered as such even though they're not is hardly new. We perceive the outside as inherently unclean. It isn't worth spending unnecessary time and energy listing everything that is wrong with this in order to see, once again, a desire to expel Arabs, either literally or by humiliating them and exposing their bodies both as sexualized objects and as carriers of disease. How familiar this all feels to a gay man, as it does, I suppose, to anyone whose unruly body has been invoked—invented, really—to naturalize social exclusion and enforce it with maximum efficacy.

(In Denmark, a controversy involving Islam and nakedness greeted the refusal of some Muslims to use group showers. To shower together in the nude, people claimed, has long been such a defining element of Danish identity that the reluctance to do so cannot be considered a simple, acceptable preference for modesty but only a sign of radical otherness and refusal to integrate into a society whose alleged openness figures in the minds of many as a collective mingling of naked bodies.)

PARTICULAR BODIES

The fact that my own body so often feels problematic to me now makes me look elsewhere for comparisons. It would be absurd to claim that everyone is a racist or a homophobe or freaked out by those who are HIV positive. Many people simply don't care or do not in any way see difference as worthy of judgment and social exclusion. But some people do, and, at my worst, so do I.

Asking himself why there is no tradition of the nude in Chinese art, François Jullien makes the following observation. In Western art the function of the human nude has been to abstract Man and figure his very essence as distinct from both the animal and the social. Why China supposedly never sought to do the same thing—or at least not in the same way—doesn't concern me here. I wonder rather how this universalizing function of the nude could coexist so comfortably with what looks like its opposite—the exclusionary uses of nakedness. The question could then be: When and where does the unclothed body cease to figure the transcendence of the human?

"When" and "where" are not innocent queries, for two main reasons. For one thing, only when it meets specific circumstances can nakedness acquire the power to particularize. Exclusion is in the eyes of the beholder, as it were, not in the naked body itself. But more important, to me at least, is the idea that such a phenomenon happens in historical contexts, and what I'm interested in is Western modernity. For Jullien, Western culture tends toward an ideal, and if the nude makes a historical reappearance in art during the Renaissance and the classical era that follows, it is because the period is also concerned with the establishment of objective and universal science. This means that the answer to the question "When and where does the naked body cease to figure the transcendence of the human?" is, in the age of reason, "When and where it is made the receptacle of unreason and, as such, the visible marker of social and political otherness."

Perhaps paradoxically, then, the development of the nude in modern Western aesthetics is symptomatic of the Cartesian operation of disembodiment that characterizes thought at the same period. In search of an ideal, Western culture turns the nude into an abstract form, "abstract in both senses of the word: of being abstracted from the posing model, and of being abstract as an essence." Therefore "the nude stands at the crossroads of two requirements related to two complementary logics: it owes its rise to the combination of unveiling (the image is revelatory) and modelizing (with a view to achieving the ideal)." This question of unveiling is, naturally, what I'm after here. And what I find striking is how modern culture may define itself as propelled by the quest for truth by means of analytic reason and, at the same time, undermine its very project thanks to its continued belief in revealed truth. The modern ideal, it seems, is perpetually undone by modern practices.

In Western art (and thought), to disrobe a body is to represent it, that is, to abstract it—to turn it into a sign or a symbol. Think of the French woman's remark about the Muslim girls who were expelled from school: "People don't get expelled from schools; *symbols* do." In this case, the symbol expelled from school represents an idea of humanity perceived as discordant with "ours." The discordance, however, may not be accommodated because our idea of humanity happens to be universal. Discordance, then, can only lead to incompatibility because it falls outside the human. Non-Western attempts at abstraction can only fail, and the only thing cultural or social others of all kinds may symbolize is that very failure.

Supposedly unable to attain the Cartesian dualism of body and mind, the racialized Muslim body becomes the "embodiment" of its idea. The two cannot be separated. But it is a body that may be humiliated, raped, beaten, tortured. Indeed it must. The Muslim body may be harmed because it is less than fully human. And it must be harmed because Muslims must be made to feel their limits and their inability to overcome their corporeality. In general, the "oriental" body is not aestheticized the way that the Western body is; like the queer body it can only be sexualized, which offers another way to deny transcendence and, consequently, the modern citizenship such transcendence supports. This is what the forced unveiling of Muslim girls in the schools of the French Republic is all about.

The profound dishonesty of the universalist argument for the unveiling of Muslim girls, and now adult women, is that, from that perspective, there is no such thing as a woman without a veil. We never think of a non-Muslim woman in a non-Muslim culture as appearing "without a veil." A Muslim woman, however, whether literally or symbolically unveiled, will always index on her body, for which the face is a synecdoche, the act of unveiling and, therefore, the veil itself. The same may be said of all such universalizing gestures designed to signal entry into full citizenship. Blacks in the United States and Jews in France will never really be free; they have been *freed* or emancipated. The past participle stands as a reminder both of their previous status and of the liberating gesture that supposedly brought it to an end—but didn't and indeed couldn't. The liberated will constantly and forever be reminded of the debt they have contracted toward their liberators, a debt that can never be repaid for the reason that the latter would no longer be able to define themselves as liberators. In other words, the liberating gesture always maintains the inferior status of the other within the culture, if not within the law. For example, how could France, no longer an imperial power, continue to define itself as the country of human rights if some people within its own borders were not deprived of these rights? In short, the perpetual indexing of the act of liberating annuls liberty itself.

In a very similar way, my body, like that of everyone with HIV, will forever index the act that led to its infection. When feeling depressed—that is to say, unfair to myself and to others—I see my infection as a sign of failure and cannot imagine how anyone else would see it otherwise. It seems that I don't just *have* HIV, I *got* it. I have become infected. The present perfect, in this sense, has always been the tense of the HIV positive. The act of my body's infection will always be linked by some people, gay or straight, to the homosexual acts in which it has been engaged, but this counts for very little in the end compared with this, a more profound indictment of my entire self as a self: I have failed to remain uninfected. This, I'm thinking, is what some try to keep at a safe distance, especially if they are gay too. But because my HIV status is as undetectable on my body as the virus is in my bloodstream, I must be made to reveal it. In my encounters with others, I too must be unveiled.

The mulling and circular thinking that characterize depression, when one is just not thinking straight, often come with a degree of self-fulfilling paranoia. Not everyone is pozphobic, it's true, but as the old joke goes, just because you're paranoid doesn't mean they're not out to get you.

THE FALLING MAN

There exist many famous photos of historical trauma and human suffering. We all know the one with the small Jewish boy from the Warsaw ghetto, walking with his hands up, as a German soldier points a rifle at him. We have seen Phan Thi Kim Phúc, the Vietnamese girl running naked down a dirt road, her body burned by napalm. And the Vietcong fighter grimacing a second before a South Vietnamese officer shoots him in the head in Eddie Adams's Pulitzer Prize–winning photo. Much nearer today is the picture of a hooded Iraqi man in Abu Ghraib prison, standing on a box, electrodes dangling from his extended arms. Heartrending and revolting as these images may be, they are not, strictly speaking, impossible to look at. Not that their ubiquity has dulled their power to shock, necessarily, but the fact that they have played such a culturally significant role has displaced their primary meaning away from what they depict to who looks at them.

Soon after the abuses at Abu Ghraib were revealed to the public, T-shirts and stickers bearing the silhouette of the hooded man on the box, with the first-person caption "Not in my name," started to appear. These images were primarily concerned with the United States and its suffering national self, not with the man whose humiliation became industrially reproduced and worn as a statement about someone else. I do not subscribe to the idea that the Abu Ghraib photos should not have been shown because doing so would only perpetuate the humiliation and torture of these men. These were sickening photos, and seeing them was necessary to turn as many people as possible against torture and against the war itself. But if the image of the hooded man could function as such a powerful symbol, it is precisely because it could not *not* be looked at, because we could not take our eyes off of it. And that's the problem. By becoming so symbolic, the individual man figured on the picture became, in a sense, severed from himself and made to stand for something bigger but also more abstract, like man's inhumanity to man rather than a person's suffering in a specific historical and political situation.

One picture that never let itself be enrolled in the service of sentimental humanism is the one of the man falling from the World Trade Center on 9/11. Many such pictures were taken that day, but few were shown, at least in the United States. The one I'm thinking of, however, became the object of a short-lived controversy after it was published in the *New York Times* the next day. Many readers were scandalized because, they said, the photo was so large that the man on it could possibly be recognized. It showed a man in a shirt and tie falling head first, presumably after jumping to his death, as so many did, to escape a more horrific death in the flames. Maybe the man could be recognized, but in the same way that the people on the flyers could be recognized. Unlike the firefighters' chaplain, whose lifeless body being carried out, as in a classic Deposition, by the very men he ministered to was pictured everywhere, the falling man could not be turned into a hero or a saint. We could not separate ourselves from him. And the picture remains impossible to behold.

But to figure out why isn't easy, for if it were possible to articulate precisely why this picture was never used as a cultural symbol, then we could easily look at it. In fact, we would have to look at it to analyze it. So I'll venture a hypothesis that I will not attempt to prove. From a purely theoretical standpoint, there is no such thing as a picture that cannot be looked at, since it is the act of looking that makes it a picture. And nothing *in* the picture itself may ever guarantee that it won't be made into a symbol, because the process of symbolization necessarily involves many more participants, human and not, and the complex web of their interactions. For example, in a conversation, once, a friend of mine referred to this picture as "the man falling from the towers." I didn't pick up on the oddity of the phrase until much later. The man, of course, was falling from one tower, not both. But our conversation had not been about 9/11 up to that point. (We were in fact talking about images of divers.) Yet I knew right away what she was talking about, thanks to the plural whose incongruous contact with the singular I didn't even notice. In fact, had she used the singular I may have asked "What man? What tower?" whereas her faulty statement all but guaranteed that I would understand it accurately. It worked *because* it was faulty. This literally inaccurate contact between a single man and the events emblematically represented by the two towers of the World Trade Center thus indicated that a cultural process of symbolization, rather than denotation, was at work in the phrase my friend had used. But has the symbol made its way into the culture at large? There is a novel by Don DeLillo titled *Falling Man*. It is about 9/11, and the title intends, I believe, to reference the photo in the *Times*. But the phrase hasn't been adopted more largely than that. I for one had never heard it before. But I understood what my friend meant. So if the symbol came about in, and for, that specific situation, it didn't come out of nowhere either. The picture's power to symbolize may have been dormant until activated, and its ability to convey truth by means of, if not quite falsehood, at least dysfunction, made for an apt testimony to our incredulous feelings in the face of an all-too-real event.

It may be more appropriate, then, to describe this particular image as haunting. And what makes the picture of the falling man haunting in a way that the picture of the hooded man isn't lies in its ability to index the horror of 9/11 as it affected not a nation, not the human race, but persons. If this picture makes us feel the unspeakable brutality of 9/11 it is because, resisting both reduction and expansion, it stubbornly refuses to allegorize what happened. We can pay tribute to the fallen, such as the Christ-like chaplain, but not to the falling. The falling, whose fall never ends, cannot bring us closure. This particular man may not be so easily abstracted from his own personhood and made to symbolize anything bigger and more abstract than himself. Instead, he reminds us of 3,000 other persons just as small and just as real.

TOWEL STORIES (II)

He had a strange habit. He had many strange habits, in fact, and he was seeing shrinks and taking meds for that. One habit consisted of showering before coming to bed but, somehow, never drying himself completely, so that he would sit on his heels for a while, naked and wet on top of the bed, until he felt he was dry enough to get his body under the covers. How odd people are sometimes. If he couldn't stand to go to bed wet, why did he come to bed wet? Why didn't he simply use his towel a bit more thoroughly? I remember looking at his small, shivering body, night after night, thinking that his mind didn't make much conventional sense at all. Then again, when I was looking at his small, shivering body, cool and warm like summer rain, it was often I who made no sense.

Both obsessive compulsive disorder and depression are manifestations of a lack of control and mastery over oneself and the world, not only because they are (understood as) mental disorders but to the extent that what propels them is circular repetition. A depressed person like me tends to ruminate, while he sometimes kept driving in circles, returning to the scene of an accident that never happened. Such circularity goes nowhere, achieves nothing, and has no purpose grander than itself. But unlike ripple effects that soften as they spread out, the circles of madness remain hard-edged, they intensify pain and inscribe it on the world. Perhaps what brought us together for a time was that we both suffered from ailments about which we felt more than a hint of touchiness and that filled our lives with shrinks, meds, and misunderstandings. It helps.

ONE DROP OF BLOOD

In 1995 the Olympic star diver Greg Louganis went on television with a book to sell and a story to tell. That evening, he didn't just reveal that he was gay, which many people, few of whom were actual rocket scientists, had suspected long before he appeared at the 1994 Gay Games, but that he had AIDS. The news wasn't very spectacular in itself. In the world of sports alone, Arthur Ashe and Magic Johnson, although both heterosexual, had preceded Louganis with their own disclosures, and the impact had been arguably greater in that, for a brief period at least, it raised the awareness of AIDS in the African American community. No, the really big news was that when his head hit the springboard during preliminaries at the 1988 Olympic Games in Seoul, perhaps spilling a little blood into the pool, Louganis was HIV positive and he knew it. In other words, what got everyone talking was not the disclosure of 1995 but the nondisclosure of 1988. Even in soft focus Barbara Walters looked disturbed. "Greg!" she admonished.

Remember that in 1995 the new treatments had yet to appear publicly, so the reaction was absolutely tremendous. TV show after TV show replayed the infamous dive in slow motion, freeze-framing it at the exact moment when the head of the homosexual with AIDS hit the springboard, and at the exact moment when the head of the homosexual with AIDS entered the pool and may have spilled infected blood in it, and at the exact moment when a doctor touched the bloody head of the homosexual with AIDS. There were scary close-ups of the wound and even scarier close-ups of ungloved fingers touching the wound. And there were pictures of the other divers, the ones who followed the homosexual with AIDS into the pool where he might have spilled infected blood without telling anyone what he knew. Louganis himself did little to stop the whole brouhaha. In fact, his autobiography opens with a step-by-step description of "The Ninth Dive" and the anguish that followed—doubtless at the suggestion of his editor, who must have been well aware of the book's major selling point—and it contains a two-page photographic insert of the hit. "Ouch!" says the caption. Although "experts" immediately dispelled any fears that so little blood in such a large pool with a lot of disinfectant added to the water could possibly have put anyone at risk, the controversy raged on for days and days. But why? What could possibly explain the masochistic urge to watch again and again a moment of nonexistent risk?

For a while, Louganis was not a homosexual with AIDS but a great champion, an object of intense national pride, his medals emblems of American dominance, and his spectacular comeback to capture the gold after injuring himself the very embodiment of the country's indomitable spirit in the face of adversity. Like every American hero, Louganis appeared both exceptional and typical. To be sure, he was far from being the only US athlete ever to triumph at the Olympics, but divers have a unique history that links them to various national narratives and visions of the world. For example, after showing athletes in all sorts of disciplines, Leni Riefenstahl chose to conclude *Olympia*, her film of the 1936 Games in Berlin, with the diving events.

The scene starts in a fairly conventional style, showing the divers on and around the platforms, preparing, concentrating, diving finally. Before long, the pace begins to pick up. The focus soon shifts entirely to the dives, many of them staged and filmed after the actual event, as the filmmaker edited out little by little all context and contingencies, including the diving boards themselves, until all that remains is pure, unadulterated bodies, sometimes even shown in reverse motion to give the impression that they are in fact taking flight, soaring toward the sun like gods rather than crashing down to earth like mere mortals. Icarus's revenge under the Nazi sun. As movement itself disappears, the athletes whose bodies close the film seem to be rid at last of all vicissitudes and materiality, in a reverse echo of the Greek statues that came to earthly life in the opening segment.

But there is no need to turn to fascist fantasies of pure beauty in order to witness the fascination that the image of a body seemingly frozen in midair exercises on collective imaginations, especially of the national kind. There exist more democratic versions as well. Many popular films about coming of age, for example, feature scenes of boys (somehow it always seems to be boys) enjoying a sunny summer day at the local watering hole—the last moment of childhood and innocence before college or Vietnam or sexual awakening splits the group of friends and ushers in adulthood and the mature life of the individual. In such scenes, the body in midair, floating and fleeting, is meant to figure that elusive moment, that intangible and timeless in-between that can no more be captured than the present itself. The near nudity, with its old allegorical association with truth, suggests the innocence that precedes the original fall (from grace), soon lost forever to corruption and, from now on, an object of nostalgia. Childhood remains everyone's paradise lost.

Pictures of this sort are also ubiquitous to an almost laughable degree in the aptly named "Escapes" section of the *New York Times*. Interestingly, the faces of the boys (girls, still held collectively responsible, it seems, for humanity's fall from grace, seldom appear innocent enough to embody blissful carelessness and its impending loss, even today, when outdoor swimming has become gender integrated) are almost never shown because, more often than not, the pictures were taken from the lakeshore or the riverbank, placing the viewer in the position of a kid who hasn't yet jumped and may still choose not to. As a result, the photos figure a sort of generic, edenic boyhood, the absent face a blank canvas on which to project one's mythic identification and to produce something like a gendered national psyche.

There are two specific *Times* stories that, because they talk about transition, attracted my attention in the summer of 2010. One, on July 18, was in the "New York" section. It was about teenage boys from the Bronx jumping into the Hudson River as boats pass by, full of people to provide the necessary witnesses to their exploits. The jumps can be dangerous and the cops try to stop the boys. But how do you stop a rite of passage without interrupting time itself? Even their fathers did it, and one kid says, "It's like a bar mitzvah . . . Now you're a man." The tradition follows "an unspoken etiquette and style" and is so ingrained in the local culture that the article made a reference to the movie *The Basketball Diaries*, which depicts a jump from the highest rock in the area.

The second article appeared the very next day. It wasn't about boys jumping into a river, but that's what the picture on the front page depicted while, inside, another one showed two little feet pressed tightly together at the edge of what appears to be a wooden dock—a child afraid or unable to jump. The piece was about that huge oil spill in the Gulf of Mexico and how it may force some Louisiana Cajuns to abandon their homes and lifestyle. What the images of the children conveyed, unmistakably so if you had read the other article the day before, was that of an ancient tradition interrupted by contamination. It isn't just into the bayou that the child may not be able to jump, but into the future.

There seems to exist a distinctly American taste for these images and for the cult of innocent boyhood that they convey. Only a national culture equating masculinity with the burdens of individual responsibility and material concerns can feel this kind of nostalgia for the carefree, collective lifestyle that is supposed to define immaturity as though it were a last symbolic remnant of the tribal societies we had left behind and must now mourn. This represents, in a way, the democratic counterpart to Riefenstahl's Nazi propaganda in which male divers do not help us mourn but rather envision, with erotic bliss, the dissolution of the individual into the aestheticized collective that we should be striving for and for which our barbaric past figures an idealized model that may actually be recaptured and reactivated thanks to the collective will to do so.

American swimming pools have also been the site of disturbing national fantasies surrounding the purity of blood, although not in consistent ways. In his fascinating history of public pools in the northern United States, Jeff Wiltse reminds us that the facilities developed at first for the dual purpose of shielding girls from the sight of boys swimming naked in local rivers and ponds (a sight immortalized in George Bellows's famous painting 42 *Boys*), and later, promoting health, hygiene, and civil behavior among uncouth working-class men, both black and white. It wasn't until the 1920s that local authorities started enforcing racial segregation at the pools—not until, that is, white women and middle-class patrons began to use them. When they first appeared in the 1880s, American pools were designed to exclude, thanks to a process of enclosure, those with whom dominant society shunned contact. Whereas half a century later, as dominant classes claimed the pools and wanted in, the facilities were used to segregate by means of *expulsion*. Either way, public pools have always been sites where social contact gets policed, be it along gender, class, or racial lines according to what specific anxiety happens to grip society at a given period. It should come as no surprise, then, that these public facilities have played such a central role in the broader policing of sex, disease, and race. Municipal pools, where private, unclothed bodies and social relations touch, are always about contact to begin with. And fear of contact, whether inside or outside the pool, was the reason that they appeared at all.

If the triumphant body of Greg Louganis at the height of his Olympic glory carried on its surface two different sets of political connotations, the democratic and the sublime (or rather, if both could be projected on the blank screen that was his near-nude body), the shocking revelation of what lurked under the surface made people remember that Louganis isn't entirely white. Born to a Samoan father and a Caucasian mother, his blood was never "pure" to begin with, never quite uninfected. He grew up a swarthy little boy under the San Diego sun, as the book's photos show, and he was often called "nigger" at school. Once a symbol for the nation, Louganis had become the embodiment of all sorts of illicit contact—racial, sexual, epidemiological. The fascination with images of the incident at the Seoul Games had to do, I believe, with the thrill of watching one's own vulnerability, of capturing the exact moment when the boundary between inside and outside dissolves and, with it, all boundaries and all manners of social order. Beyond the thrill, however, lies the need to represent risk—especially unseen or even unreal risk—in order to repel it symbolically again and again. When it comes to inducing fear of contact and persuading people to act out on that fear in the realm of everyday social relations, risk carries more potency than danger in that it shifts the focus to individual behavior and away from the threat of external forces.

Usually gawked at wearing very little, or nothing at all in *Playgirl* once, Louganis seemed not to be hiding anything from us. Naked as a newborn babe and looking almost as innocent, he was the picture of health and beauty. But the attractive young diver turned out, in the end, to be a sort of monster. His unclothed body was really a veil. And as in horror stories, the thrill of abjection is saturated with race and sex and dangerous bodily fluids that won't stay contained. With Greg Louganis who, like Rock Hudson before him, looked so truthful, innocent, and wholesome but wasn't in reality, had America invited some kind of cultural vampire into its national living room?

And then there was the story of two-year-old Caleb Glover, an African American kid born with HIV and adopted by white parents. In the summer of 2007, as the family was vacationing in an Alabama RV park, the parents were told that Caleb, whose HIV status his mother had revealed in a casual conversation, was not allowed to use the facility's grounds, showers, and pool. The local and then national media were soon on the story, and before long a band of AIDS activists invaded the RV park and took a swim in its pool with little Caleb in tow. Is it because the story took place in the South and because Caleb is black that, of all the amenities to which the little boy was denied access, it is the pool specifically that seems to have caught people's imagination and triggered their outrage? "Sweet Home Alabama" was the somewhat condescending title of the article in the issue of *Poz* magazine that featured Caleb on its cover alongside white, HIV-positive swimmer and reality TV celebrity Jack Mackenroth in a swimming pool.

The title of Louganis's autobiography is *Breaking the Surface*. The clever play on words (redundantly illustrated by a cover photo of the diver taken in midair but "placed" underwater next to a rather tasteless touch of red hue) echoes the phrase "breaking the silence" often used for similar testimonial writings and refers all at once to the sport of diving, of course, to his injury at the Seoul Olympics, and to the numerous disclosures that pepper the book in an attempt to present a coherent identity to the world. In his own words: "I want to start living my life the way normal people do, without having to watch every word, without having to remember what I've shared with whom. I want never again to feel compelled to hide out in my house in the California hills, avoiding situations in which I have to edit what I say and lie about my life."

But Greg, darling, this is exactly what "normal people" do and how "normal people" live—except for that bit about the house in the California hills perhaps. No matter how naked the body and how open the heart, there always seems to be something lurking under the surface, always a deeper, more naked nakedness to be unveiled, a truer truth to be revealed. Someone somewhere will make sure of that in order to retain their power over you, and they will skin you alive and torture the nonexistent truth out of you if they have to. So it may be in our best interest to think of our disclosures as stories rather than truths, because if the human body is a representation to begin with, there will always remain layers to peel off of it, more pain to be inflicted.

Disclosure

SHAME AND EXPERIENCE

Like so many others, I first reacted to my diagnosis with shame, which had the advantage of allowing me to experience a wholly novel situation thanks to an affective framework already well-known to me. As the queer scholar Leo Bersani has noted, "A potential sexual shame is inherent in being HIV-positive. For the overwhelming majority of HIV-positive gay men, to acknowledge being infected amounts to a sexual confession: I have been fucked." Even now, I can argue with myself until I'm blue in the face that I didn't do anything wrong and that I have nothing to be ashamed of anyway; people can feign disbelief when I tell them that I have been struck with a paralyzing sense of failure and unworthiness that I still find difficult to shake at times; they can look puzzled on learning that I slid into depression not on hearing the news but one year later, once my viral load had plummeted, my T-cell count edged up, and everything looked good: all attempts at restoring a supposedly therapeutic sense of self and integrity are futile. I may now have become a regular at the hospital's Department of Internal Medicine, but the truth is, from the get-go, my own, deepest, most personal experience of HIV was social, an outside–in dynamic that I perceived as a familiar feeling of dispossession. Contemplating myself as other was not a new phenomenon for me, and I could embrace this familiar feeling of disjunction with an odd sense of reassurance.

On a more general level, this will doubtless sound obvious if one considers that experience is not something the self does by itself but a form of knowledge and is, therefore, always mediated. It is nonetheless telling in that respect that one's first consciousness of having HIV is, as is the case with any other ailment, attached to a diagnosis; that is, not to the illness itself (which, in my situation, cannot in any case be experienced apart from the social discourses that make up the disease) but to its legibility by and intelligibility to someone else—even if this someone else is also me positioning myself outside the disease, the old, healthy version of me that I lived with for much too long to ever completely cease to be—my inner, young Barbara Stanwyck. (For this reason, to become ill is always a kind of breaking up of the self.) Even beyond past and potential infections, there is no experience of HIV or AIDS that isn't relational. Shame told me that. For feelings of shame indicate that we may experience our own sense of self only as vulnerability and openness to others—just as the experience of my own nakedness takes place only with (the possibility of) someone else seeing my naked body or touching it, whether kindly or not.

THE DOORSTEP OF SHAME

That time in the ER I recounted earlier (a short paragraph that took me days to write), that day when I found myself facing another person's absolute, irreversible contempt for me, illustrates what a dehumanizing force shame can be. Being an *object* of disgust made me feel like less than a human being, but seeing myself with someone else's eyes allowed me to double up into more than one. To be a human being means to be no less but also no more than one, and shame's dehumanizing power consists in upsetting such a delicate balance from two sides at once. Worse even, it makes us aware of how precarious something as basic as our humanity—not our life but our humanity, what makes us different from other living things, such as grass or chickens—turns out to be. That unforgettable knowledge can kill you or it can make you mad.

It was absolutely crucial for Annie Ernaux's working-class mother to send her daughter to a private Catholic school. But for Annie, who would grow up to become a teacher and a writer, it marked the beginning of a profound sense of social alienation. In her book *Shame*, she recounts a scene in which her sense of being split into two incompatible selves becomes manifest. She is returning in the middle of the night from a school trip to a religious festival. A teacher drives Annie home, along with other students who live in the same part of town. The girl knocks on the locked door until, finally, her mother wakes up and, to her daughter's horror, appears in the door frame wearing a nightgown soiled with urine. It was common for some people in those days, as Ernaux explains, to wipe themselves with their nightgowns, but such knowledge about bodily functions was never meant to be shared with people outside one's own group. Annie is of course mortified and feels utterly humiliated in front of her more elegant school friends: "I rushed into the store to stop it all. It was the first time I saw my mother through the eyes of the private school."

Other than the dual positioning that characterizes shame, as one sees oneself as if with the eyes of another, it is the open door that I find especially telling in this passage, the play between inside and outside, private and public identities, and the need to choose one side for fear of completely losing any sense of who and what we are. The reversal of inside and outside represents a giant conceptual leap yet requires but a tiny step in actuality. As one's place in the world can stop making sense literally in no time, the first reflex often seems to be to rush in and "stop it all." And shut the door. But an open door is also an invitation of sorts. The question is, to whom?

FORGET YOUR HEALTH

When you're HIV positive you also know what it feels like to be HIV negative. You remember it. This HIV-negative, healthy body that was once yours is still somehow with you or near you but no longer you, not really. In fact, not unlike a younger age, it appears sometimes as if it were incarnated by others. Rosalyn Diprose reminds us of Maurice Merleau-Ponty's distinction between remembering and forgetting, the former being a kind of figuration that allows us to distinguish the past from the present, the latter a way for the past to be concurrent with the present but without our having any perception of it. "But," she adds, "memory and forgetting are ideal functions that change nothing. Rather, like the relation between truth and lies, there is a passage between memory and forgetting, forgetting and memory." Diprose wrote these words as she reflected on the colonization of Australia and the harm done to Aboriginal populations, but I find them resonant here and in other contexts as well. Haunting, I believe, represents such a passage. It is a form of perception of the past that, if shapeless and essentially affective, nonetheless signals that the past and the present cannot be separated. In fact, I am tempted to say that the shapelessness of it—and of affect in general—signals that we are standing too close for comfort. When HIV-negative guys and I relate to one another, I see my past and they see their possible future. It isn't particularly pleasant for me either—I do not look back on my healthier days with any particular fondness—but it is that or no relation at all.

Poz guys whose treatment is working often describe themselves in on-line ads as "healthy," a more appealing answer to "clean" and less technical a term than the paranoia-inducing "undetectable." No doubt "healthy" is used in the hope that neg guys will not be scared away. In many cases they will be, though, just as sure as if you had described yourself as ravaged with oozing sores and purulent lesions. You might as well call yourself bubonic, frankly, it wouldn't make any difference. The phrase *healthy poz* has no practical meaning because it relies not on objective medical facts but on a fantasy—health—that excludes us by definition. Although I am not "strictly" speaking sick (as of this writing), something in me keeps me from describing myself as healthy. First, I must affirm my solidarity with others who are in fact sick and dying of HIV disease. Second, it would suggest that there really isn't much difference between having HIV and not having it. There may very well be more similarities than differences, but these differences do exist, and it would be illusory, and dishonest, to deny them. Third, there is much to gain from this doubling up of oneself as both healthy and sick.

A friend told me once that he was a bit puzzled whenever I referred to myself sometimes as having AIDS rather than as merely being HIV positive. (I don't really do it anymore; it's just too over the top and no longer of any tactical help to me. Not that I have a problem with being over the top, far from it in fact, as the anger that pervades parts of this book may suggest, but I think that I have achieved everything I could hope to achieve that way in matters of HIV.) Given that the friend in question is about my age, this isn't too surprising. Gay men of our generation remember the different stages of the epidemic and the importance of using certain terms rather than others, either as a matter of factual accuracy or to serve political needs. But once the treatments arrived, full-blown AIDS, as it was once called, was no longer a stage of no return in an inexorable process of degradation that led to death. Indeed, it became possible to return from it. Since I was at one point teetering on the fateful threshold of two hundred CD4 cells, the official boundary between having HIV and having AIDS, I too have returned. Yet to say that I no longer have AIDS would be absurd. I have AIDS, and the new treatments are keeping it in check for now. As a result of these new developments in care, the term *HIV/AIDS* became almost universally used to indicate that the difference between the two is no longer so meaningful. Now it's just HIV. AIDS is gone. Except, of course, in the press, where it still makes for catchier headlines.

You may have noticed, however, that I keep using all these different phrases—HIV, AIDS, HIV/AIDS—throughout this book and that I seldom do so with any apparent consistency. As you might have guessed, this is a matter of what kind of effect I want to produce. But it also testifies to my desire to avoid being trapped and seeing my experience captured within preexisting discourses of knowledge that could only reduce my life and preempt the possibility of dynamic and creative contacts with others. At a deeper level, though, to be infected with HIV is to testify to the porosity of borders, be they literal, as in national borders, or figurative, as in the boundaries of bodies or individuals. Borders are always figurative, of course, in that they are never tangible but mere effects of the differential play of what they articulate. In the end, this inherent untenability of boundaries is what one discloses when disclosing an HIV status (even a negative one, in that it implicitly recognizes the possibility of ceasing to be negative). This is why people are often more scared by the disclosure itself than by the virus.

I will relate a specific example in a moment, but let me say this for now, using the terminology proposed by Emmanuel Levinas. When I disclose my HIV status, people tend to react to the saying (the openness to the other) rather than to the said (the closing of the self onto itself). The "it" that could be the object of a "said" is, in the case of HIV/AIDS, an effect of its multiple enunciations and, as such, far too unstable an object. Diprose writes in her beautiful and beautifully titled book *Corporeal Generosity* that for Levinas "generosity is the passivity of exposure. . . . Beneath the community of commonness grounded in the said of language is the community of saying, of exposure to alterity." And she goes on to quote another philosopher, Alphonso Lingis: "Before the rational community, there was the encounter with the other, the intruder. The encounter begins with the one who exposes himself to the demands and contestations of the other."

To disclose my HIV status is thus to expose myself at least twice: first, because I reveal or unveil something that, as a disease, is of a corporeal nature, and second, because I am forcing the other to take a social position with regard to my body. But which one will it be? To pretend that it is really to the said (HIV) that they're reacting allows others to have or give the false impression that they are really rejecting the disease—and who could blame them, right?—but not the person who happens to have it. Focusing knowingly on the saying of disclosure would be to acknowledge that contact has occurred, that the HIV positive and the HIV negative have entered into some sort of community, and that the border between the two is porous. And that, it seems, is a little too much to ask. Yet a reaction of hostility betrays that one has in fact been affected by the saying, that some kind of encounter has taken place, and that something of HIV has been passed on. Hostility thus always betrays denial.

DISCLOSURES AND SURFACES

To disclose something is a way of relating, both in the sense of telling a story and of establishing a relation with someone else. Either way, it is a mode of being with others and therefore has to do with contact, be it accepted or denied. Whether one longs for such contact or recoils from the mere idea of it, disclosures involve surfaces. We seem to bring out to the surface what had been hiding below it. When it is an illness that one discloses, or anything understood to be physical in nature, such as an ethnicity or a disability or a sexual longing, this contact often feels like disrobing and exposing oneself, leaving one's skin open to the touch of others, a touch we both fear and desire. This sort of vulnerability, coming from the disclosure of something we once felt safer to hide, feels especially thrilling in that we are placing ourselves at the fluctuating and very dangerous limit between humiliation and desire. What will the other do to my exposed skin?

OBAMA'S DISCLOSURES, FOREVER DEFERRED

The power of disclosure to prevent contact sometimes works by demanding that a disclosure be made and, at the same time, postponing it forever. Not unlike unveiling, disclosure is a mandate that cannot be fulfilled without undoing the power of those whose *project* it is to demand disclosure and transparency. Like any project, this one would cease to exist once completed.

The pervasive sense that some people have of Barack Obama's irreducible otherness, the deeply felt conviction that, somehow, he's just not like us, is easy enough to account for. The reason that so many Americans feel that way about him is literally plain to see: the man is black. But for most people who harbor such feelings of unease and contempt toward their president, the source of it cannot be stated so bluntly, at least not in public and not in front of just anybody. In some cases such racism may not even be felt at a conscious level. Whichever the case, be it societal norms regulating speech or lack of individual awareness, the feeling must be transformed in order to become utterable. Obama's perceived difference must therefore be explained not by what can be seen yet cannot be spoken—he is black—but by what cannot be seen yet must be spoken—there is something about him that we don't know. His supposedly foreign birth and Islamic faith adopted in an Indonesian madrassa, his imagined postcolonial hatred for America and white people, what have you . . . all these beliefs stem from the idea that Obama is hiding something and must have something, anything, to disclose. The fact that he eventually made his long-form birth certificate public will not change that. No one suspects the president of being a one-man terrorist sleeper cell yet, but I'm sure that jump isn't too big for some.

The catch, though, is that Obama's words may not be believed. Blame it on the duplicity of the Muslim or on the inscrutability of the Orient. The man makes too many speeches, but they're somehow just a little too eloquent for a country of plainspoken, tell-it-like-it-is folks. He is "overexposed," but we never quite know anything about the "real" Barack Obama. His words work like veils, always concealing things instead of revealing them. And when Republican leaders make comments such as "When he says he's a Christian I take him at his word," they don't need to add that his word means nothing and that, no matter what Obama reveals about himself, no honest disclosure has in fact ever occurred. If duplicity is a defining feature of Muslims, even when unveiled they cannot be trusted to be showing us the truth. And even after the financial backers of the so-called Ground

Zero mosque became known (and they were never unknown), opponents of the project were still asking who was "behind" it. Muslims cannot *not* have an ulterior, inadmissible motive, and objective proofs to the contrary are but smoke screens with no truth-value whatsoever. From that perspective, revelations conceal the truth, unveiling masks it.

Not all forms of social exclusion work in the same ways, of course. Someone's ethnicity, skin color, or socioeconomic status may be visible enough not to require any other proof of that person's supposed inferiority. Yet, in certain historical circumstances, especially in disenchanted cultures where the visual plays a central part in the construction of truth and knowledge, the invisible is often an object of fear and a source of anxiety. Jews changing names and light-skinned blacks passing have provided, at times, salient examples of this phenomenon. So today have secret bisexual men on the down low, especially if they are men of color toward whom racial aversion may not be too overtly stated and must therefore be displaced. In such cases, unveiling and disclosure (as well as "coming clean," "speaking out," "coming out," etc.) often become associated with the idea of social integration, for which they are said to be a condition.

Both, however, are avatars of the same operation: to deny the intractability of inequality by giving the impression that the have-nots actually have something—something to hide—and that it must be revealed, unveiled, disclosed for the playing field to be even. And it makes little difference if "have-not" isn't to be taken necessarily in its strictest economic sense. It remains a structuring trope, perhaps *the* structuring trope, in a system motivated and propelled by economic inequality. If Obama were to reveal that he really is a Muslim after all or that he was born outside the United States, his legitimacy as president would be undone and his otherness confirmed. But when having something to hide is made to define certain categories of powerless people, *not* disclosing these "facts" confirms that powerlessness. Obama's position, therefore, remains illegitimate no matter what he says or doesn't say.

CHAT (1)

I must have said something, because he sensed it. "poz?" he asked. I typed back "yup," wondering whether this was the right context for a virtual Gary Cooper impression. "i'm not but it's no big deal," he replied. "like i said i lived in sf for years so hiv isn't new or scary to me. comes with the territory." I can only assume that HIV must have in fact been old and boring, because I never heard back from him and never made it to his territory.

CHAT (II)

Him: "it doesn't mean we can't chat"
    Me: "it doesn't mean we can't fuck"
    Him: "lol true"
    The chat ended soon after that.
    The fucking never started.
    (lol)

ADVENTURES IN ONLINE CRUISING

It is surely not a surprise if laws so often mandate that one's HIV status be disclosed before engaging in certain sexual practices, for there is something in the very act of disclosing that, in the absence of concerted attempts to the contrary, makes it nearly impossible not to see the object of the disclosure in negative terms. This is the logic of the confession, with which our notions of disclosure tend to be entangled and that actually performs the sin or the crime into existence. When confessing, rather than sharing, his or her pathological status, a person with HIV becomes disciplined—meaning both known and policed—and, thanks to this joint operation of the clinic and the police, eventually cast out one way or another. To disclose one's HIV-positive status is, in essence, to come clean about being unclean. I do not, however, use the phrase *cast out* to imply that people with HIV are systematically ostracized by all the people to whom they disclose their status. This would be an absurd claim, and it has not been my experience. Yet to confess is a way to open up and shut down at the same time, if only because the act of confession seeks to define each interlocutor as an autonomous individual distinct from the other, each one the protagonist of a different story.

We have entered Foucauldian territory here, so it may prove useful to quote from *The History of Sexuality*. In the following passage, Foucault describes what he calls "the internal ruse of confession," by which the dissemination of power in the modern era gives the erroneous impression that to speak the truth is intrinsically liberating while silence confines:

> The obligation to confess is now relayed through so many different points, is so deeply ingrained in us, that we no longer perceive it as the effect of a power that constrains us; on the contrary, it seems to us that truth, lodged in our most secret nature, "demands" only to surface; that if it fails to do so, this is because a constraint holds it in place, the violence of a power weighs it down, and it can finally be articulated only at the price of a kind of liberation. Confession frees, but power reduces one to silence, truth does not belong to the order of power, but shares an original affinity with freedom: traditional themes in philosophy, which a "political history of truth" would have to overturn but showing that truth is not by nature free—nor error servile—but that its production is thoroughly imbued with relations of power. The confession is an example of this.

Thanks to its link with the modern democratic ideal of transparency, disclosure seems to pertain to the unimpeded circulation of information and thus takes on the aura of progress and freedom from authoritarian power. In reality, it replaces authoritarianism with authoritativeness, a form of power that Foucault tied to what he termed the will to knowledge.

Now consider this: as of this writing, thirty-six states in the United States criminalize seropositivity in one way or another, mostly by making it a crime not to disclose one's status in certain sexual situations or, in one-third of these states, by considering it an aggravating factor in other offenses. In some states, a conviction will be accompanied by placement on a sex offender registry—sometimes for the rest of your life. This, in turn, mandates that you disclose your status as a sex offender every time, for example, that you look for housing and employment or move into a new neighborhood. Being thus sentenced to disclosure for life after an initial failure to disclose is so constraining that, the legal scholar J. J. Prescott has noted, it feels a lot like prison and ends up fostering secrecy rather than openness. Being HIV positive, once a death sentence, has become a life sentence, a never-ending work of policing. What's particularly Kafkaesque about this is the fact that such a life sentence was made possible because of the virus's simultaneous association with and dissociation from death. Lifelong disclosure may be the form of punishment that has replaced death, but the HIV positive, caught in a double bind, must be punished one way or another.

In many ways, the inevitable physical death that HIV infection once signified in pretty much everyone's mind has now been replaced by a vicious, pernicious social death, all but ensuring that if people don't die of AIDS, somehow they still do. In his seminal study *Slavery and Social Death*, the sociologist Orlando Patterson outlines two kinds of social death, the intrusive kind, in which outsiders are depersonalized before being incorporated as nonbeings, and the extrusive kind that strikes "an insider who had fallen, one who ceased to belong and had been expelled from normal participation in the community because of a failure to meet certain . . . norms of behavior." The HIV-positive person as outcast falls in the second category.

Thus, to mandate HIV disclosure in the context of a sexual encounter does not serve the purpose of sharing facts and promoting safer sex but, rather, is designed to obscure facts and minimize the possibility that *any* sex act, be it safe, unsafe, or uncertain, will occur at all. Framing HIV disclosure in terms of legal mandates about informed life-and-death decisions, for example, hinders the facts about undetectable viral load and actual risks of transmission. And because it is very difficult to become or remain friends with someone who has thus rejected you, mandatory disclosure also nips in the bud a potentially very creative variety of social contacts that sexual encounters, even if just considered, may bring about. (And I mean "considered" in both senses: envisioned as a possibility and valued as a legitimate mode of human interaction.)

To the extent that, in optimal treatment conditions, HIV disclosure carries any practical usefulness at all for the listener, it is only in that it empowers him or her, as truth telling subjugates the speaker. Mandatory HIV disclosure, then, has no other purpose than to distribute power unequally and to produce injustice. As is the case with torture, the truth of disclosure matters less than the act itself. The work of the police may appear to concern only sex here, but its aim always has a broader, more comprehensive social reach. And it always fails because confession can never escape the fact that it is an act of relating and is, at least potentially, inseparable from the very contact it seeks to abolish.

But who needs mandates? I once had an exchange of e-mails with a guy in Los Angeles whose profile I had seen online and who looked interesting, for whatever reason. The conversation was going well (he had even attended med school at Michigan), and we were about to make dinner arrangements to see if things would also click in person. Boys being boys (or whatever), we had also talked about what we were "into," as the phrase goes. We agreed that there would be no unsafe stuff and proceeded to make a list of fun things to do should we hit it off. This sort of letter to Santa may sound like the typical gay, cut-to-the-chase attitude that so many straight people pretend to find abhorrent. It is true that the serendipity of human encounters may be one of the greatest and most pleasurable aspects of sex, especially gay sex I might add, but let's be honest, sometimes you know what you want, and if you're in the mood for a greasy old chili dog, sole meunière just won't do, no matter how exquisite.

In my case, though, coming up with a plan of action is also a way either to ensure that I will have no legal obligation to disclose my HIV status if I don't want to or, if I do want to, to increase ever so slightly the chances that the other guy will still want to go ahead and play. That time, I was vaguely hoping for something a little more developed than just a hookup, maybe a little dating and hanging out too, and I didn't want to jeopardize future possibilities by giving the impression that I had been less than truthful at the outset. And this is one of the cruelest things about HIV disclosure. Either you say something, and you run a high risk of killing the possibility of a sexual encounter, or you keep quiet and you get together with the guy, but you may have ruined the chances of transforming a hookup into anything more durable.

Anyway, this guy didn't sound like Mr. Perfect either, so I told myself I wouldn't be losing that much. Not to mention that I was in L.A. for a while, and guys were a dime a dozen there, and far less provincial than in Ann Arbor. And come on, he was a doctor! So before we even met, I told him. I reminded him that we had decided to be safe anyway and, just to be, well, safe, I explained what having an undetectable viral load means in terms of risk. (I actually like the metonymic slippage "being undetectable." Like "dormant" in the early years, it can make you feel like a spy. At the very least, substituting the person for the virus brings out the issue of HIV as a social as well as medical one.)

Here's the answer I received from the good doctor: "hey david, thanks for your honesty. unfortunately, i have to say that i would be uncomfortable with playing. i know that safe play would most likely prevent anything. however, being a healthcare professional, i know that anything is possible. i apologize for being very shallow about this, but it's not something i am willing to risk. i hope you understand. k***"

In all fairness, it is true that no matter what you list in your letter to Santa, you can always end up with a surprise in your stocking. That's the magic of sex, I guess. Unless you're a strict fetishist, things may occur that were not in the script, no matter what you think you want. Yet I found myself so hurt by that guy's rejection, which hit me like a profound injustice against me and my body and my life and my . . . I don't know, everything, that it pretty much killed my cruising (and more) for a long and painful time. It was all I could do to stop myself from sending him the angry reply that I composed and refined in my head for days and that sounded something like this: "hey k***, as a so-called healthcare professional, you don't know shit. an empirical mind such as yours should be aware that for a certain thing to happen the right conditions have to be met. if they aren't, then the thing will not happen. a rational person would never write a sentence such as 'anything is possible' because, outside of a tex avery cartoon at least, it is demonstrably false. your rather baffling attitude, therefore, can only be attributed to one or more of the following explanations: you are shockingly misinformed; you are bigoted; perhaps you are afraid of coming into contact with patients. whatever it is, i am grateful that you are not my doctor. but for the sake of others, i urge you to consider a career move into retail, where bullshit is almost a guarantee of success. oh, and one last thing: when did the burden of understanding fall on *my* shoulders?" I came up with several versions depending on what profession I happened to find the most contemptible that day.

Especially irritating in the context of HIV and sex is that people who reject you on a completely irrational basis will often ask for your understanding. That is, for your own acquiescence to discrimination against you. Clearly, they use the word to mean something like compassion or sympathy—as if they were the putative victims of *your* intolerance—but they hope nonetheless to capitalize on the rational sense of the term (reinforced here by the claim to speak as "a healthcare professional") and apply its legitimating power beyond the realm of reason. To describe an emotion as understandable seeks to make it reasonable rather than emotional. But I calmed down, and in the end my actual answer was more measured than the one I dreamed up. I replied that no, I couldn't say that I understood but that I was getting used to people's unfounded fears. And because I really couldn't let him off so easily, I finished with the rather devious send-off: "good luck trusting future partners who will tell you they're not hiv+." And he didn't want to sleep with me for fear that I would leave him with a poisoned gift! Well, I guess I did anyway.

Most people who claim that they will not engage in sex with HIV-positive people have in fact done so and will continue to do so as long as their partners don't disclose—because these partners choose not to, or are afraid to, or, as is the case with many people who are infected, because they just don't know it. Oftentimes, the topic isn't broached at all; sometimes it is preempted. In online ads, for example, the shorthand "ddf," for "drug- and disease-free," may be used to indicate that one claims to be HIV negative and expects the other to be as well ("ub2"). I particularly like the newer, self-affirming and blame-inducing (the two are linked) "Neg and I intend to stay that way." (So did I, sweetie.) And one now encounters with increasing regularity online profiles that include the last date of the person's negative test results. It would be interesting to ask if the date refers to the day the blood was drawn or when the person received the results, but my zeal has its limits. I guess we all decide to trust each other to know and tell the truth.

The practice of announcing and dating one's negative test results may have developed because it gives the appearance that the claim can be backed up by evidence. Yet it is just as pointless as claiming to be ddf. We know that HIV transmission is most efficient when the viral load is exceptionally high. This happens twice in the entire course of the disease: when one is nearing death (and perforce unlikely to be sexually active) and immediately following infection, when one is by definition sexually active and, interestingly, when the basic, cheaper test, which detects antibodies to the virus rather than the virus itself, will come out negative. So when people tell you that they are HIV negative as of this morning, it could just as well mean that they are in fact highly infectious.

I once called a guy on what seemed (to me) an odd contradiction in his online profile. To the question "Safer sex" (a far more useful bit of information to provide than HIV status) he had selected the reply "Always." Yet on the list of "Things he's into" he included "Barebacking." This is in fact a very common occurrence on such sites. "Very simple," he explained. "When the guy is 100% percent sure he's clean I don't use condoms, but otherwise I always do." Any sign of irritation or bafflement on my part could have jeopardized the hookup so I kept quiet, but further observation (sometimes I don't know if I'm cruising or collecting data anymore . . .) led me to the conclusion that, for certain people on some gay sites, barebacking is not understood as inherently risky; it all depends on the other guy's status. Well, yeah, sure, but . . . Leave aside for a minute the fact that the Internet in general and cruising sites in particular are hardly places to turn to when looking for truth (I remember this guy who used to hit me up with creepy regularity, and each time he did his penis had grown by an inch; surely he must be in the Guinness Book of World Records by now), the basic thing is, a negative status is often far less certain than a positive one.

So why do people choose to believe someone who tells them they're HIV negative while knowing full well that such belief is unsure at best and utterly irrational at worst? And why refuse to have sex with people with an undetectable viral load even if you are perfectly aware that it would convey no risk of transmission whatsoever? I suspect this has to do with the symbolic charge of "HIV" and "AIDS," which are so saturated with meaning that one may react to them only with affect (fear, disgust, and the like) or force of will (the will to reject, the will to remain uninfected) rather than with rational thought. Yet the stories I have told didn't occur in a culture organized primarily around symbolism, such as certain tribal societies or totalitarian states, but in a culture of reason. Why such incoherence then? Because when our body and its integrity are involved we leave reason aside.

We can think about our body and about the bodies of others, but we cannot seem to think with it.

At a simpler, more practical level, the answer to these questions is likely to be that cruisers don't necessarily believe the other person. I am not qualified to undertake the sort of sociological research that would support my claim, nor do I know of anyone who has, but my intuition is that "ddf" and "negative as of . . ." are, as I suggested, ways to preempt all discussion of HIV because the topic is such a killjoy. I thus speculate that the purpose of mentioning information that cannot be, and indeed is not, blindly believed has nothing to do with risk management but is intended instead to remove the very idea of risk from people's minds during sex.

The queer theorist Eve Kosofsky Sedgwick recalls the case of a teacher in Maryland who was fired for disclosing his homosexuality. The appellate court overturned the rationale for the initial decision (a teacher should not disclose his homosexuality), but agreed that the teacher should not get his job back because he had *not* disclosed his homosexuality when he first applied for the position. The case is old now (1973) and wouldn't play out quite the same way today, but it remains relevant in that it gives us an example of "disclosure at once compulsory and forbidden," as Sedgwick puts it. This is just the sort of double bind in which HIV disclosure finds itself caught: You must disclose your status, but I don't want to hear it! The question, then, is why insist on an approach that is so demonstrably faulty? Out of naive faith in the powers of reason and individual responsibility? Possibly. Or should we conclude that the failure of policing discourses is intrinsic to the way they operate, hence generating more and more policing? Are the two explanations incompatible? Foucault would say that they are not.

But don't get me wrong. The contradictions and shortcomings of power, no matter how indispensable they are to its operations, also provide us with opportunities to act on the very structures that oppress us. Who cares really if what people write in their online profiles sounds dumb or contradictory or even AIDS-phobic as long as we all get laid in the end? Should we take such blatant failures of etiquette—forms of tactlessness, in a sense—as outright rejections? Maybe not. In the words of the literature and culture scholar Ross Chambers, "Flaunting is, par excellence, the gesture of visibility that requires reading." What these online cruisers present to other cruisers, whether consciously or not (it doesn't matter), is the possibility to read overt mentions of HIV as covert invitations not to care about it. Failure of propriety is thus crucial here. Speaking in a different context, Chambers writes of AIDS witnesses: "They have to get themselves read, but without compromising their wrongness, the means by which they signify, which is what would occur if they made themselves too readily readable." Indeed, to state directly in an online profile that one doesn't particularly care about a partner's HIV status may drive some potential playmates away because they will assume that you are yourself HIV positive while attracting others for the same reason. Simultaneously flaunting and flouting individual responsibility, statements of, and request for seronegativity that no one seriously believes may in fact constitute subversive appropriations and resignifications of policing discourses for the purpose of ignoring their mandates and continuing, as Douglas Crimp once wrote, "to have promiscuity in an epidemic."

To return to the good doctor, the guy was sexually active and, since he never bothered to ask, was also willing to play with someone without any mention of HIV, albeit safely, since we'd promised Santa we'd be both naughty *and* nice. Yet he couldn't bring himself to do it once he knew. How could I have been so naive? How could I invoke the freeing power of truth telling? In the end, it isn't HIV per se that is the problem, or even the lack of knowledge about the risks of transmission and how to minimize them, but, as is always the case in any don't-ask-don't-tell situation, knowledge itself—in this case the knowledge that the other person is infected, naturally, but, more important, the knowledge that you are capable of rejecting a person for no good reason. In the end, this is what I may have passed on to k***, and this is as impossible to get rid of as the virus itself. I wonder if he will ever disclose to anyone that he did this to me—and that he did it as "a healthcare professional." "prolly not," as we say online. And while my small revenge brought me some degree of satisfaction at the time, the relief proved short-lived. I was hurt, so I decided to hurt back, and today I am not so proud of what I did, whether politically or ethically. But the saddest thing in the end is that we didn't have sex. What a waste, really.

ON THE QUESTION OF BAREBACKING, VERY BRIEFLY

Barebacking is a topic that I feel both compelled and reluctant to discuss in these pages. Compelled because so much HIV scholarship has now turned to it that it would be a mistake to dodge the issue altogether in a book such as this one; reluctant simply because I have little to say about it in the end, my opinions on the matter being as fluid, so to speak, as the practice itself. Some queer scholars, most notably David Halperin, seek to wrest the discussion of barebacking from the grip of psychology and its pathologization of gay lives. Others, such as Tim Dean and Bersani, make ample use of psychoanalysis, not to pathologize of course, but to probe the ambiguous politics and complex ethics of what has become known as bug chasing and gift giving, the consensual sharing of HIV. Gregory Tomso understands the practice as a form of resistance against neoliberal regimes of health and life, but the ample use of the rhetoric of kinship and reproduction in heavily ritualized communal practices of sharing semen point in a very different political direction. Still other scholars focus on the specific question of bareback porn and the studios that specialize in it. In other words, queer thinking on barebacking tends to replicate the internal diversity of queer studies itself, which comes as no surprise.

As for me, what can I say? Personal discomfort with the practice has nothing to do with my lack of deep engagement with the issue or my inability to take a stand on it. I find the idea of sex without condoms a little disturbing but not repellent, and short-sighted but not stupid. I understand that some gay men see it as a deeply meaningful form of sharing, articulating community sometimes with an especially reactionary rhetoric of male heroism, as Dean describes in detail, or with mystical overtones, in which Bersani sees a form of asceticism and a way to think of intimacy without an ego. Fine. But we must also remember that barebacking is a term that encompasses a broad range of sexual practices and motivations (something none of these scholars fails to acknowledge, I must say), from safe sex fatigue to a desire for enhanced pleasure, from the darkly ritualized to the merely expedient, from subcultural expression to personal preference. Having little interest in kinship or spirituality myself and feeling naturally disinclined to think that sex should be a matter of opinions, I shall refrain from passing judgment on people who, for whatever reason, prefer to fuck without condoms while I choose not to.

To those who are prompt to apportion blame, however, remember that gay meeting websites specializing in barebacking often are a way for HIV-positive men to find one another and avoid rejection from people like you, regardless of what actual sex acts come of it, if any. What's more, unprotected sex is essentially the norm among straight people, yet I hear few voices condemning the heterosexual lifestyle as a whole for being irresponsible, self-destructive, and even insane or, thanks to rising health care costs, for forcing the rest of us to shoulder the consequences of the reckless, antisocial behavior of people who obviously hate themselves.

For the purposes of this book, then, I will state very simply that while barebacking represents in many ways a fascinating and important topic of inquiry that may intersect in fruitful ways with some of the ideas I try to develop, I don't think that a detailed discussion of it would contribute anything especially pertinent to my own reflections on sharing and contact as I understand them here.

CODA TO THE STORY OF K***

I once presented and discussed some of what precedes and some of what follows to a group of graduate students in Chicago, whose work dealt with gender and sexuality topics. Of all the instances of HIV disclosure mentioned in the text they had read ahead of time, the ones they were almost exclusively interested in were, predictably, those that occurred in sexual contexts. I say "predictably" now, but at the time it took me by surprise.

A few weeks before my visit, they had invited another gay scholar who had told them that ethics and sex had nothing to do with each other, and they were intent on continuing that conversation. What about k***? Wasn't my anger against him motivated by ethical considerations, by the fact that he had been unjust and had wronged me? I disagreed. I still do. Yes, I had felt hurt by the rejection, but because it wasn't the first time I'd been rejected on the basis of my HIV status and because I'd reacted more philosophically to earlier instances, it seems unfair to claim that rejection is always unethical. If, as I surmised, k***'s silence about the question of HIV might have been a tactful invitation for me to keep quiet as well, it was I who failed to demonstrate comparable tact and thus ruined the connection. Couldn't it be also that some people just reject others less than tactfully?

Yes of course, reactions such as this one can hurt, but are they necessarily unethical or, as some activists claim, politically unacceptable? The fact, for example, that some people find serosorting—choosing sexual partners whose serostatus is the same as one's own—discriminatory when HIV-negative people do it but justified if you're HIV positive (presumably because the former amplifies an already existing discrimination) indicates only that the practice doesn't have an inherent ethical or political value. In the end, I tried to argue with the students that there was no fundamental difference between rejecting a potential sexual partner on the basis of HIV status and tending to be attracted (or not) to people of a certain ethnicity or body type. *That* they could relate to, and that's pretty much where things stood.

As you can imagine, I felt the rippling effects of that painful conversation for days. It's not that I felt particularly embarrassed for having been caught off guard and unable to address an interesting question in great depth. It happens. But because the students who argued with passion and eloquence were young gay men for whom, I imagine, the issue resonated far beyond the realm of philosophical inquiry, I had missed an opportunity to make a very simple point—namely, that what we do with our minds and what we do with our bodies overlap without necessarily being the same.

Everyone gets rejected at some point, and you tend to deal with it fairly well because you too reject people. That's the way it goes, it's just sex. I know it and these students knew it. But we also knew that this was different, that there is something about certain manners of rejecting someone who is HIV positive that isn't quite right. Were they hoping that I would absolve them for things they themselves had done and weren't too proud of? I don't know. Maybe. But it was clear that all of us were grappling with a certain failure of reason, wondering how benign or harmful that failure could possibly be.

How we determine risk and safety is often a matter of perceptions shaped by social forces and discourses rather than the result of an objective evaluation of the facts. That much has become clear after 9/11. In other words, I find it hard to blame individuals who behave unjustly with others in the name of personal safety because their decisions do not emerge from a cultural vacuum and cannot be simply discounted as the thoughtless acts of fools. HIV presents us with another context in which reason's shortcomings when one deals with other people's bodies become evident. Shaming and appeals to intelligence in hopes of getting people to act reasonably are thus bound to fail. I do not mean to exculpate pozphobic people altogether (as if, for example, individual Nazis couldn't be blamed for killing Jews) but, rather, to turn our critical eye to systemic, political problems. My point, then, isn't that k*** did something ethically wrong or just stupid when he rejected me—he was tactless at worst, I think—but that to look for a rational account of his reaction and mine isn't the most beneficial way to go about it. Desire is far too complex and unruly an emotion to fit neatly into ethical and political categories for one to rely on faithfully when certain situations arise. We and our desires deserve better, I think.

TOUCHINESS

A fairly young guy hit me up once, and after our e-mail conversations confirmed our mutual interest, I told him. As he had recently settled in the area, he said he was definitely interested in making friends but that sex was now out of the question. I must have been feeling particularly touchy that day, because I sent him to hell. So he turned the tables on me, telling me that he was the one now being rejected but that, despite that, he was not upset with me. Lovely. HIV-negative people often find it so obvious to refuse to sleep with HIV-positive people that they do not even see what they're doing as a rejection. This kind of blindness to the other's point of view always characterizes one's identification with the norm.

But when he informed me that he had only recently started having sex with other men, it dawned on me that I had directed my anger at someone who didn't deserve it, someone who had enough on his sexual plate already and could not reasonably be expected to deal with an HIV-positive partner in the way I would have liked, not right now anyway. Each of us had, in essence, failed to realize how touchy the other one was for his own particular reason—I about our different HIV statuses, he because his lack of experience made him feel vulnerable in relation to the more formidable, battle-scarred gay man I must have become in his eyes.

That's what so odd about touchiness—something always lurks below the surface that, as spatially counterintuitive as it may sound, stands in the way of contact. Depth is what's in the way. Touchy people tend to withdraw and, literally in this case, refuse to touch each other. To protect one's integrity means to construct our skin as a shield against others rather than as the open invitation that it should signify. Only when things are brought up to the surface, that is, when the safeguards offered by subjective depth are at least momentarily forsaken, can contact occur. Not that it would always work so easily, though. What made the difference here is that, as it turned out, the guy and I both had something to feel touchy about. When he understood my touchiness thanks to the realization and acknowledgment of his own, he was able to give me the opportunity to perceive his touchiness through mine. It requires the realization that subjectivity should not be protected and the willingness to put one's self at risk for shared touchiness to turn into mutual touching.

REASON TO EXCLUDE

The exclusion of the infected must be forceful and resolute. It must appear to be based on objective knowledge and not irrational fear, because it needs to veil the fact that, by definition, the uninfected is vulnerable—to infection. In fact, every rejection will be a reminder of that defining vulnerability and, therefore, the more you reject people with HIV the more unsafe you'll feel. (And the more unsafe you feel, the more often and forcefully you'll reject. That's both the point and the operating mode of the police.) This sort of rejection endows itself with all the trappings of reason and puts forth the notion of a responsible, autonomous individual making the right decisions to ensure his or her own bodily integrity. ("Neg and I intend to stay that way.") Waver and you're screwed. The person who rejects, however, doesn't realize that reason has already been infected—with irrationality and magical thinking, with affects (such as fear, hatred, contempt, admiration, desire, etc.), and with the complex and ever-changing meanings imparted to bodies in social situations. These various forms of infections, subjective and internal as they may feel, testify to the fact that some kind of encounter has already taken place. The self has willed nothing, somebody has rejected somebody for nothing—other than for the sake of rejection.

Now I wouldn't be completely honest if I didn't disclose something else: that I, too, once rejected a guy because he was HIV positive. Or to put it more accurately, I didn't reject this guy because he was HIV positive—as if *he* were responsible for the rejection, which the phrase hypocritically implies—but because I was afraid of coming into contact with him. I wasn't even brave enough to be brutal about it. This was the kind of act of cowardice that e-mail and IM chat let us enjoy with impunity, the way a face-to-face meeting or even a telephone conversation never quite could. Instead, I wrote the guy a long, convoluted reply, telling him that, in all likelihood, I had already slept with poz guys but that this was the first time I would be doing it knowingly and that there was no telling how I would react, blah-blah-blah . . . Bullshit, basically. He didn't bother to respond, and I never heard from him again. Frankly, I can't blame him. I was trying to reason and I acted like a fool. And how could I blame him anyway now that I am him? But I've never forgotten this. Even before my own diagnosis, the guilt that I felt at having possibly hurt him (or not, I'll never know) has stayed with me as the trace of our failed encounter.

THE STORIES OF AIDS

To disclose that one is HIV positive, especially within the logic of confession, sheds retrospective light onto what now seems to have been a narrative all along; in fact, several narratives. This is true of every kind of disclosure, of course, but I'll limit myself to the one we're all here for. There is the narrative of the illness, from infection to suffering to death maybe, or perhaps endless deferral in the serialized stories of what is called chronic disease. People often want to know how you became infected, how exactly it all started, and sometimes they even ask. They want to know what the future holds for you. There are elements of suspense too, now that treatments have displaced certain death to less fortunate corners of the world. How long can you expect these particular meds to work? Then what happens? Does the treatment have side effects—subplots, one could call them? And there is also the story of the epidemic, with its heroes and villains and its international intrigue. There is the research narrative, half whodunit and half treasure hunt. There are the stories of sin and redemption, of rises and falls, falls and rises, that have framed deviant sexualities for a long time.

The stories may not all be compatible with one another, and they tend to be full of holes in any case. After all, different people tell them for different purposes and to different putative audiences—one of these audiences being themselves. It can all be very confusing but also rich in possibilities. Much fun can be had with gaps and discrepancies—as implied in the double sense of the French verb *jouer*, to play but also to be loose. To begin with, if HIV disclosure is a narrative act, it logically follows that it must be subject to the rules, presuppositions, and various parameters that make up narratives, such as genre conventions with their power to organize social relations, susceptibility to transgressions, shifting contours and interrelatedness, but also style, register, complex and specific conditions of utterance, historical context, multiple interpretations, readability, viral transmission as in gossip and rumors, even the death of the author.

But these constraints are also too many not to allow for playfulness. I am not so naive as to think that I can escape the stories of AIDS; they have become far too entrenched in our collective reactions to the epidemic and unavoidable if we are to make sense of it. Indeed, we don't try to uncover the meaning of these stories but, rather, produce these stories—and produce them as one would fictions—to make up the meanings of HIV and AIDS. These are the stories that I tell, directly or indirectly, when I disclose, and the stories that people like k*** tell themselves—or hurl back at me—when they hear the news. They are not lies, however, but more like games of seduction and desire that allow me to oppose, by inhabiting them, these stories that I cannot escape yet cannot let determine me and my relations with others entirely. If I don't want to find myself disciplined by my disclosure— that is, if I don't want to find myself trapped within disciplinary regimes of knowledge and my "truth" captured by discourses—I have no choice but to use my stories as seductively as I can. This is one reason that I keep referring to this sort of disclosure as a form of sharing. To share, in that sense, is a matter not of unveiling some kind of truth but of making and remaking knowledge together in order to serve our needs, as different, situational, and ephemeral as they may be.

ACADEMIC TALK

Today, in Western countries, where effective treatments are easily available to most who need them, to disclose one's HIV-positive status is not as easy a proposition as some may think. If "HIV is no longer a death sentence," as the ubiquitous phrase goes, what exactly am I disclosing when I say "I'm HIV positive"? How am I disclosing it, that is, what accompanying statements are necessary? What contexts, what situations, what timing, what interlocutors come into play and affect the disclosure? In fact, why am I disclosing it at all? Why would I risk turning myself into an object of your knowledge?

Thrice (but my heart didn't race as fast after the first time) I opened a talk this way: "I'm HIV positive. There, I said it. Easy enough." A rather blunt and unusual attempt at seduction perhaps, but one nonetheless, since I had an audience to convince and bring over to my side. Things got tricky after that. The problem, first of all, is that I'm not sure exactly what "it" is. Ask anyone—well, almost anyone—and they'll tell you the same thing: the most annoying aspect of coming out, and perhaps its most salient feature, is that you have to do it over and over again. No matter how unambiguously and often you come out, you never seem to be out once and for all. After a while, the big news just becomes a big pain in the ass, and "it" isn't made any clearer by its many, indeed endless, iterations. In fact "it" changes all the time. But couldn't this also be a good thing, rather than a mere annoyance? If coming out—or disclosing, in the case of HIV/AIDS—is a never-ending process of relationality and negotiation, doesn't it spare us the risk of leaving ourselves open to all sorts of bad things, such as, say, belief in self-identity and other such policing devices?

To write an essay, especially an academic essay, on the politics and poetics of disclosure that is itself an act of disclosure means inevitably to raise questions about the limitations and potentials of the genres that give form to our inquiries. Can a talk given at a conference, an article in an academic journal, a book published by a university press be what it is about without losing as a result the distance that is supposed to guarantee its scholarly status? Should the critical apparatus stand safely apart from its object? Can it? And what happens if it doesn't? Is this necessarily a self-defeating proposition? How can the marginalized tactically inhabit certain genres in order to subserve their own interests rather than those of the very institutions of power that marginalize them? These are the sorts of questions confronting those of us working in fields, inherited partly from feminist scholarship, sometimes called affect theory and personal criticism.

If we understand and practice our trade as an avenue for egalitarian modes of exchange rather than as a relay for power, then its institutions may help us form a view of the intimate simultaneously within and against the power dynamics of the confessional mode. It should be possible also to give a more personal, literary form to what is, in essence, a theoretical reflection on abstract concepts. In the end, it is all a matter of what kind of community we intellectuals want our writing to inhabit, how closely we want to think alongside our readers and equals, and for what purpose.

So here I try to blend the personal and the scholarly and implicitly to act on their generic separation, not to juxtapose them and leave each intact in the end. Academics and people living with HIV—I am both—have nothing to gain from these distinctions. The categorical blurring (or confusion of genres) that I propose here is not an arbitrary decision on my part but, rather, a reflection on and of the experience of living with HIV and the modalities of its disclosure. To make this experience fit into preestablished cognitive categories would mean, in a sense, to betray "it"—this "it" that I want to see, that I need to see, as resistant to disciplinary knowledge, the way a virus may become resistant to treatment. What I seek to disclose in the end is the inevitable mutual contamination of body and thought thanks to the act of sharing.

A BRIEF HISTORY OF HIV/AIDS DISCLOSURE

If HIV and AIDS have a history, so, logically, does their disclosure. The hypothesis may sound absurd, but if AIDS had remained completely and consistently undisclosed it would not have a history. This suggests that we cannot separate the history of AIDS from that of its disclosure and that the latter is not simply a marginal detail in the epidemic. The HIV/AIDS coming out is a genre inscribed in a chain of other, preexisting genres—the confession, the news announcement, the legal disclosure, and naturally, the gay and lesbian coming out with which, for obvious social reasons, it shares more than its performativity. Because of its generic lineage, the linguistic act of coming out is relational, not just because it must involve at least one interlocutor, but also because it indexes and recycles all these preexisting genres. The meanings of HIV disclosure rest on contextual contiguity, in a synchronic fashion. But I want to propose the idea that meaning emerges and varies diachronically as well. What a disclosure of HIV-positive status means depends on what it (has) meant and what one imagines the future will bring. Yet because past and future always remain out of reach, they cannot possibly provide a firm foundation on which to build anything lasting. (The same goes for the present, naturally, since it has no tangible existence and, like a boundary, acquires the appearance of existence from the pull of what it divides.) Coming out can therefore never perform steady identities, which would find themselves undone from within by the always unstable process that would seek to bring them into being. (I call this process unstable in that it necessarily involves relating to something other, which it evokes or references or reuses.) A performative statement is always supposed to constitute a first in the sense that it ushers in something that didn't exist before, but if it generically conjures earlier statements, it is at the minimum a second. If a statement is not original, how, I ask you, can it possibly be originary?

But the HIV/AIDS coming out has a history of its own, as well as generic ancestry. For one thing, even though I, as a gay man, have experienced the disclosures of my HIV status after and through those of my homosexuality, I am aware that "coming out" may not provide a conceptual framework that can fit everyone's needs. Furthermore, as the realities of living with HIV have changed, so have the identities and cultural relations performed by the disclosure of one's status. I start there and roughly outline four periods. The term, however, may be a slight misnomer, since these "periods" have overlapped and often coexisted in ways that signal how AIDS, a pandemic of historical proportions, continues to resist all easy inscription within the disciplinary categories of history and geography. My purpose is to give a sense of a process by which certain social attitudes came to occupy the social forefront and to produce dominant AIDS discourses and marginalize others.

In the very early years of the epidemic, coming out could be extraordinarily difficult; that is to say, it was necessary. People with AIDS were often spoken for and spoken about, usually in unflattering terms, to say the least. They were diseased pariahs, patients different from other patients, medical mysteries, punished by God, potential murderers, poisoners of wells, modern-day Dorian Grays, Draculas, and Mr. Hydes. Harking back to previous centuries, these categories said very little about actual people with AIDS and a great deal about the fears, anxieties, and self-perceptions of the cultures that produced such identities in history. In France, for example, where ambivalent anti-Americanism and rationalism have been time-honored national pastimes, some dominant cultural voices emerging from political, scientific, and intellectual circles made a point of producing countercategories to the ones perceived to saturate public discourses of AIDS in the United States or Africa, the regions most identified with the disease at the time. The French public was soon told that people with AIDS were not pariahs, not different from other patients, and certainly not punished by God, since France is, as we all know, a staunchly secular republic steeped in the belief that reason and science can solve all our problems and where God has no legal powers to punish anybody. The good thing was that, as early as the mid-1980s and thanks to this sort of rhetoric, France had made it illegal to discriminate against people on the basis of HIV status. Yet in the end, in accordance with French universalist values, people with AIDS were nothing; so they had no social specificity and no identity, two concepts often denounced as "Anglo-Saxon" in the first place. All that these discourses said was that France was not like the United States or Africa. Whether people with AIDS were stigmatized or actively unstigmatized, this all served the same purpose: to shame them or to cajole them, but always into silence and invisibility.

Not surprisingly, the second period came as a reaction against the first, and not just on the part of the individuals directly affected. Gay voices hardly resonated beyond gay communities back then. But as it became increasingly clear that the epidemic would not stay confined to marginalized or distant groups, the newly anointed "general public" needed to know and needed to be reassured. (What it needed to know, mostly, was that sociological categories, be they racial, sexual, or class based, were "real" and that they could not bleed so easily into one another.) During this period, AIDS disclosures, whether pre- or postmortem, often had to be attached to celebrities in one form or another to find a significant echo in the culture at large. Rock Hudson, Rudolf Nureyev, Anthony Perkins, Arthur Ashe, and of course Greg Louganis are a few examples. In France, once again, things happened a bit differently, because of strict privacy laws and a stronger cultural split between public and private spheres, in particular when it comes to sexuality and illness. With the exception of a few rumors, some accurate and some not (Foucault and the movie star Isabelle Adjani come to mind, respectively), people who publicly disclosed their illness became celebrities because of it—provided that they already enjoyed some degree of symbolic capital. Few people knew of Hervé Guibert, Pascal de Duve, or Cyril Collard before they wrote books or made films about AIDS. Now they were on TV, on magazine covers, and in theaters near you. Gifted, romantic, and doomed, they enjoyed widespread sympathy inasmuch as they were hypersingularized and kept at a safe distance from the "general public." Articles lamenting the tremendous losses that AIDS was inflicting on the rarefied (and distant) circles of art and culture were common at the time. The romantic artist, in that sense, is the benevolent flipside of the diseased pariah; both figures are equally potent forms of rejection from the rest of us regular folk. AIDS was a shock whose ripples many were hoping to keep from reaching their own shores.

The third period saw the arrival of a highly visible brand of AIDS activism, spearheaded by ACT UP with its spectacular tactics and media savvy. All of a sudden—or so it seemed—people with AIDS were no longer "entertaining" us with their unusual gifts and celebrity status; they invaded the New York Stock Exchange and St. Patrick's Cathedral; they "zapped" the offices of pharmaceutical companies, forcing them to lower their prices; they publicly shamed politicians; they marched in the streets and posted eye-catching placards all over city walls; they also made the evening news, whether invited or not. They were often respected and admired for their courage. They were young and they were sexy. More important perhaps, they were no longer just individuals; they were a community, and it was as a seemingly real community that people with AIDS were now critiquing and challenging that other, manufactured, community known as the "general public." This was a difficult time.

Then, the good news came. In 1996, fifteen long years into the epidemic, word rang out of Vancouver that new treatments proved effective in prolonging the lives of people with HIV/AIDS. Although the overall perception(s) of the disease didn't change overnight—far from it, in fact—people in the global North did start to get better, and deaths from AIDS started to plummet. As a result, activism began to wane. (There were other factors.) ACT UP–New York, torn by internal political dissensions, was already gone, and other chapters vanished one after the other. Queer Nation, whose conceptual influence lingers to this day, seemed to have been little more than a flash in the pan as an organization. ACT UP–Paris has been more resilient, but the group was left wondering how it could reinvent itself as it was progressively disappearing from public view, its membership and political influence in free fall. Its leaders' attempts to demonize barebackers failed to register in the mainstream and were often met with skepticism and hostility within gay circles. In the wake of the new situation, large information and prevention campaigns disappeared. The "general public" ceased to be scared or admiring or even interested. The epidemic seemed relegated to distant developing countries, where such scourges are said to be a dime a dozen anyway. In the affluent North, people with AIDS were no longer diseased pariahs or romantic artists or brave activist heroes; they were people taking pills and going on with their lives. They were nothing. And that's pretty much where we are today, for better and for worse. Silence, once equated with death in ACT UP's most famous slogan, had returned, and coming out—the breaking of the silence—became fraught with a whole new set of difficulties.

FOUNDING MOTHERS

Soon after starting this book and under the pretext of research, I found myself doing something I hadn't done in ages: I devoured memoirs, poetry, and works of fiction written about AIDS in the late 1980s and early to mid-1990s—the darkest years of the epidemic in the West. Some of them I had read before, at the time, but the whole thing had gotten too draining emotionally, and I'd burned out on these books. Now, I couldn't put them down. Paul Monette, David Feinberg, Amy Hoffman, John Weir, Sarah Schulman, David Leavitt, Jamaica Kincaid, Rebecca Brown, Gary Indiana . . . everyone. Good, not so good, it didn't matter. I went through a period during which I would hardly ever read anything else, during which I couldn't stand reading anything else. One day, I handed a $20 bill to a waiter in a bar and almost asked him to give me shingles. I kid you not. Soon, I started dreading the anxiety that would inevitably arise as soon as I'd read all these books, but I wouldn't slow down. I told myself I was looking for a great passage to help me make this point about tact or that point about disclosure. It was all for work, I said to myself.

Sure enough, I did find a lot of interesting stuff. Adam Mars-Jones, for one, does mention tact all the time, but it doesn't count; he's British. Reading Leavitt's novella "Saturn Street," about doing volunteer work in L.A., reminded me with some unease that I did no such thing when I was living there in the early 1990s and that I chose to keep the epidemic at a certain distance. And there's the humor. Often, the most harrowing among these books are also the funniest, at least those written by gay men. In these texts, as was the case in real life, wit, sometimes bitchy and sometimes self-deprecating, provided tropes whose legibility was, like shame, a common feature of the community that also shared the experience of the epidemic, and it worked as a sort of substitute for an immune system now damaged. As Oscar Moore remarks, "Now that I have no physical defences I find myself with very few mental defences." John Weir, in a fictional version of his real-life friend Feinberg, writes:

> Zack looked like I felt: unprotected and furious. He was pushy about his self-loathing. "I'm so gay," he said, "that even the high school drama club wouldn't take me." Actually, he wasn't that gay. He was *posing* as a queen. He was exhausting, I guess, but I never got tired of him—not until he started getting really sick and his

cushioning irony wasted away, leaving nothing but his cutting remarks.

Troping is life. Remove it, and relating becomes difficult at best because all that is left is raw suffering.

Yes, these books gave me much to think about, but how, given the unbearable stories they told, could they make me feel, good? The truth, as usual, crept up on me until I could no longer ignore it and felt a little embarrassed about being so blind to my own motivations. What I was really looking for was the community I had lost. Reading these books allowed me to return to a time that was awful, yes, but in which AIDS was central to our collective life as gay men in a way that I now miss. When I returned to the stories written back then, I was looking for friends to give me shelter—to do what so many gay men will no longer do.

LOOK BACK IN ANGER (WHEN AIDS WAS ALL THE RAGE)

One of the things I miss the most about early AIDS activism is anger. Today, anger has become one of the most maligned emotions, singled out of proper sociability thanks to the usual alliance of stigmatization and pathologization. In a classic case of double bind, the "angry person" finds himself or herself accused of excess and lack at the same time, of expressing too much too loudly and, also, of failing to deal maturely with the so-called real issues that outbursts of rage always seem to mask. Anger is rude, inappropriate, inelegant, and tactless. In other words, we think of it as the *cause* of certain people's marginalization rather than its outcome.

The French phrase "les mots ont dépassé ma pensée" (literally: words went beyond my thoughts) implies that emotion, making its way into speech, clouds thought with something both in excess of and foreign to it. People collectively defined by their corporeality and emotions are often depicted as angry and thus politically delegitimized. We know the angry feminist, the angry black man or woman, the angry queer. Anger, it seems, defines those who cannot or will not think. But ACT UP's politics or rage demonstrated once more that the opposite could be true. Anger about AIDS led to the sharpest, most trenchant understanding of the epidemic, and it made possible a wide range of actions that saved lives and brought us closer to a resolution of the crisis. Still, many today claim that anger necessarily destroys people and disrupts human relations. Bullshit. AIDS does that, not anger.

Today anger, instead of being seen as an understandable reaction in certain circumstances, such as rejection and discrimination, is framed simultaneously as a psychological and a social disorder—exactly as homosexuality once was. One of ACT UP's greatest merits is to have shown that anger was not only healthy but also quite effective at solving problems. As the epidemic raged, so did queens.

UTTERING AIDS

Sociological studies of HIV disclosure in the United States reveal how difficult this act remains for many people living with the virus. And how complex a process. The authors of one such study were surprised to hear a New York man working "in an AIDS service agency" admit that, in sexual contexts, "I tell the truth only half the time." And they add, "Other men and women as well, in discussing the experience of being infected with HIV, repeatedly said that one of the hardest decisions they faced was whether to reveal the truth, to lie, or to speak in code to sexual partners and others in their lives." What I find particularly striking in this observation is that HIV disclosure doesn't appear to fall into a clean binary—either to tell the truth or not—but, instead, along a far more nuanced gradation of possibilities. As one would expect, the complexity of disclosure extends to the many different ways in which it is received. Responses to disclosure can be coded too. For example, "Not a problem" usually means "Oh, man, I really need to think about this," and "I need to think about it" means "No." When the authors of the study ask, "Why is disclosure, for many, among the most difficult aspects of being HIV positive?" the answer has to do with the availability of effective treatments. If you are lucky enough not to have to worry primarily about health care issues, the social is almost all that's left. That is always a messy affair, and disclosure triggers it all.

If coming out is always performative, coming out with HIV today often doesn't appear to perform anything, at least not anything that may be delineated with much clarity. The element that once made coming out both socially difficult and politically useful but that is now missing is of course death, the all-but-certain end point, until recently, of the AIDS narratives and the purveyor of their meanings. What, in the absence of imminent danger and violent social exclusion, could warrant the urgency of a disclosure? "I have something very important to tell you: I have to take a pill every night before going to bed." Lacks a little something, doesn't it?

I don't mean to oversimplify the matter, let alone to ignore the fact that, for many, things have not become all that easy. Even I, from my privileged position as an academic in a liberal college town, have witnessed firsthand the punch an HIV disclosure can pack. For one thing, not all the people I disclose to are peers. This is especially true of sexual partners. (But who *are* the peers of an HIV-positive person, when familiar social identifiers no longer provide reliable predictors of people's reactions?) And even in the global North and a few other regions that have successfully made treatments available to many and reduced AIDS-related deaths in significant numbers, personal circumstances vary enough to make for very different experiences of HIV disclosure—or nondisclosure, or the many statements in between. And by "personal circumstances" I mean a person's situation as it relates to matters of class, economics, religious, or other community standards, and so on. In many contexts, to disclose remains fraught with tremendous risks and endowed with great performative power indeed. I may live in prosperous Ann Arbor, but Ann Arbor sits a mere forty-five minutes from Detroit, in many ways a different world.

Even in what, for short, I call "the gay community," to be or to become HIV positive today is implicitly perceived as a hindrance to the progress of what, for short, I call "gay rights." It's easy to understand why. If gay rights testify to our full membership in the general public that had invented itself as an AIDS-free entity, political integration can be achieved only by severing our ties to HIV and AIDS.

Interestingly, political claims that had gained much traction as a result of the epidemic and its devastation are understood separately from AIDS, now that homosexuality has become more and more normalized. The crisis, its tragic toll and the courage gay people showed against devastation and injustice, played a crucial role in legitimizing the gay community as a mature political actor, but AIDS turned out to have been a bit like growing pains. As rights-oriented gay politics turns toward the future, living traces of the collective past are often met with impatience, to put it mildly. Indeed, one of the most perverse effects of the political focus on marriage rights is that it places at the core of "our" fight a practice and lifestyle—monogamy—long championed as the safest barrier against the spread of the virus, and this makes current gay activism constitutionally hostile to those of us with HIV. If anything, AIDS, like promiscuity and drug use, with which it is so often equated, as Kane Race has so brilliantly shown, is, to many, an embarrassing reminder that homosexuality may not be all about getting married and having children after all. Some gay activists would rather see the AIDS focus shift to populations, such as Africans and, in the United States, African Americans, perceived to be at risk precisely because they haven't yet reached the liberal-democratic, consensual mainstream with its emphasis on individual responsibility as the bedrock of full citizenship. In one way or another, whether by means of privatization (as now) or radical cultural othering (as then), the act of HIV/AIDS disclosure has been rendered politically irrelevant. AIDS theorists once warned about what they called the "degaying of AIDS," the everybody-can-get-it rhetoric that shifted the focus away from the social exclusions that still fueled the epidemic. The problem today seems to be the deAIDSing of gay that has made the gay community inhospitable to dissonance.

If camp, the misfit's humor, is itself a kind of playful dissonance because it makes the archaic resonate out of historical context, have I made a costly mistake by using it for resistance? Have I banished myself to the outer recesses of my own community by striking a pose so obsolete that it made me appear not just pre-1996 but even pre-Stonewall? Have I merely made an error in calibration by failing to understand how inappropriate my efforts would be in a small Midwestern town, or is the situation similar in bigger cities? My personal observations tell me that being HIV positive in a city where many others are as well increases the chances of finding a sense of community with them, but still marginalizes you in relation to the gay community at large.

On the thirtieth anniversary of the known epidemic, the journalist Mark Trautwein, a long-term survivor, remarks, "As the epidemic grew through the 1980s, all gay men lived with AIDS, whether infected or not." Indeed, once upon a time, to be gay was to define yourself in relation to AIDS. You defined yourself in relation to many other things, of course, and these things varied among people and groups, but AIDS was there for all. You had it, you knew someone who had it, you could get it, you tried your best not to get it, you were afraid of it, you fought it, you wondered what you could do to fight it, you felt guilty for not fighting it, you made sure you ignored it, and so on.

Of all the pills I've had to swallow, the bitterest may well have been the realization that to "come out" as HIV positive often has the opposite effect of what I, a gay man, expected it to have, that is, an entry into a messy, frustrating, but nurturing community. If the circumstances are right, to come out as having HIV may bring a person into an HIV-positive community, but for many gay men it can be devastating to come out and find ourselves repelled by the welcoming community the act was once associated with. And without a community, it is one's sense of self that becomes threatened. Disclosure, legally mandated or not, always contributes to making HIV exceptional. In the epidemic's early years, however, the prevailing attitude among sexually active gay men was to assume that every potential partner was HIV positive and to act accordingly—meaning to have (safe) sex with the other guy, not to shun him. Disclosure was not a relevant issue in sexual matters then, and as a result safe sex became possible because your partner's status was thought to be positive by default. Today, if you assume that every potential partner is HIV negative unless he discloses otherwise, which has become the new norm, not only do you discriminate but you also put yourself at greater risk of infection. Such a transformation of gay community dynamics is mind-boggling. By embracing the ideology of health once used to oppress queers, we have turned against ourselves.

As for HIV-positive heterosexuals, they often do not find that the coming-out metaphor provides them with a useful conceptual framework, because it never has in other contexts and isn't associated with a community. The studies I am aware of make no mention of this, but it could very well be that, in addition to misperceptions about gay solidarity, homophobia may play a part in straight people's reluctance to talk about coming out. It is as if, in the context of HIV, the metaphor itself conveyed infection—infection with homosexuality or the inevitable suspicion of it (directly for men and indirectly for women). Be that as it may, it is also the case that for some gay men with HIV comes the added distress of forsaking a familiar and reassuring tool in the face of a new challenge. To put it bluntly, if you are HIV positive today, the safest way to remain a full participant—and when I say full and safe I mean sexual—in the gay community is to be closeted (about being HIV positive), and this constitutes a reversal so shocking that it cannot be contemplated without pain, anger, and, literally, unspeakable sorrow.

WHERE'S THE POLICE WHEN YOU NEED 'EM?

Why should I miss the identity categories performed into existence by the act of coming out? Surely not just out of campy fascination with obsolete forms and genres. Early AIDS theorists had read their Foucault. We know Foucault's critique of confession. We also know of Rancière's definition of the police as what produces and enforces radical distinctions for the purpose of creating inequality and social control. And we are quite aware that the genres on which the HIV disclosure piggybacks have often been used historically to police people and assign them fixed places within and without a disciplined social order. Indeed, these genres represent something like the concrete enforcers of a series of interrelated discourses (in the Foucauldian sense): religion, medicine, law. Again, coming out is a never-ending process of repetition: as it repeats certain genres, it repeats with them the power structures they were conceived to sustain. Think, for example, of the disciplinary power of the mandatory disclosure to previous and future sexual partners. The HIV-positive person must speak *out* so that the virus may stay *in*. To keep it all in would be to risk contaminating others. This is why forced disclosure, when all is said and done, represents a form of enclosure. So why do I, as a gay man living with HIV, seem to long for the social categories that, as an intellectual, I have been criticizing as oppressive and debunking as untenable in the first place? The short answer is: because it is difficult not to be anything.

Clearly, silence, while tactically useful in certain situations, cannot offer an acceptable political option in the long run, even as a form of resistance against legal and public health mandates. The AIDS pandemic is still tied to social inequalities and injustice. Silence still equals death in the end. Conversely, to attempt to reinstate the old identity categories—or to invent new ones, for that matter—cannot constitute a viable political endeavor either. The potential of disclosure to outline concrete modes of equal social relations may thus be found instead in its dynamics rather than in its outcome. What if, in other words, the politics of disclosure was a matter of utterance?

An utterance is a complex linguistic act made up of different elements and of how they relate to each other: a statement, interlocutors, and circumstances of time and place. As such, then, utterance cannot be isolated as a stable object of empirical knowledge, and, the linguist Emile Benveniste has taught us, it can never be reproduced. The HIV disclosure, understood as utterance, must constantly recur but, unlike the statement "I'm HIV positive," never *à l'identique*. For instance, I first presented working versions of this section in front of audiences. At this point in the presentations, it was the third time that I had made the same statement since the opening sentence of my talk, and each time the utterance was different, either because I simply made the statement at three different points in time (it was no longer a disclosure after the first utterance) or, not so simply, because I used it in hopes of creating different effects in the recipients in relation to a specific stage in my argument. This iterative dimension of the HIV disclosure is thus the sign of a perpetual reinvention of social relations—relations between interlocutors, between interlocutors and statement, between interlocutors, statement, and situation, and so on. Understanding disclosure as utterance, then, means that none of the elements involved in the process—people, statements, situations, and beyond—may stand still long enough to be captured, that is, to constitute, or be constituted as, steady categories. In fact, categories find themselves undone in favor of endless dynamics. To a large extent, I believe this also works in the case of a written disclosure such as this one.

Like many others, I have disclosed my HIV status, or opted not to disclose it, for various reasons and with different, often crisscrossing motivations. Most will sound familiar to anyone who has come into contact with the facts of HIV disclosure. Issues of transmission, sexual safety, and other health-related matters always arise. Sometimes, especially in the beginning, I was either looking for emotional support or alleviating stress, as speaking out can do. Often, the goal was the preservation of a preexisting relationship that could have suffered from a lack of openness. Or from an excess of it. But creating new relationships has also been an important factor in some decisions to disclose or not. Whatever the situation may be, all these motivations foreground the relational dimension, not just of disclosure, but of living with HIV. To disclose is thus a way to bring others as full participants in that experience. And this, in turn, means that two crucial factors come into play: my needs, first of all, and my ability to "read" situations and interlocutors to gauge as best I can what the response is likely to be.

WHAT I SAID AND HOW I SAID IT

The disclosure, as I made it to close friends immediately after my diagnosis, did more than transmit a basic piece of information. It also implied: You are my friends, I am your friend, we matter to each other, and I need your support right now. It hardly felt like a disclosure at all, really; this sort of friendship doesn't police. The statement, at the time, didn't need to be completed by much else, and the fact that it often wasn't (what else could I say at that point? I was stupefied) conveyed a certain sense of urgency located outside the statement per se—perceived, although not explicitly heard. And this sort of indirection is precisely what made the urgency of it all the more available to social connection, or sharing, because it had to involve, on the part of my interlocutors, a mode of reading at once more proactively engaged and more receptive. Friendship, which allowed such contacts to occur in the first place, also found itself prolonged yet transformed—reiterated would be the right word. With friends, you don't confess; you share. And sharing necessarily involves gaps, lacks, and silences for people to latch onto. (What I'm trying to figure out is, If friendship makes it possible to share, is the reverse also true? Does sharing make friendship—or some kind of friendship—possible?)

The same news, given to another friend, with whom I had had sexual relations in the not-so-distant past, acquired an additional level of unspoken signification: it would be a good idea for him to get tested, in case he hadn't been in a while. Because that friend was, like me back then, a foreigner in the United States, but one who hadn't yet obtained his green card, parts of the conversations initiated by the original announcement also dealt with the unique intersection of the political and personal aspects of HIV and AIDS within the larger international contexts of the pandemic and immigration—in this case the risk of sudden deportation and its consequences. (The Obama administration has since rescinded that rule from the Reagan era.)

I sent e-mails to sexual partners I wasn't close to—provided, of course, that I knew their e-mail address, which wasn't always the case. Yes, I did it to obey the law but also because Ann Arbor is a small town in many ways. I felt it wiser to tell them than to take the risk that they may learn it from a third party. I also felt concerned about their well-being, but I must admit that I didn't feel any particular urge to take responsibility for their actions. That said, I had the option to do this anonymously and still comply with the law. I opted not to because in each of these cases where I could identify and contact the man in question I felt safe enough to do so openly—and I had to protect myself. Was there also some reluctance on my part to depersonalize the question of risk, to sever its attachment to a specific memory, a specific person, a specific body, a specific face—a specific contact? It's possible. I don't know.

When, several weeks later, I broke the news over the phone to friends overseas, I was able to complement the basic statement with reassuring news, namely, that I had begun treatment and that it was working very well. Indeed, that was why I had waited before communicating with some people I could not have face-to-face contact with. Because of the physical separation, I also prefaced the statement with something self-referential such as, "I have something to tell you but let me reassure you right away, it isn't as serious as it sounds." My efforts at reducing unwanted noise, however, were not always successful, reminding me that I could never be in full and sole control of what I was saying, that listeners, too, determine meaning. One such friend, for example, replied that he was relieved to hear that everything was going well, but that I should never, ever again start with "It isn't as serious as it sounds," because the phrase had produced exactly the opposite of the desired effect. Thinking back on this with greater clarity now, I realize how thoroughly unsurprising this is . . .

In at least one case, a friend expressed some disappointment that I had waited so long to tell her, thus foregrounding the importance of the time factor in the act of utterance. I explained my reasons—that I wanted to tell her but be simultaneously reassuring—yet I couldn't help but notice, once again, how utterances are subject to noise. What was it exactly that disappointed her when she learned I hadn't told her right away? Did she feel a sense of betrayal, thinking perhaps that true friendship always requires transparency? No, not like her at all. Did she have the impression that I may not have trusted her completely? But trusted her to do or say what? Trusted her not to disclose it to others who, by her act of withholding, would find themselves less close than we were for not being "in on it"? Is it unfair to demand of our friends that they keep secrets from their friends? We expect the truth from our friends and torture it out of our so-called enemies. We demand it from our parents and from our children, from our leaders and from our teachers. Is there anyone from whom we do not demand the truth?

I mustn't forget to mention that sometimes I opted not to disclose. (I usually don't to complete strangers, of course.) There were, and continues to be in some cases, situations in which saying it would have been too taxing. Too taxing for me, I mean. I would have had to explain and to educate. The focus would have soon turned to *their* sadness, *their* fears, *their* anxieties. In the early months especially, I had no desire to be someone's therapist or teacher.

Yet I am a teacher after all, and just as I've always found it better for all involved that my students know I'm gay, I soon came to realize that I couldn't simply put aside the question of my HIV status either. Well, I could, I guess, I just didn't want to. But how to do it? With homosexuality it's easy. That's pretty much become part of these kids' lives, and many of them are quite open about being gay themselves, especially boys in French classes. More often than not, homosexuality is a perfectly speakable matter in a university classroom. HIV is a different story, though. I knew I couldn't rely on shared cultural codes and playful winks that, given how far HIV seems to be from these kids' preoccupations, had little chance of being picked up on. So I kept waiting for an opportunity to arise so that I might pretend to be spontaneous about something I had been mulling over for a while.

Once, a gay undergraduate student of mine wrote a paper about that very topic: for the first time, a close friend of his, also gay, had just told him that he was HIV positive. The paper was so over the top in its emoting (lovely kid, really, but what a drama queen . . .) that I saw an opening. It became possible to talk first about someone other than me, build on a student's work, and inject some humor into the whole situation by gently mocking him and me. It was the end of the class period, and I was returning the papers. "You know," I said out loud as I was walking around the classroom, "what you're talking about isn't that tragic." I made sure that he was OK with an open discussion of the topic, which he was. (Drama queens are also exhibitionists.) "Sure it sucks, but your friend isn't going to die, you know that." As I reached his paper down the pile, I came closer and asked, "So you know only *one* person who is HIV positive?" "Yes," he replied, and as I was now standing right in front of him I shook his hand and said, "There, now you know two," and went on giving the papers back to the other students as casually as if I'd just expressed a preference for Madonna over Lady Gaga. I'll never be able to ascertain the ripple effect of what happened that day, but I thought I had done pretty well and, for once, I walked home with a bounce in my step as I passed the usual signposts.

My friend Rostom, to whom I told that story, finds this sort of disclosure violent because it often stuns the listener and leaves him or her with no opportunity to respond or even react other than with shock. If I understand his objection well, the problem is that everything begins and ends with the disclosure and leaves the speaker, me, in full control of the terrain. After all, I used "you" and not "I" as the subject of my statement and focused it on the student's own knowledge, which is my job. On the one hand, I see why this could represent a case of disclosure that, like a door slamming, encloses itself as well as myself (and therefore the listener) and forbids all possibility of contact. On the other hand, reclaiming control of one's own HIV disclosure, as bound to fail as such an endeavor may be of course, is nonetheless understandable and in many ways necessary. Moreover, one could argue that no matter how blunt the disclosure it still continues its work, adding to the statement itself the relational dimension of utterance. In the end, the ripples spread gently even if throwing a rock in the water seems violent at first.

The tension between overreaction and underplaying is significant. Overall, early instances of my disclosure were often (but by all means not always) met with roughly two types of reaction, related to the historical periodization I outlined earlier and evidence that there is some overlapping going on here. One could be labeled "pre-1996," the other "post-1996." (But just as I did earlier when periodizing, I am positing for clarity's sake categories that are in reality neither cohesive nor autonomous.) In the first case, the recipients would be shocked, extremely upset, and even scared. Either they were old enough to have known the early years of the epidemic and had their views so affected by that experience that it overdetermined their immediate reaction; or they were misinformed about the current and overall far less tragic reality for many people of living with HIV in the global North. The other reaction was pretty much one of confident dedramatizing, more often than not out of genuine concern and a desire to be reassuring. Nothing too serious to worry about. To be HIV positive these days is no longer such a big deal, what with all the incredible advances in research. The cholesterol approach.

The truth is, I too oscillated between the two attitudes at first—a sure sign that there was something unsatisfactory about both and that the reliance on one or the other gets determined in each situation and for tactical purposes. What may have appeared as casual dismissal on the part of some may, in the end, have been less matter-of-fact than a matter of tact. But allow me to repeat it: to tell me, as they did at the hospital, that it is unlikely

I will ever die of AIDS implies that I am no different in that respect from someone who is not HIV positive. No, I probably won't die of AIDS; but no, AIDS is not like cholesterol. Again, I'm categorizing, or dichotomizing, a bit unfairly. My friends were, just like me, trying to navigate between two poles, and, by and large, they did it very well, making statements they knew couldn't be fully believed, but making them nonetheless with complete sincerity. (This, incidentally, could be an interesting definition of tact.) Just as was the case with my disclosures, the multiple meanings of my friends' reactions could not be located strictly within their statements. That's what made them (the friends *and* the statements) tactful in the first place. Anyway, how can the experience of testing positive for HIV be a satisfying one for most people? The two kinds of reactions, then, were the outcome of a specific generic ancestor of the HIV disclosure: the announcement.

In certain specific contexts and if certain conditions are met, the identifying marker of the announcement is enough, and no additional statement is required for the disclosure to take place. In his memoir of a relationship with a man who eventually died of AIDS, Fenton Johnson describes the moment when things between the two begin to grow beyond the merely casual and sexual. Larry, Fenton's lover, realizes that the time has come to tell:

> "There's something you ought to know," he said. In the mid-1980s,
> in San Francisco, among gay men there could only be one thing I
> ought to know, and I'd sensed it already. A delicate vacancy around
> the edges of words; his careful and limited use of the future tense,
> my intuition that my particular life script called for me to be taught
> some lesson by love, and my knowledge that such learning often
> comes hard.

This passage is of a place and of a time: San Francisco's gay community in the 1980s. The time, the place, the people all conspire to produce the necessary conditions for the disclosure to be understood without needing to be stated—unlike in my classroom. Elements in the larger situation of utterance but exterior to the statement per se are such that they are enough to produce meaning. Larry did speak, of course; it would have been inexcusable to exclude him from the meaning-making process of disclosure, and he had more to say: "He spoke the terrible facts aloud—HIV-positive, still healthy, no symptoms, T-cell count still high, above 800, almost normal. He had yet to tell his parents because, after all, they were aged, who could know what might come to pass."

In gay memoirs and novels of the worst years, from the early 1980s to the mid-1990s at least, HIV disclosure—or for that matter the sight of unmistakable signs that made words unnecessary sometimes—is often accompanied by a blunt expletive rather than conventionally tactful behavior. I even came across a manual of gay etiquette that recommends a plain "Oh, shit!" as a perfectly appropriate response. In such contexts, tactful avoidance of the topic of HIV and AIDS makes little point because there is no difference in kind between the interlocutors. I'm speaking of course of the years when gayness and AIDS could not be easily dissociated, making it impossible for the listener to use tact to create a bond with other listeners at the expense of the man with AIDS. The "delicate vacancy around the edges of words" may have been a manifestation of tact, but it was no avoidance. It was a form of encoding and a telltale sign that something was left unsaid (literally unarticulated) and that we all know what that was. The kind of eloquent silence, like language itself, produced a community and resulted from it at the same time.

Things are different today. Unstated disclosures are still possible, and they happen all the time. But because of that deAIDSing of gay I mentioned earlier, signs need to be more specific than simply being gay in a big city in a certain decade. The jargon around barebacking or other practices may be an indicator that a person is HIV positive. So can your bathhouse of choice or the bar in which you decide to meet for a first date, at least in a city large enough to offer you options. Leaving the question about HIV status unanswered in your profile on a cruising site is another example. In other words, nondisclosure discloses, not unlike the telltale signs of closetedness. The subtlety of these signs and the fact that they probably cannot be understood by most gay men who are not themselves poz (or directly in contact with poz people and cultures) show how far HIV as a social force has been pushed toward the outer reaches of the gay community—the margin's margin.

But let me return to the issue of announcement. If I were to try and elicit different responses from my interlocutors—neither panic nor dismissal—I would have to find ways somehow to disclose without announcing. I did, and I'll give you a few examples.

In one case, a friend was telling me, in a somewhat confessional mode, of her own medical problems and how they were affecting her mental well-being. Because the reason for the conversation was to ask me for advice, I weighed in with my own story. "When I found out I was HIV positive . . . ," and so on and so forth. Intended to convey empathy, the statement, this time, was framed not as an explicit announcement but as an exemplum, that is, as simultaneously singular and relational. And it is by foregrounding the relational without sacrificing singularity that I was able to prevent the two unsatisfactory responses I had witnessed before. Indeed, what was so unsatisfactory about them was that they could be read as forms of rejection, even if they were not at all intended as such. I was either going to die soon or I was going to live just like everyone else. Again: no, I'm not, and no, I'm not.

If in this case I seized an opportunity that I hadn't foreseen and made a disclosure that I hadn't planned on making just then, it is quite a different story with my next illustration. I wanted to tell the friends present that night. At the appropriate time in the conversation, I (sort of) seamlessly mentioned that I'd had an unusually long bout of diarrhea lately (I'm not sure when it is appropriate to talk about diarrhea in a social setting, and I apologize for being a tad inelegant here as well, but we are after all discussing an illness, let's not forget), so naturally I worried since I'm HIV positive and all, but it turns out there's no connection, so everything's good. This is what I could call sounding shockingly matter-of-fact, an apparent contradiction that really renders, accounts for, and confronts the affective ambivalence I have been describing. By embedding the statement within another, larger narrative that seemed to contain the main item of information—a bout of diarrhea—I produced a jarring effect intended to prevent pre-1996 overreaction and, more interestingly, to prod the listeners into confronting their own possible post-1996 desire to be casual about the news. (I couldn't predict which one, if any, would occur; that—and much else that makes up an utterance—was beyond my control as speaker.) "Did I hear this right? How could I not be matter-of-fact about it if he is? But how can he be so matter-of-fact?" Ripples. Considered in the larger context of utterance, the possibility of casual dismissal by the listeners became part and parcel of the news. The jarring effect brought speaker and listeners, all of us friends, into a gently unsettling relationship, in which casual dismissal became a source of discomfort when, in theory, its purpose is supposed to be the exact opposite. Comfort—defined in this context by the ability to rely on one of two readings to the exclusion of the other—found itself altogether undone as a basis for relationships, which, in turn, became redefined as the sharing of difference, or empathy. Could the HIV disclosure, then, be a way to establish contact that neither relies on the preexistence of stable identities nor seeks to produce them? A form of *faire signe* rather than interpellation perhaps?

THE PURLOINED LETTER

My friend Michael is fond of letters. He likes to write them and to receive them, which never ceases to impress his mailman in Mexico City. It was only fitting that in this case I would want to tell Michael in writing that I had tested positive for HIV. Because of the campiness of the whole enterprise, which I found ideal for HIV disclosure to a fellow homo, I also wrote it as I imagined George Sanders would have, or Eve Arden—in a detached, world-weary style. I mentioned my last visit to New York for Rufus's show at Carnegie Hall, when Michael still lived in the city. I explained what an unforgivable faux pas it would have been for me to ruin everyone's fun with such dreadful news. And I even included the letter in a Christmas package alongside the CD and DVD of Rufus doing Judy, as well as a few movies. In fact, in my letter I devoted the largest amount of space to all that. The HIV issue was purposefully framed as a digression away from matters of genuine import, such as the enduring and endearing popularity of "The Trolley Song" among adult homosexual men.

Michael was visiting relatives in D.C. for the holidays, so that's where I sent the package . . . which Michael left behind as he flew back to Mexico, not realizing that it contained a letter, right there under his eyes. For months I didn't hear back from him. Well, I did hear from him, but not about *that*. I knew then that the letter had become lost somewhere, but where? What to do? Send it again? Settle for a more prosaic phone call and ruin something I had so thoughtfully planned? Until one day I received an e-mail from Michael, and its subject line wasn't the title of Hope Lange's obituary in the *New York Times* or any other matter whose singular urgency usually motivates Michael to use modern communications technology. After a long long time in limbo, my disclosure had finally reached its recipient, and its accidental delay, followed by a flurry of conjectures and (mis)interpretations, not only dramatized the very nature of writing but also transformed an act of disclosure into a story in its own right, one whose importance must be located in the in-between space of relationality itself.

SO AM I

I'll move on now to a more complex example of disclosure—that of the first time I knowingly said "it" to someone who was also HIV positive. For I'm not the first person to be HIV positive. I'm finagling with my argument a little here, since I didn't say "I'm HIV positive" that time, but rather, "So am I." My interlocutor and I were involved in a discussion about our adventures and misadventures in online cruising. At one point, he said, "I've tried putting 'HIV+' in my profile, but it didn't exactly help me get laid." You'll recognize the anti-announcement tactic I had used myself: to embed a seemingly secondary but possibly more central statement within a primary one that may become relegated to the status of context, equalizing center and margin and tactfully leaving the listener with the freedom to choose on which piece of information to articulate the rest of the discussion. The larger context of our conversation provided me with enough clues to understand that my friend's revelation also implied a question: "Are you HIV positive too?" Then, after I made sure that he was indeed HIV positive and not talking about some strange sociological experiment, I said "So am I"—a statement worth lingering on for a while.

"*So.*" So what? This "so," the HIV-positive status, does not constitute a stable object of knowledge, since the experience of living with HIV results from various social determinants. Clearly, medical "facts" that appear similar on the surface have very different significations and consequences in different cultures or different parts of the world. To be HIV positive in a country where you are likely to die as a result is just not the same "thing" as to be HIV positive and have access to first-rate medical care, as I do. To live in a rural area can turn a routine visit to your HIV specialist into a long and costly expedition. To be HIV positive and African American means that you have been caught up in a racist system that often precludes equal access to resources and that you belong to a demographic group with a shockingly low life expectancy. Not "so" for everybody. And there are personal factors as well. Does one have a network of friends? A supportive family? And so on. My interlocutor, although younger, had lived with HIV for much longer than I and once, on a later occasion, started a sentence with, "In my day . . . ," a phrase I couldn't have used at the time, since I had been diagnosed for a little over a year and my day was another day for him. Older than him in age, I was a callow youth in HIV time. And now that people who recently seroconverted have started to turn to me for advice and support, I too have acquired the aura of a veteran. But advice is one thing and knowledge is another. They overlap only if you understand them as situational processes of sharing and exchange. In other words, what we share—"so"—is neither fully known nor fully knowable.

"*Am*." In this particular instance, the use of the verb "to be" doesn't carry a stable ontological dimension, at least not in the traditional sense. If, according to the Cartesian model, categorization is supposed to be the precondition of thought and thought the precondition of being, then the sharing of an unstable, unknowable, uncategorizable trait, and one so fraught with affect—"so"—cannot support the kind of being grounded in the sort of rational thinking that the *cogito* proposes.

"I"? Really a "we," not only in the context created in and by this particular sentence, but because no "I," not even that of "So am I," may be articulated apart from a process of exclusion. The implied "we" includes the one other "I" that one is *like* but inevitably indexes all those other I's that one is *unlike*. As the philosopher Judith Butler explains it, referring to the notion of lesbian identity but in a deconstructive way that I find legitimate to generalize:

> To claim that this is what I *am* is to suggest a provisional totalization of this "I." But if the I can so determine itself, then that which it excludes in order to make that determination remains constitutive of the determination itself. In other words, such a statement presupposed that the "I" exceeds its determination, and even produces that very excess in and by the act which seeks to exhaust the semantic fields of that "I." In the act that would disclose the true and full content of that "I," a certain radical *concealment* is thereby produced.

If disclosure-as-utterance results in the undoing of the categories involved, then the "I" of "So am I" doesn't refer to the speaker as an autonomous individual but to an ephemeral, relational entity existing only in and for as long as the context of the utterance; the fleeting citation of an institutional discourse of "subjectivity" rather than the expressive sign of a voluntarist self. The interlocutors may be part of the process, but, by the same token, the process is also part of them. Disclosure operates in a liminal space of touch or contact whereby entities make and unmake themselves and one another and, therefore, are revealed not to be entities at all. An HIV disclosure, like any other disclosure, always reveals more than one thinks and what the statement says.

"So am I," then, constitutes a relational gesture resting on no fixed categories whatsoever, including the subject. For "I" is not the first person to be HIV positive. To return to my initial statement—"I'm HIV positive"—and without having to undertake a full deconstruction of the subject, I must remember that, at the very least, this "I" always indexes its relationship with a "you" and that this "you" can exist only in relation to an "I." The HIV disclosure, understood as utterance, is thus a form of ontological contamination in that it necessarily reminds all involved that everyone has an HIV status and that it is a matter of difference and not distinction. This form of sharing is what I could call disclosing without identity.

My interlocutor in the last example also told me a while later that HIV-negative people cannot understand what it's like to be positive. On the basis of personal experience, I profoundly believe this to be true. To meet another person who is HIV positive often feels like sitting down at long last after being on your feet for an entire day. In a 1984 novel, Paul Reed describes one such meeting using a different metaphor: "Andy shook his hand and smiled. He had expected to feel some apprehension, but he felt a vague relief, something like coming home after a long trip." The nature of such apprehension, when it occurs, is itself a factor of discomfort, for it signals a reluctance to acknowledge a bond with a peer and, with it, the social reality of one's own status. That discomfort too finds relief when the meeting turns out to have a liberating effect rather than a confining feeling of identity.

But although my friend's statement, that HIV-negative people cannot understand what it's like to be positive, seems to entail an identity (to be positive) whose experience is only accessible to some, it also implies that this identity is in fact a community formed by two relationships: one with other positive people and one with negative people as well. To be positive is to be positive like and, at the same time, to be positive unlike, each term automatically undoing the other in a never-ending process of relating; that is to say, of telling and connecting. The ultimate outcome of the HIV disclosure is to reveal nothing, in the sense that "nothing" is what a relational dynamic, or community if you want to call it that, is all about. I must now revise my earlier statement: if coming out as HIV positive performs nothing, it may be because it performs "nothing"—that is, nothingness itself. And that's really something.

SMALL TALK

My first very public instance of disclosure was at an academic conference. It wasn't around drinks, mind you, but as part of my presentation and in front of a sizable, if very friendly, audience. That evening, a bunch of us were smoking outside the hotel when one of the boys mentioned in passing something about "taking my meds," just like that, in the middle of a story to which the detail had no meaningful narrative connection whatsoever. In relation to the story's events, the act of taking the meds occurred in proximity to the plot but had no bearing on it. The protagonist stopped whatever he was doing and took his meds. Then the action resumed. That contiguity was, in turn, structurally mirrored in the telling of the story, where the information was equally irrelevant. The narrator interrupts his story, mentions the taking of the meds, then resumes where he left off as if nothing incongruous had occurred.

The result was too jarring to be a mere *effet de réel*, and although these meds could, in theory, have been just any meds, I immediately interpreted the combination of the first person and the familiar abbreviation (among gay men, still, "my meds" doesn't mean the same thing as "some meds"), along with the contextual proximity to my paper, in which I'd alluded to the same act, and the digressiveness of the utterance, which mirrored my own, as a tactful HIV disclosure and a gesture of solidarity. Of course, nobody jumped in with a "Wait, wait, wait! You took what?" and to make sure I wasn't imagining things, I later asked another guy who was there if our friend had indeed said what I thought he'd said. (Ripples.) We agreed that indeed he had. In all likelihood, the whole group had picked up on it just as we had and as our friend was hoping we would.

Today I'd be hard-pressed to tell you what the original story was about, and I'll bet you anything that no one who heard it remembers it either. The story wasn't the point. The insignificant detail, the aside, the footnote, had engulfed everything else, and what remained was an act of sharing and *faire signe*—a first-person singular that produced a first-person plural. That was the point. To disclose tangentially without making a big announcement. Instead, the collective dynamic of small talk left plenty of room for sharing important things in and as a group.

THE STORY OF THE RACONTEURS

OK, I'll give you one last story, one in which things went very wrong.

As is the case with every rock concert these days, you would get to see the Raconteurs at the Fillmore in Detroit only after waiting in gender-specific lines, at the end of which you were asked to show the contents of your pockets and agree to be patted down. I didn't mind one bit. It hadn't crossed my mind, however, that the small pillbox attached to my key ring could attract so much attention. Surely, there must be better places to hide drugs than a pillbox. The bouncer unscrewed the top of the small, metallic cylinder and dropped the contents into his hand. With his big, clumsy fingers, he unwrapped the small piece of tissue with which I got into the habit of cushioning the pill after I realized it would otherwise crumble.

"What is this?" he asked.

(FUCK!) "Medication."

"Yeah, but what is it?" he insisted.

(FUCK! FUCK! FUCK!) "It's called Atripla."

"I don't know it. Let me call the medic."

(FUUUUUCK!!!)

Some uniformed guy came by—the medic, clearly, although he looked like a cop—and he didn't seem to know what the pill was either.

"What is this?" he asked.

"It's called Atripla."

"Never heard of it. What is it for?"

I had become really upset by then. I was caught off guard and felt a bit embarrassed as a result, unprepared to have to disclose my status in a place where I'd come to enjoy a kick-ass rock 'n' roll band, and I felt utterly powerless. Out of spite and feeling the increased pressure (and embarrassment) that comes with blocking a line, I decided to make *them* feel uncomfortable with the whole situation. To this day, there's something about rock concerts that always makes me feel like a teenager.

"It's for AIDS," I said defiantly. ("HIV" just wouldn't do for those fuckers.)

"What'd you say?"

Remember that we were in the lobby of the theater at the time. The opening act was already onstage and, between the loud music and the crowd, the place was filled with noise—in both senses of the term.

"It's for AIDS," I repeated a bit louder, increasingly unsure that my defiance was such a bright idea after all, yet unable to back down without feeling defeated and even more humiliated than I already was.

"It's for WHAT?"

I started yelling: "AIDS! AIDS! I HAVE AIDS!!!"

The whole thing had turned absolutely ghastly. The medic must have decided it was better to trust me. (What kind of idiot would yell "AIDS!" in a crowded theater for no good reason? Presumably, the same kind of idiot, come to think of it, who would hide illegal drugs in a pillbox attached to his key ring, but never mind.) He gave me back my meds with an expression that seemed to say, "All right, all right . . . Jeez, dude, keep your skinny jeans on." With my cheeks on fire and what felt from the inside like the look of a madman in my eyes, I immediately walked to the bar and ordered a cocktail. Like me, it was shaken, not stirred. Actually, it was an ordinary rum and coke in a plastic cup, but you get the idea. Long story short, to make matters worse, I never even got the bouncer to pat my butt.

Hoping to match power with power, control with control, I recognized in hindsight that all parties involved in that ridiculous incident had somehow been forced to relinquish something. Deciding how to come out, where, when, and to whom, often gives the illusion of control, as if coming out, and being whatever it is that one is after that, could possibly be effected on our own terms only. That's a grave mistake that consists in confusing tactics with strategy. According to French thinker of the everyday Michel de Certeau, only those in control of the terrain can strategize. But no one is ever in sole control of the contacts we establish with others. Furthermore, to believe that it is possible to master the afterlife of the messages we put out, or that of the gifts we give, is to rely on nonrelational notions of subject and object and on the assumption that language *is* the reality it seeks to convey—the illusion, in other words, that each element involved in the complete process of utterance of a given message is untainted by the other elements. But even if I could accurately predict the exact effects that my statement will have on a given audience, how can my message be entirely mine if, each time, I tailor it according to its recipients and factor in the time and the place? My message is mine, yes, but it is also not mine. To believe otherwise is to entertain fantasies of purity and power. We must, in other words, always welcome our lack of control with open arms. And when that happens, I strongly recommend having Jack White around.

COMPATIBLE DISCORDANCE

Modes of HIV transmission are so caught up in a web of cultural taboos and fantasies that sticking to objective facts, we are told, offers the best way to manage our fears, protect ourselves, and organize our social and sexual relations. I would like to focus on this now: not, however, to illustrate how we envision our relations with others on the basis of known facts but to argue, first, that how we choose to relate to others provides us with a framework for shaping the facts of HIV infection, and second, that the complex dynamics of disclosure play a central role in this process.

In the early years of the epidemic, as you may or may not remember, the lethal combination of medical impotence, ethical lapses, and political wrongdoing made it crucial for anyone involved to gain the upper hand in the realm of discourse. But discursive, and therefore political, ascendancy can best be achieved rhetorically by building on preexisting patterns that most people are expected to recognize and accept as being beyond discussion. From its inception, then, the AIDS crisis has been framed by a seemingly endless series of familiar binaries meant to give a reassuring appearance of clarity to the epidemic and to benefit different constituencies. The goal was to provide both those directly affected and the others with a useful, perhaps even life-saving, road map. Among these "choices" are health or illness, truth or lies, facts or myths, knowledge or ignorance, science or superstition, tolerance or bigotry, and so forth. Superpose them, and the true and the right, the rational and the ethical begin to fuse. I want to argue that these binaries, no matter how negotiable their lines of articulation and how strategically useful they may be, for example, against denialism and egregious discrimination, fail to account for the far more complex experience of living with HIV. Furthermore, because their purpose, whether stated or not, is to capture the infected and the uninfected as two incompatible categories, such binaries end up producing their own kind of denialism and discrimination. I believe that we need to rethink HIV disclosure outside regimes of truth, with their implacable oppositions, to address the murkier complexities of experience and to open up possibilities of contact between the directly affected and the indirectly affected.

For people whose concerns are not primarily of a professional nature, the desire for facts has to do not with an ethical commitment to truth, not with a philosophical investment in knowledge, but with control—control over oneself, over others, and, more important, over the boundary between self and others. To many people, a rational approach may seem like an obvious choice when confronted with medical matters. In the context of HIV, however, what makes reason appealing is not its promise to bring about results but its deeper structural workings. Western reason functions according to two movements that appear contradictory. The first consists in discerning a collection of discrete facts; the second synthesizes these facts into a larger coherent truth. Separating and totalizing: this dual dynamic structures what can be called "a world of reason," a world that claims to be universal but from which some people must be excluded in order to protect and preserve its integrity. From this we can deduce two things: first, reason discriminates in both senses of the word; second, fear of contact, often discredited as irrational—the second or "bad" term of those binaries—is in fact a foundational element of rational thought. Because we understand contact as a kind of contamination that threatens to undo the categories on which the entire edifice of reason stands, any analytic system of thought is inherently hostile to contamination by otherness.

I just suggested that it would be interesting to look at what happens if we superpose these binaries in the context of HIV and AIDS: health or illness, truth or lies, facts or myths, knowledge or ignorance, science or superstition, tolerance or bigotry. . . . The superposition, of course, has been going on from the start of the epidemic. Still, the mutual incompatibility that separates the two sides of each pair doesn't pertain only to this specific context. It is at the core of what we call Cartesian thinking—the idea that one thing cannot both be itself and what it is not. In less modern times, something like this was known as the principle of noncontradiction. Either way, reason rests on this idea. But truth, health, and tolerance, for example, may be, and often are, easily juxtaposed in a variety of rational discourses and represent different policing devices operating in different areas of a culture but always in the service of the same system. Doesn't this imply, then, that reason is always in contact with the corporeal and the moral, each domain contaminating and spoiling the other?

I'm arguing here against the supposed autonomy of reason, but I don't mean to conclude that, in the context of HIV infection, all reason ought to be abandoned in favor of craziness, or that the epidemic ought to be approached primarily through the prism of affect. What I mean is that truth, facts, and logic alone cannot account for life with HIV, and that whereas discrimination is supposed to guarantee the integrity of rational thought, the experience of HIV keeps getting reinvented in relation. Discordance, in other words, need not presuppose incompatibility, even if the apparent contradiction in terms that is the phrase *compatible discordance* does suggest a kind of "ill logic"—the ill logic of contact, whether feared or welcome.

This is where the issue of disclosure comes into play, and where some notions of pragmatic linguistics come in handy. If the experience of HIV is a social one, then it is premised on disclosure, that is, on the externalizing of something kept inside until then. Whether or not the HIV-positive person discloses his or her status doesn't change the fact that the issue of disclosure signals one's entry into the social, regardless of how the issue is resolved. As soon as a person learns of being HIV positive—and this usually happens when being told—disclosure becomes at least latent, and to imagine or predict other people's reactions to a possible disclosure is enough. Moreover, disclosure is based on rational concepts of truth, authenticity, and good faith—a kind of small autobiographical pact, if you like. As such, it pertains to an ideological apparatus of knowledge—knowledge of and about HIV infection—and constitutes a crucial element in establishing facts. Disclosure is indeed about telling the truth and making facts visible to others. But involve others, and things get complicated right away.

The novelist Harold Brodkey, who died of AIDS in 1996, tells how his doctor urged him to keep his disease a secret, like "the overwhelming majority of middle-class AIDS patients." Increasingly inclined not to follow this advice, Brodkey later concludes: "The overwhelmingly powerful thrust of bourgeois life is to lie, is to hide things. A house, an office, is a stage set. I think that much of what is hidden is chosen arbitrarily, family by family, person by person. Having secrets and confessing them is what deep attachments are about. Telling the truth is never wholly recommended, however." A crude but not entirely inaccurate way to describe this phenomenon would be to call it typical bourgeois hypocrisy. The problem with this interpretation is that it still posits inauthenticity as an unwelcome deviation from the ideal of truth and thus leaves that ideal untouched as such. I prefer to think that, in the bourgeois system, truth and authenticity are not the absolutes that many of us are led to believe but only discriminating devices thanks to which people are triaged between those who have power and those who don't. Paradoxical as it may sound, the fact that we always demand disclosure of others rather than of one's peers (even when it is the very demand of disclosure that constitutes the others as other) implies that the values socially held in such high regard that they remain unattainable—absolute truth and authenticity—apply only to those one seeks to exclude. In the name of truth, one tortures, unveils, and demands complete disclosure.

That's not all. Disclosure, while expected to be an honest and true statement of facts, remains nevertheless, by virtue of being a matter of communication, subject to interpretation (or misreading or outright denial and disbelief, etc.). In short, much depends on the addressee. The primary purpose of disclosure, it seems to me, is neither truth as a basis for action nor the understanding of how certain facts affect the speaker's life and subjectivity. Rather, because disclosure, as the word implies, always concerns the relations between an inside and an outside, its ultimate stakes are the ordering and reordering of the addressee's world and the protection of its integrity—or health or sense of justice. (In modern Western culture, all three—integrity, health, and justice—are conceived in direct relation to each other.)

What's in a disclosure then? And what is it that makes disclosing such a complicated process? For there to be disclosure, obviously, you need a speaker and some sort of informative statement. You also need a context or a situation of address in which the utterance is possible, and you need an addressee to receive the statement. First of all, the speaking self must be identifiable. Anonymous graffiti proclaiming "I am gay" in a men's room stall, for example, cannot be called a disclosure—only a tease, at best. The interlocutor, however, needn't be a single, identifiable "you," since no "I" may be uttered without positing at least the theoretical existence of a second person, and a disclosure need not find its recipients right away; think of written, or narrative, disclosures and of the peregrinations of my letter to Michael. A disclosure, in this case, is separated from an actual situation of address. What this implies, though, is that if the speaking self must be identifiable, identification depends on the prior existence of something like a social or cultural echo chamber in which the statement may be received. Logically, then, the possibility of the echo precedes and predetermines the possibility of the utterance. In other words, the identity of the self, perceived to be the condition of disclosure, is really its result, or, to be exact, of the foundational possibility of disclosure. Sharing and relationality are thus not outcomes of disclosure but its conditions.

What sort of statement may then constitute a disclosure? One necessary condition of disclosure is that what it states must be unknown or assumed to be unknown by the addressee. If I tell my friends, "I am gay," I'm not disclosing anything, I'm just boring them. But is it sufficient to reveal just any heretofore hidden fact? No, it isn't, for whatever gets disclosed needs to have been experienced by the speaker as something negative or potentially problematic, something worth hiding, or enclosing, in the first place. I can inform you, for example, that under my sweater I am wearing a plain white T-shirt, but that would hardly qualify as a disclosure, unless wearing a plain white T-shirt had previously been constructed by our society and experienced, that is to say, recognized, by me and you as somehow undesirable. Now, anyone who has ever seen Marlon Brando in *A Streetcar Named Desire* knows that this just isn't true. What is all this telling us, then? That disclosure is as much a matter of outside–in dynamics as it is of inside–out and that, therefore, some sort of prior "knowledge" about the object of the disclosure and its value in the culture was shared by all involved—the knowledge that it is "a bad thing." In Foucauldian terms, HIV and its disclosures may pertain to such heterogeneous fields as medicine, politics, morality, and so on, but these fields make up, in the culture, a discourse of HIV. This discourse plays a role in all the elements involved in the sort of utterance we call a disclosure.

Certainly, disclosure is manifested by the externalization of something the speaker had in his or her possession, as it were, like a secret about himself or herself. (Strictly speaking, the statement "This guy is gay" is a kind of disclosure, as the term *outing* implies, but because it's not in the first person it functions in different ways.) But think of the classic opening: "I *have* something to tell you." If that "something" can be the object of a disclosure, then its initial enclosure needs to have been experienced as socially mandated because of a negative value that it supposedly has had outside the self first. (In reality, this negative value is inseparable from the constitution of the self and therefore always inside it as well.) Simply said, for the secret to be lived as a secret it must already be constituted, in a way, as an object of some knowledge within the culture. This means that every secret is an open secret, every disclosure a confirmation. When something is disclosed to me, necessarily for the first time, when for the first time, I lay my eyes on it, it already bears my fingerprints. The fact that knowledge is always shared in that way is what makes it a possible source of anxiety. This is how shame works, for example, and what accounts for its being so contagious. And this also explains why some favor a "don't ask, don't tell" approach to matters such as HIV or homosexuality. With all that in mind, then, a more appropriate prefacing statement to a disclosure would be, "There is something I have to tell you." This "something" is now located "there," outside the boundaries of the self, and the verb "to have" now points to an external obligation—something previously shared in the culture and organized discursively—rather than to a personal possession of the speaker alone.

In other words, what feels as though it originated within the self and told us not just something but something about that self was in fact imported from the outside and implanted inside the self in order to make it a self and give it a sense of its limits. Disclosure, like shame, appears to play a foundational role in the constitution and experience of selfhood. In this view of things, what, in modern Western culture, we understand as subjective interiority really begins and ends outside, just passing through the subject, as it were. This process simultaneously makes someone a subject—by endowing a person with depth—and threatens to undo that subjectivity at any time.

What I have been describing is a process of disclosure that, following Foucault, I have called confessional—a policing device with which modern forms of power produce both, and at once, power and the categories over which it exercises itself. The two sides are thus constitutive of each other. Inside and outside, subject and object, and the dynamics between them— all come about at the same time. Self-identification as HIV positive; the awareness of HIV as a bad thing; the issue of disclosure; the identification of the listener as distinct and superior: these do not in fact happen in sequence but simultaneously. The appearance of sequencing is a narrative effect of reason and betrays the necessity for reason to seem unspoiled by what it divides and conquers.

Not all disclosures are confessions, however. There exist other ways to say something that, for one reason or another, must be said. My own experience with disclosure, haphazard and improvisational as it has been, represents my attempts at finding these other ways. If one understands, and embraces, disclosure as *sharing*, new tactical possibilities may open up, as each element involved in the process—statement, interlocutors, and the social context of the utterance—finds itself reinvented with each iteration, and always in relation to, or affected by, the other elements. Each time an utterance occurs, a small world is created that can be acted on because it is within arm's reach. Accepted in that sense, the disclosure of one's HIV-positive status may be an opportunity for the big, oppressive world of reason to reassert itself, to be sure, but it may just as well be practiced, by all involved, as a reminder to the uninfected that they too are active participants in the much narrower worlds of experience. For what is being shared in the end? Not the "thing" itself that is the object of the disclosure but everything else that gives that thing meaning. To share, in a way, is to enable all involved to partake fully and equally in a community through meaning making, a process understood as collaborative and ephemeral. In the pandemic, to be HIV negative means to live *near* HIV, in contact with it and with the people who "have" it, and, while we cannot deny that some people have HIV and some don't, discordance need not be perceived as incompatibility but as nearness.

THE BATTLEFIELD OF THE BODY

What makes Annie Ernaux's testimonial narrative *Happening* so eloquent in its engagement of the complex inside–outside dynamics of disclosure is that it involves an unwanted pregnancy and an abortion, specifically a clandestine abortion taking place at a time when the procedure was illegal, stigmatized, and often dangerous. As Ernaux reconstructs not just a past "event" (the book's original French title is *L'événement*) but the cultural, or shared, conditions of its occurrence, the issues raised by her disclosure, issues at once personal and political, find themselves inscribed onto the narrator's body by the very culture in which the story unfolds. What could have been a confessional and exclusionary statement of individual disclosure becomes inscribed in the relational dynamics of utterance, moving back and forth between the everyday and the catastrophic, past and present, history as event and history as process, until the readers, as happens with all compelling testimonies, find themselves entangled inside a story that concerns them too. In a sense, Ernaux's story allows whoever reads it to move from the shared conditions in which the event occurred to the shared conditions that frame its utterance.

Written in 1999 and published the following year, the book opens in the present, when the narrator goes to the Lariboisière hospital in Paris to await the results of her HIV test. Ernaux seems to describe everything and everyone around—the shops and passersby along the boulevard, the hallways of the hospital, the people and objects in the waiting room. To Annie's amazement, a link is established between a supposedly intimate sex act and a very public place: "I kept picturing the same blurred scene—one Saturday and Sunday in July, the motions of lovemaking, the ejaculation. This scene, buried for months, was the reason for my being here today.... Yet I couldn't associate the two: lovemaking, warm skin and sperm and my presence in the waiting room. I couldn't imagine sex ever being related to anything else."

The nearness of the personal to a larger context sets the "real" story of the book in motion—not a story of HIV, at least not directly, since the test comes out negative, but of a clandestine abortion that occurred many years earlier, when the narrator was a young, unmarried student. The book's opening section begins with a hint: "I got off at Barbès métro station. Like last time, men were idly waiting, clustered at the foot of the elevated train"; it ends more clearly: "I realized that I had lived through events at Lariboisière the same way I had awaited Dr. N's verdict in 1963, swept up in the same feelings of horror and disbelief. So it would appear that my life is confined to the period separating the Ogino method from the age of cheap condom dispensers." We notice, of course, the word *verdict*, whose connotations signal the existence of the sort of judgment necessary for there to be disclosure. But more important, perhaps, is the location of the narrator's life between two cultural markers that have framed her sex life and that of many others and anchored her self outside itself. As it turns out, sex always was "related to anything else." Sex, supposedly an expression of the private self, always takes place in the shadow of unexpected consequences, under the watchful eyes of others, and its intimate nature always makes it a matter for disclosure. (When I say "always," I'm referring, of course, to the specific culture in which the story takes place.)

Ernaux describes the writing of her story as clandestine, making the book itself a disclosure of sorts. The specific instances depicted in it are thus impossible not to read as *mises en abyme* by which we, readers, may gauge our own reception of the narrator's story. At least two of these embedded disclosures provide us with useful signposts. The first one involves the character of Jean T. A married student with revolutionary ideas and a member of the then "semi-clandestine" organization Family Planning, Jean seems like an obvious person with whom to share the news of an unplanned pregnancy and the desire to terminate it. He can be trusted and he could help. But the reaction of the narrator's schoolmate surprises her: "His face instantly took on an intrigued, thrilled expression as though he could picture me with my legs wide apart, my vagina exposed. . . . He asked me who the father was and how long I'd been pregnant." Later, he invites her over to his place for an informal dinner, and, as she is doing the dishes, he tries to convince her to have sex with him.

There's a lot to unpack here. Jean's knowledge of Annie's secret endows him with a form of sexual power over her—or at least, that's how he sees it. His desire to reconstruct a narrative chain of events—who's the father? how long has it been?—plays a crucial part in this knowledge-power play. It allows Jean to position Annie as a separate object of a knowledge *he* now has. The same is true when he visualizes her having sex—or rather when she visualizes him visualizing her having sex. Whether he actually does or not is of no importance as long as she's feeling watched, reified. It is in that sense that disclosure is not inherently liberating but may, in fact, constitute a mode of subjugation all the more powerful in that it appears self-inflicted. Indeed, Annie doesn't really blame Jean, and the book doesn't present this hypocritical revolutionary as a bad guy. It isn't he who gives Annie her new identity but a larger, impersonal system that produces categories and gives them meaning:

> I didn't think that Jean T had shown contempt for me. In his mind, I had moved on from the type of girl who might say no to the type who had undoubtedly said yes. At a time when this distinction was paramount and dictated boys' attitudes toward girls, Jean T was merely being pragmatic, confident that he could no longer get me pregnant since I was already expecting.

Annie has become transparent. She has had sex. This is what is known about her. And it serves as the basis for certain social relations, namely, the traditional assertion of a man's power over a woman: Jean sees Annie doing the dishes and he wants to fuck her.

The next instance of disclosure presents a kind of reverse image of the first. O., another student, is not an obvious choice of interlocutor. Unlike Jean T, she is known both for her reactionary politics and for her inability to keep a secret: "I knew she was greedy for secrets which she treasured and then bestowed on her peers, making herself worthy of interest for a couple of hours. Moreover, because of her bourgeois, Catholic upbringing and her observance of the Pope's teachings on contraception, she was probably the last person I should have turned to." Why tell her then? With Jean, we have already established that one's professed political values are not a reliable predictor of behavior, so why not tell O.? Moreover, her desire to learn secrets marks her as a kind of outcast, and thus a kindred spirit, since knowing secrets is precisely what makes you "in on it," as the phrase goes.

But O. doesn't simply allow Ernaux to emphasize a point that was made clearly enough with Jean T a few pages earlier. The second episode, rather, is bringing *us* into the picture, along with our own responsibilities as recipients of the disclosure. In case we had neglected that dimension of the book itself, and how it involves us, Ernaux soon makes the connection explicit. After describing how Annie loses all control over herself in the hospital where she has to go after suffering complications from the abortion, the narrator brings us back to the present of her storytelling. Her choice of words places the traumatic experience of 1963 and 1964 into a direct parallel with her writing in 1999, a move that necessarily extends to her interlocutors then and now: "The same situation will probably occur after this book is published. My determination, my efforts, all this secret, and even clandestine work—no one has been apprised of the project—all this will vanish overnight. I shall have no more power over my text, exposed to the public just like my body was exposed at the Hôtel-Dieu Hospital."

About her disclosure to O., the narrator adds, "I realize this: I had to reveal my condition, regardless of people's beliefs or possible disapproval. Because I was so powerless, the act of telling them was crucial, its consequences immaterial: I simply needed to drag these people into an awed vision of reality [la vision effarée du réel]." Whether Ernaux intended *effarée* to mean "stunned" or "scared" I don't know, but either way the word signals how disclosure can also undermine certain power relations. By inviting Annie's interlocutors—and, implicitly, her readers—into an uncomfortable proximity, Ernaux is using disclosure in a distinctly nontherapeutic way. Rather than attempt to heal or normalize the traumatized self through expression—an attempt she knows to be futile—she seeks instead to traumatize the norm. And us, since all recipients of a disclosure—its echo chamber—are always potentially complicit in its normalizing function, which they are called on to amplify and propagate.

Using disclosure to bring the excluded back into the system that produces exclusion allows Ernaux to unmask the inner workings of that system, turning the ideological power of disclosure against itself. The speaking self, which seems to emanate from the *story* as if naturally, is thus always inscribed within the *history* that produces this thing we call a self. As she so often does, Ernaux surrounds her first-person narrator and what happens to her with a cultural context, especially popular culture because it is what is the most widely shared. This use of recognizable cultural artifacts enhances our sense of nearness and underscores the fact that each interlocutor involved in the process of utterance is a condition of the other's existence. But the narrator also notes that, "compared to such people embodying normality, I had become an outcast in my own eyes [par rapport à eux, à ce monde de référence, j'étais devenue intérieurement une délinquante]." This remark reveals a lot. It shows how disclosure, far from being a kind of externalization allowing the excluded to reintegrate into the group, is in fact the very process by which exclusion becomes internalized and accepted as an inherent quality of the person, not as the effect of cultural forces that it really is. In other words, what the disclosure discloses, in addition to what the disclosure denotes but inseparable from it, is the context of utterance that makes a statement a disclosure. Trauma, as a result, no longer appears as a sort of breakdown, a chasm between a person and her sense of self, but rather as a continuation of the social into the self in the mode of subjection.

It will come as no surprise to readers familiar with Ernaux's work that this subjection should bring back a theme that runs through almost her entire body of work: the unresolved question of her origins as a working-class woman. As if reduced to mere flesh by her unwanted pregnancy, the narrator feels expelled from the world of abstract concepts she had managed to enter as a university student. Suddenly unable to focus on her thesis on "women in Surrealist writing," she doesn't experience her feelings of powerlessness as a temporary psychological effect of what is happening to her but, instead, as the inevitable return of the working-class body she'd hoped she could leave behind. The fetus she carries does not represent a hopeful future but her shameful, unending past; the abortion is experienced as the termination of the forward-looking narrative of bourgeois advancement. It is, in a word, as if her *embourgeoisement* had been a form of disembodiment she wasn't entitled to:

> Somehow I felt there existed a connection between my social background and my present condition. Born into a family of laborers and storekeepers, I was the first to attend higher education and so had been spared both factory work and commerce. Yet neither my *baccalauréat* nor my B.A. in liberal arts had waived that inescapable fatality of the working-class—the legacy of poverty—embodied by both the pregnant girl and the alcoholic. Sex had caught up with me, and the thing growing inside me I saw as the stigma of social failure.

Now that she is pregnant, the past has returned in the form of reembodiment. And with this return of her body, thought itself no longer seems possible:

> Connecting different spheres of knowledge and incorporating them into a structured piece of writing was beyond my strength. . . . Now the "intellectual heavens" were out of reach: I was wallowing down below, my body overcome by nausea. One moment I would be longing to regain my powers of reasoning once I had gotten rid of my problem. The next moment I believed that the knowledge I had acquired was but an artificial structure that had definitely collapsed. In a strange way, my inability to write my thesis was far more

alarming than my desire to abort. It was the unmistakable sign of my silent downfall. . . . I had stopped being "an intellectual." I don't know whether this feeling is widespread. It causes indescribable pain.

In this passage, the narrator's traumatic experience of the loss of her ability to reason appears inseparable from an experience of time that, too, is traumatic. Because it is abstracted from the material and the contingent, reason thinks itself as universal and therefore atemporal. Time is the domain of the contingent by definition, since to touch each other—*cum tangere*—is to experience one's limits.

But as Brodkey reminds us in the context of AIDS, "logic and intelligence depend on a future." The present makes no sense. In fact, the present alone makes nothing at all, since making posits a future. By abandoning the idea of a future, I also turn my back on reason. (Remember my earlier point about worrying as time gone mad.) In Lynne Huffer's words, "The future—as a retrospective, teleological act of meaning making that distances itself from nonmeaning—is the stance reason takes . . . as separate from unreason." This implies that reason too exists in relation to time—and bourgeois time at that, at least in the modern context. Reason looks forward and, to the extent that it repudiates the past as incomplete at best, if not downright barbaric, it is inseparable from modern notions of progress. The future, then, is part of reason's internal logic, while the past gets assigned to those expelled by the enforcement of reason as a social norm. To experience a disruption in temporality is to experience unreason, and this is just what happens to Ernaux's narrator. The abolition of the future is represented by the abortion, and the return of the past manifests itself as the double trauma of unreason and loss of social status. The issues of knowledge, power, and the class system soon come together in a different way in the small apartment where the abortionist, whose legitimate job is as a nurse in a clinic, is depicted with sympathy as a sort of witch. As she helps young mothers in her official capacity while terminating pregnancies on her days off, her clandestine work figures, in a way, the dark side of modern science—a form of knowledge that may be unrecognized, untold, and archaic (undisclosed, really) but as essential to science as shame is to pride. Wondering what could motivate the woman, the narrator concludes:

Clearly, money was a strong motive but she may also have felt she was helping women. Moreover, for someone who spent all day emptying the basins of the sick and the new mothers [des accouchées], enjoying the same authority as doctors who barely noticed her, practicing in a two-room apartment in the Passage Cardinet must have given her a secret thrill. Consequently she charged high prices—for the risk, the expertise that would never be acknowledged and the feelings of shame she was to inspire in women afterward.

Risk, shame, secrecy . . . paradoxical as it may sound, the abortionist and her client form a bond that is all the more intimate for being depersonalized and remaining unarticulated (and, at the time, undisclosed). It represents a form of intimacy that, while literally probing, differs from confessional disclosure, in that it does not rely on the recognition of a personal subject through self-expression and judgment, but precisely on its effacement: "She attended to her business [Elle prenait les choses en main] with quiet determination. Without being overly familiar—she didn't address me as '*tu*'—or inquisitive—she asked no questions—she focused on the essentials of the job: the date of my last period, the price, the technique used. This emphasis on practicality was strangely comforting. No feelings, no morals."

Emphasizing the larger relevance of her personal disclosure, Annie, who, you remember, studies literature, remarks on the absence of direct depictions of abortion in novels: "Although abortion was mentioned in many novels, no details were given about what actually took place. There was a sort of void between the moment the girl learns she is pregnant and the moment it's all over." And the present-day Annie extends this observation to the visual arts: "I don't believe there is a single museum in the world whose collections feature a work called *The Abortionist's Studio*." These mentions of art and literature remind us that if disclosure does not merely constitute an informational use of language but, rather, organizes social relations through what is nonetheless an act of figuration, then it bleeds into the aesthetic. It seems that disclosure is in many ways a matter of culture. This explains why revelations that have the power to breach the contours of recognized groups, such as social classes and the sexes, are often dismissed as lacking in taste. The fact that a disclosure, in a confessional mode, can be both socially mandated and culturally inappropriate because of its unseemly subject matter indicates that its purpose is to exclude, that is to say, to enclose the other as other or, if you prefer, to enclose outside, so to speak, as in a prison or a mental institution, for example, or other such sites that bring together physical confinement and social exteriority. Ernaux can thus describe her own testimonial disclosure—and perhaps all testimonies that successfully circumvent the confessional—as part abjection and part social irritant:

> I realize this account may exasperate or repel readers; it may also be branded as distasteful [taxé de mauvais goût]. I believe that any experience, whatever its nature, has the inalienable right to be chronicled. There is no such thing as a lesser truth. Moreover, if I failed to go through with this undertaking, I would be guilty of silencing the lives of women and condoning a world governed by male supremacy.

The original French phrase "taxé de mauvais goût" is especially telling if we understand it here in its literal meaning. Taste pertains indeed to taxonomy. Its objects are ranked, categorized, classified in ways not so different from the objects of science. And just as that of science does, the organization of taste in the modern era pertains to the development and enforcement of a new social order. Both, in a word, belong to the same paradigm.

It is indeed in the hospital that class and the female body converge most violently. Until word gets out that she is a university student, Annie, who is suffering from complications after the abortion, is treated like trash by the doctors and nurses who assume that she couldn't be anything but trash. She is lying naked and vulnerable, her legs spread open, not knowing what is going to happen to her, and the smug young surgeon who is about to operate dismisses her anxious questions with a joke: "I'm no fucking plumber." The joke, like all jokes, is a community builder, but, in this case, it is made for the benefit of the other medical personnel present and at the young woman's expense. The original French phrase refers to a well-known punch line by a popular comedian at the time, and its societal dimension feels even more potent. The impact of that remark will never end, forever searing social inequality into Annie's subjectivity, a subjectivity at once made and unmade, as with torture, through bodily humiliation: "In my mind [en moi], this sentence continues to split the world in two, ramming home the distinction between, on the one hand, doctors, and on the other, workers or women who abort, between those who rule and those who are ruled."

The idea that the body of a young woman may constitute the site on which to inscribe and perpetuate a system of domination extends in the book thanks to another aspect of the historical contexts that frame the story itself and its writing decades later. In the early days of 1964, the Algerian war for independence has been over for just a year and a half, and the aftermath of France's defeat is amplified both by the ongoing revelation of acts of torture that its military and police have committed and by the return of young draftees often shocked into stunned silence by the atrocities they had witnessed and perhaps engaged in. Lest we forget, the book references *The Umbrellas of Cherbourg*, the 1964 film about a young, unmarried woman who finds out she is pregnant after her boyfriend has left for the war. In the movie, the war remains unseen, its brutality only alluded to in the young man's haunting letters. She has the baby; he returns from Algeria suffering from what we now call post-traumatic stress disorder. The two eventually marry—only not each other.

In one of the parenthetical remarks, in which she comments on her own writing and establishes parallels between past and present, Ernaux notes, "As I am writing this, I learn that a bunch of Kosovar refugees are trying to enter Britain illegally [clandestinement] via Calais. . . . Today smugglers are vilified and pursued in the way that abortionists were thirty years ago. No one questions the laws and world order." Once again, clandestinity allows her to bring disparate events into contact: abortion and AIDS, Algeria and the former Yugoslavia. . . . But the implicit parallel between the torture of prisoners by the French and the systematic use of unwanted pregnancy through rape by the Serbs also brings the oppression of women and that of migrant workers, colonization and globalization, into uncomfortable proximity. Could the same be said of writing and reading?

The movement toward the past, along the diachronic axis of memory, takes us back to the present, as the narrator finally returns to the little street where she once had her abortion. Between the opening scene at the HIV clinic and the closing of the book, Ernaux hasn't just moved diachronically but also synchronically, establishing contact, not only between events, but between events and their contexts. Depicting the injustices of the past, she has reminded us of those of the present, our present. Her disclosure, if we hear it and accept it, is not a matter of confessing but of sharing. Her "awed vision of reality" has become our vision, her reality our reality. If her identity has been spoiled, then ours has too. Ernaux's personal stories make communities on the ruins of her first person—and ours. Understood as sharing rather than confessing, once more, disclosure becomes an act of witnessing that does not isolate the speaker from the listeners but, instead, brings all of us into a form of community: it dis-closes us. In the end, it is we the readers who find ourselves unable to disengage our sense of self from the collective histories of others. We may very well, in fact, be reading Ernaux's book at a time of war too, a time of torture and secret prisons where Arabs are humiliated into confessing crimes they may or may not have committed. And we, too, become entrusted with the work of witnessing and with the mission to undo the exclusionary power of clandestineness, humiliation, and confession.

DYSCLOSURE

I have no particular interest in coining critical neologisms, but the discussion of the two types of disclosure—confession and sharing—may be summed up more efficiently if I do.

Disclosing does not emancipate people anymore than unveiling does, and it does not produce equality. Take the well-known conundrum of open homosexuality. Yes, coming out is a necessary, liberating gesture, but one of its effects is to draw visible boundaries around the "object" of homosexuality and thus facilitate its policing. Paradoxical as it may sound, to disclose homosexuality is to enclose it as a discrete object that may be more easily identified, policed, and severed. The so-called out person has in fact moved from one form of enclosure (the closet) to another (identity) from which it is far more difficult to extricate oneself. And it has done so by means of disclosure. Disclosure is thus not the end of enclosure but the beginning of a spiral of policing and control. Indeed, if something we disclose becomes immediately reenclosed, then it becomes subject to disclosure once more, and then again to reenclosure, and so forth. To succeed as policing devices, then, enclosure and disclosure must fail repeatedly.

Against this oppressive logic, I propose to think of disclosure as sharing, that is, as a form of relational dynamic premised on equality. I call this process *dysclosure* to expose the inherent dysfunction of confessional disclosure and in the hope that, even though we cannot escape the police, it might help us think of ways to harness some of the emancipatory potential of the act of speaking out.

IF YOU THINK of testimonies of trauma as forms of disclosure—broadly defined: the making public, with great difficuty, of something "bad" or harmful to the self—then the reality of closure, and its stubborn refusal to come to an end with the act of disclosure, becomes apparent. Charlotte Delbo famously described the returnee's feeling of having died in Auschwitz. For Jean Améry, someone who was tortured stays tortured. Susan Brison testifies to having been "murdered" by a rapist. Disclosing doesn't end anything, doesn't erase anything of what's happened. Dysclosure thus pertains to survival more than to life.

DYSCLOSURE ACCOUNTS for the fact that one cannot disclose once and for all and be done with it. Every time I disclose I disclose a different thing, and

the process changes me as well. I provided many examples for a reason—
because each testified to the invention of a small world and each time anew.
Each disclosure represented a whole experience of living with HIV, not a
piece of the puzzle.

Terrified at the idea of informing his mother of his positive status, David Feinberg simply cannot understand why this turned out to be such a
difficult task given how seasoned he now was at the exercise:

> I'd practiced telling on everyone else: the census taker, Marlin
> Perkins of Mutual of Omaha's *Wild Kingdom*, last week's trick, the
> counterperson at Arby's, my proctologist, my third cousin once
> removed in Tampa, dead Laura Palmer of *Twin Peaks*, encased in
> plastic, the woman who stood beside me in the half-price TKTS
> line (I told her to skip *Cats* and try for *City of Angels*), the editors of
> *The New Yorker*, the men who installed my carpet from Macy's, and
> my father's grave. I'd sent telegrams, rented billboard space, used
> the electronic zipper in Times Square, leased skywriting planes, and
> written personal testimonials printed in *The Village Voice*. I'd added
> my seropositive status to my résumé. I'd become so adept at telling
> that it was almost second nature when I met a prospective gentle-
> man caller, hat in hand, bent at the waist, then springing up with a
> flourish, arm extended, my personal calling card gently placed into
> the receptacle of choice.
>
> Why was Mom such a stumbling block?

Dysclosure has no future, no logic, no reason. It has no past and no
memory either. Its social and political potentialities are entirely in the here
and now, and therefore cannot be called potentialities. It would be foolish to
think that when someone discloses his or her HIV status, an entire system
of thought premised on the self-enclosure of discrete elements collapses.
Dysclosure is literally useless beyond itself and the relationships it reinvents
with each iteration. I understand that some may have a hard time seeing
this as political, but that's perhaps because they're not HIV positive.

I HAVE SOMETHING to tell you and what I have is yours. If I share my HIV
status with you, I still keep it whole, not just some of it. I cannot sell it, cannot
exchange it, cannot give it away. So why bother, right? What dysclosure tells
me is that HIV is not something I and other HIV-positive persons have. It
is an experience transmitted by, among other things, HIV-negative people.

THE QUESTIONS that arise when wondering about the nature of that "something" I have to tell you, about what the mysterious "it" of "I said it" actually is, have to do with knowledge and therefore with truth. If dysclosure is concerned with the aimless creation of new and contingent truths (that is to say, truths produced by and for the duration of ephemeral contact in small-scale worlds, what earlier I called small talk and point of view) rather than with the revelation or discovery of universal ones, then such creation represents a form of oppositional bricolage. It consists in using whatever bits and pieces of stuff I have at my disposal, here and now, to make up something that serves my interests in the midst of a bad situation. When it comes to HIV, I'm not a doctor. I do not have, nor do I wish to have, the kind of apparatus that would allow me to deal with a unified and unifying truth.

Truth making as bricolage pertains to community dynamics. It works in situation and in relation. Small truths are neither incomplete nor reduced versions of a larger, universal one. Similarly, small talk is neither an incomplete nor a reduced version of discourse. Such a process of bricolage is not taking place within the universal, like a synecdoche, but at a short remove from it, in amused contemplation of its ruins, its ultimate dysfunction.

DYSCLOSURE is my improvisational way of facing the torture of disclosure.

DYSCLOSURE messes up all sorts of limits, and the one that separates the private from the public is a particularly interesting one to look at, I think. What constitutes the object of a disclosure—a thing's disclosability—is always understood to be private in one way or another. It is mine to disclose, and I understand that its entry into the public sphere literally doesn't go without saying. I am apprehensive of disclosure because I expect it to be a painful process. My heart races, I hesitate, I stumble against the words. Is it even a good idea to disclose? Will I embarrass myself and make my interlocutors uncomfortable? But keeping it all inside is also painful. If it wasn't, I wouldn't feel the urge to disclose. Either way, it seems, there appears to be something inherently painful, something not quite right, not about the object of the disclosure, but about privacy itself. Contrary to what social norms would have us believe, something doesn't get enclosed because it feels bad, but, rather, it feels bad because we have enclosed it. And unlike a secret, which ceases to be secret once it is told, the private doesn't become public when publicized as long as the system that rests on the division of the two spheres remains in place. In fact, to disclose something confirms its private nature, whereas revealing secrets affects the power dynamics outlined by its knowledge and lack thereof.

Pain is always an experience of limits. This means that, even though it is inarticulable, it articulates. And what it articulates, in this case, is the division between the private and the public. If pain feels real and beyond argument, then what triggers it—the public–private division—must be just as real. From the viewpoint of power the only thing that matters in the end is that something—anything—be the object of enclosure and disclosure so that limits may exist. Pain distracts us from the fact that the object of our disclosure does not have any inherent value, but that its value—always negative—is produced by separation and inequality as principles of power.

It should come as no surprise that what Elaine Scarry wrote about torture in *The Body in Pain* may apply to other forms of disclosure. The two are intimately linked, as torture "bestows visibility on the structure and enormity of what is usually private and incommunicable, contained within the boundaries of the sufferer's body." With what she calls the "spectacle of power," "The physical pain is so incontestably real that it seems to confer its quality of 'incontestable reality' on that power that has brought it into being. It is, of course, precisely because the reality of that power is so highly contestable, the regime so unstable, that torture is being used."

A PRACTICAL APPLICATION: "Undetectable" is impossible to disclose as such. To begin with, admitting undetectability sounds like a contradiction in terms. To state that your viral load is undetectable makes *you* detectable. You've blown your cover. At a more complex level, *undetectable* is the third term rendered unspeakable as a third term in discourses of HIV that the positive–negative dichotomy so tightly frames. If I choose to respond to the question "What is your status?" with "Undetectable," I intend the word to mean "You can't get HIV from me." Yet because one cannot disclose nothing, I know that my interlocutor will understand "undetectable" as meaning something other than "HIV negative" and will, in all likelihood, resignify it as "HIV positive," since this is the only other "HIV negative" is supposed to have. "Undetectable" is meaningless within a system in which meaning is believed to be produced by a strictly binary opposition rather than by a multiple play of differences. In such a system, "positive" means "not negative," "negative" means "not positive." The two are mutually exclusive, and that's all there is to it. As is the case with "ill" and "healthy," in the confessional and diagnostic practices of what Foucault has called biopower, the positive/

negative dichotomy simply redoubles that of disclosure and enclosure.

I would thus like to hypothesize (with great caution and moderate optimism) that to insist that "undetectable" represents a legitimate response to the status question may have a small destabilizing effect on the system of enclosure/disclosure and thus constitutes an act of dysclosure.

WHO, OR WHAT, is the dysclosing subject, the "I" that speaks out? It would be reassuring to think, as many prefer to do, that becoming infected with HIV modifies a person, adding a virus, subtracting health, but not putting the person's status as individual into question in any fundamental way. Yet it is also possible to experience infection as a kind of trauma, and as with other instances of trauma, testing positive for HIV often comes with the feeling that one is no longer the same person one was before. If "I" will never again be without HIV, whoever "I" was without HIV no longer exists. In that sense, the body with HIV doesn't belong to an individual who, at some point, was infected; it belongs to another individual whose sense of self we cannot posit apart from the "event" of infection. And the event, in that sense, doesn't represent an external entity that will affect a previously constituted self but the simultaneous making and unmaking of the self.

This feeling is not universal, however. It depends largely on how sensitive one is to what other people will think. This is why disclosure, whether one decides to go ahead with it or not, rests at the core of HIV experience from the start. One's sense of self is always relational, and one cannot be HIV positive outside the social parameters that give "HIV positive"—the phrase as well as the experience that one cannot separate from the phrase—its meanings. To put it differently, in the absence of physical symptoms, an illness can be experienced only as and through its pathologization, that is, the convergence of social forces and discourses that literally make sense. But if one's sense of self with HIV doesn't stem from an internal quality, if it is shaped or formed by my coming into contact with what and who is outside the self, then this *sense* of self—its meaning and its sensation—is first felt on the body's surface as a kind of touch. If my experience of my own body is a social one, my social being has a corporeal dimension. Dysclosure—closure always vulnerable to dysfunction—may then be understood as a form of nakedness and as the nakedness of form.

The change from one self to another does not represent a radical break, however. Old self and new self are not consecutive but concurrent. I likened dysclosure to survival earlier: both split the self. I am the same person with

HIV as I was without because I have the same memories, the same friends, the same body. I am a different person in that these memories, these friends, this body can now be a source of pain and discontinuity rather than give me the reassuring sense of my own contiguity with the world. I may look at them from different vantage points or subject positions. If contiguity defines what Barthes has called a reality effect, then the defamiliarization that HIV infection entails makes one's own self feel somewhat unreal.

Who I am with HIV is thus in constant flux, shifting as the meanings of HIV that continue to circulate in the world without my direct involvement in them intersect with those I make every time I disclose and put my body on the line. This is what dysclosure is: the ongoing redefinition of the self-with-others, plural, a self beside itself, in a situation of nearness to itself—close but never fully there. By dysclosing, then, I may forsake the pleasures and tactical benefits of duplicity, but I gain those of multiplicity.

The duplicity afforded by nondisclosure mirrors, in a sense, the binary structure of confession as well as its hierarchy, which is why being duplicitous about one's HIV status is, if not completely useless, at least of limited use, especially in those cases in which silence is not an option. Dysclosure, the openness to the multiple, is located between confession and silence.

TOWEL STORIES (III)

Some relationships have no future, but this doesn't mean that they have to end. Maybe all they need to do to survive is exist in a never-ending present. I grew to love his contagious slowness. Even though it was for him the result and the source of painful anguish, I saw it as a perpetual deferral, a yet-to-come that never comes. Isn't a person's "shortcomings" always where contact occurs? Isn't it lack that leaves room for you, that beckons you and invites you to come nearer?

But I threw in the towel in the end. It was sad of course, but fortunately there's a song for every occasion. This one's about a slow boat to China.

Taste

INTIMACY IN PUBLIC

The stories in most of the old AIDS books that I read while writing this one take place in cities—the usual suspects: New York, Los Angeles, San Francisco, but also London and, to a lesser extent, Paris—and they tend to present a specific experience of the epidemic that was, back then, organically connected to urban social dynamics. The city, in other words, doesn't provide a mere background to the stories; it is as much a part of them as the disease itself. This can mean many things, and it does. It tells us much, for example, about a time when AIDS was primarily associated with male homosexuality and male homosexuality was primarily associated with cities, not only in dominant discourses but also in the minds of gay men who, despite what many preferred to think, didn't live completely beyond the reach of normative social forces. But the imbrication of personal lives and places of great demographic shuffle also reminds us that cities, like epidemics, are cultural sites where the division of the private and the public appears at its most tenuous. It isn't that cities render any kind of privacy impossible. Anonymity in the midst of a crowd, for instance, provides, I think, a kind of privacy. What cities do, rather, is redraw the lines that separate the public from the private in such a complex way that they efface their dichotomous articulation by redefining privacy not as a social norm but as a need-based, tactical engagement with specific situations.

There is this passage in Sarah Schulman's *People in Trouble* in 1990. The novel is about AIDS and—this sets it apart from many others—it recounts the trajectory that propels individuals toward collective action in a fictionalized version of ACT UP. In the passage, two lesbian friends discuss the love affair one of them is having with a straight married woman: "They were having one of those intense conversations that New Yorkers carry on in public places and still have privacy because everyone around them has heard it all before." In the same way that you can do pretty much anything you want in the backseat of a New York City cab because drivers have seen it all before and nothing shocks them anymore, it is the public repetition of certain actions or conversations, their extreme visibility, that makes them unremarkable. Sharing, in other words, can allow individuals to carve a safe and free space for themselves.

In *What I Did Wrong*, John Weir takes on more directly the defining role that the modern concept of privacy plays in the distribution of power and how this affects gay men in particular. The narrator, a writer, is breaking up with his lover, Mark. The main problem? "He [Mark] liked his privacy." When the narrator's old friend Zack says on their first meeting "Sleep with a writer, wake up in print," things make sense: "I saw what he meant. Zack knew he was always in public. He had grown up in the floodlights, like me. Because he was Jewish, and gay, and odd, his acts and inclinations had always been on display. People were constantly pointing him out." This, of course, isn't the case for gay men alone: "Well, women don't have privacy either. They find out fast that they are being watched, and Zack and I were judged as harshly as girls from the time we were kids. 'Why are you a fag?' people asked. 'What makes you such a fag?'" Acknowledging the very publicness of homosexuality from the get-go, Weir ends up questioning what has been the very backbone of gay politics since Stonewall and perhaps the one thread that, since then, has tied together strands of gay politics with very little else in common: the foundational act of coming out: "Keeping things to myself was out of the question. I was everyone's business starting at age ten. I don't know what people mean when they say they're in the closet, or when they talk about someone else being in the closet, or when they claim they have come out of the closet. What closet?" He goes on: "I never had any privacy. Yet I dated gay men who thought they had a private life."

The book was written years after many of the events it describes took place; it was published in 2006. The critique is unmistakable from today's vantage point: gay politics geared toward the acquisition of individual rights are misguided and cannot serve our interests because they start off by accepting as a given that the social value of individual privacy is on our side when it was really invented at our expense. Among the many reasons that cities keep attracting new generations of queers in times of greater social tolerance and Internet connections, the flight from social, sexual, and affective isolation may not be the main one anymore. But was it ever? Or is it that cities have always given us the opportunity to act on all sorts of barriers and to open up the possibilities of contacts with people we didn't even know we were ready to embrace?

ACCOUNTING FOR TASTE

The concurrent and mutually reinforcing appearance of modern sciences, the Reformation, and the gradual empowerment of the merchant class led Western culture to give birth to a new kind of Man. By "Man" I do not mean "male" but, rather, the new, universal self that was to become the centerpiece of Enlightenment philosophy grounded in secular reason. But as we know full well, the body of Man was far from abstract and universal, its corporeality stubborn and resilient. Drawing on Renaissance ideals of bourgeois balance and moderation, it was indeed male—as well as Western, Christian, and, with the eventual appearance of new racial, medical, and sexual categories, white, healthy, and heterosexual. It was as though once we had opened up human bodies and stared at what was inside them, once we had shed light on what had been hidden till then as if under a rock, we were forced to establish a radical distinction between Man, a universal, abstract concept, and the messy particularities of his body. Bodies were opened before, of course, and their insides were stared at, only not with the same kind of knowledge-producing gaze. Was an autopsy ever used as the subject of a painting before Rembrandt's 1632 *The Anatomy Lesson of Dr. Nicolaes Tulp?* I don't know, but I doubt it.

Despite the best attempts by deconstructionists, feminists, postcolonial critics, and others, the offspring of the Cartesian dualism of body and mind have been with us Westerners to this day, no matter how much the unpredictable messiness of our material and affective lives keep bearing witness to the vibrancy of opposite forces. Thinking premised on the existence of distinct categories continues to police our daily lives in many ways, multiplying and cleverly adapting to the specific demands of history so that its oppressive effects may not be perceived, and especially opposed, too clearly. The divisions between the public and the private and subject and object, the two-sex system that the historian Thomas Laqueur famously wrote about in his book *Making Sex*, parallel sets of supposedly distinct identities such as those defined by sexuality and race, and so on—all these modern sets of distinctions owe a serious debt to Cartesian thinking and its resilience in the texture of daily life. Of course, taxonomy and the principle of non-contradiction, for example, predate Descartes by centuries as tools for articulating knowledge and thought. But in their modern reinvention, these categories came about as new questions about the human body were being raised and different things were demanded of it. Simply said, they rest on an operation of disembodiment and are propelled by a desire for purity and a general fear of contamination, of which the contamination of thought by the corporeal remains the template.

To be sure, I am painting a picture in broad brushstrokes here. No thinking ever takes place away from the material conditions of physical life, contradictory social interactions, and, more largely, history that inevitably make all thought impure and more open to play sometimes than it intended to be. Reminding us that "the word *contagion* means literally 'to touch together,'" the literature scholar Priscilla Wald notes that "one of its earliest usages in the fourteenth century referred to the circulation of ideas and attitudes," especially of the nefarious kind, and that "the medical usage of the term was no more and no less metaphorical than its ideational counterpart." Fear of contact clearly predates modernity, as does the corollary idea that safe boundaries seek to guarantee the integrity of something we would now call identity against encroaching otherness and alteration. What we are facing today, however, constitutes much more than a simple reencoding of ancient fears, even if it is that too; fear of contact has become a foundational characteristic of the times rather than a mere attribute of them. When Wald specifies that, once, neither usage of contagion was a metaphor for the other, she implicitly indicates that no operation of disembodiment had occurred. When we call ideas contagious today, we intend to draw on disembodied disease connotations. In the fourteenth century, that shift was yet to happen. And one of these operations of disembodiment is my focus now: taste.

Sometime in the eighteenth century, taste undertook a process of metaphorization and acquired a new meaning, shifting from the strictly gustatory (taste of and for food) to the aesthetic (taste for art). This becoming-metaphoric of taste was not an overnight event; such things usually aren't. It found its source in Italian Renaissance painting, with its development of the single viewer's perspective. It soon reached a particularly interesting form in the still lifes of food in Dutch painting. That movement was later reevaluated in the nineteenth century, that is to say, on the other side of the various revolutions that gave the bourgeoisie its political power. (You'll remember, of course, that the Netherlands was where capitalism took shape, and that the nineteenth century was when it finally triumphed, for good, I'm afraid.) The still life, or *nature morte* (French for "dead nature"), is worth lingering over a bit, in that it can help us understand how a metaphorical turn, such as the one from the gustatory to the aesthetic, from food to art, may ground specific forms of political power and social relations, moving from the aesthetic into other domains of people's daily lives. To provide the legitimating transcendence once ascribed to God, nature had to be killed and physical life stilled, that is to say, severed from the contingencies of the social.

In the still life, actual food on actual tables is replaced by *representations* of food and tables. (The food was usually not prepared, however. At the time, that would have been too directly evocative of bodily functions and gustatory taste and, therefore, considered poor aesthetic taste.) As a result of such representations, the circle of actual bodies, sitting together, as a group, at the table and sharing food, makes way for a totally different, dichotomous structure separating the individual subject and the object of the gaze as two mutually exclusive entities performed into existence by the aesthetic act of looking. The binary may still form collectivities, however, but ones that are more akin to classes. What I mean is that, by looking together at the same object, which it thus constitutes as a single, radical other, the group seeks to acquire the very self-sameness, or oneness, of the object against yet through which it defines itself. By this operation the heterogeneous group becomes a homogeneous class. Or hopes to. The process is always doomed to self-defeat, however, since oneness on either side of the divide is only an effect of a denied relationality. If the oneness of the object is a projection, that of the subject that mimics it is a sort of reverse projection.

Reading my colleague George Hoffmann's fascinating study of Reformation satire, I realized that if France did not ultimately become a Protestant country—a close call, according to him—the confrontation didn't leave the country unscathed either. Not only were Protestants attacking what they saw as Catholicism's excessive "fleshiness" and people's "disorderly appetites," they also sought to replace a profoundly collective religion with one rooted in an individual's personal relationship with a god whose earthly embodiment in the person of Christ was only temporary. (As Hoffmann shows, the Catholic belief that the presence of Christ's body in the host was real and not metaphorical was fertile terrain for Protestant mockery and even fueled accusations of cannibalism.) The shift from a self that was produced by and within the intricate relational network of a social institution—the church—to one resulting from a binary confrontation with an abstraction found a way to survive the Reformation's failure to win over France. Abstract spirituality may not have carried the day, but abstract reason did—and so did a certain class system. In the end, it was through secular culture that reformed notions of the disembodied self made their way into Enlightenment philosophy and what remains to this day one of the most puritan, body-averse lefts on earth.

I use the term *class* here in its taxonomic sense—the sharing of a definable feature—but also, following the sociologist Pierre Bourdieu's analysis in *Distinction*, in its political sense—a system of exclusion and domination. Indeed, the separation of subject and object through the metaphorical turn of taste implies, indeed creates, a hierarchy. In the old embodied model (eating), taste is a quality that defines both food and commensals; all have a material existence. Whereas in the abstract, aesthetic model, only the subject possesses taste; the inert object doesn't—at least not in itself, not until the subject's gaze becomes involved. Cartesian reason and Kantian judgment may lean in opposite directions in relation to the object—the latter toward and the former away—but they both require that there be a distance between subject and object. The *possession* of taste is precisely what, in the modern bourgeois system, justifies the relegation both of the object as object and of supposedly inferior subjects by defining each in terms of lack. In other words, taste made metaphorical is also a trope for the capitalist system of economic class domination, in which to have or not to have is the question. More than a trope for the system, it is really its cultural foundation, anchoring it firmly within people's daily lives.

In a circle, however, where everybody looks at and is looked at by everybody else, each member is always and simultaneously subject and object. The two do not, cannot, articulate a radical distinction, or stable categorization, since each position faces the other as its coconstituent, and both owe their existence to an ever-changing group dynamic that is recognized as such. This form of defining heterogeneity is what I like to call a group. Of course, a group may very well constitute a class too. After all, who may eat with whom, around the same table, is often quite strictly determined and, in certain cultures, subject to many rules and taboos about age, rank, and gender, for example. But the fact that each member of the circle always occupies more than one symbolic position at any given time keeps undermining the very basis on which to establish a binary power structure. Nothing I can think of best represents what I mean than the typical Chinese restaurant table, with a *zhuan pan* at the center—what we call a lazy Susan—allowing dishes to be shared by all, and the reliance on others to refill one's own bowl. Even though how and when to turn the *zhuan pan* is subject to strict rules of etiquette, the mess—pluralism, I mean—can make the uninitiated a little dizzy. But people do other things with their bodies, not just eat. And these other things may also be done in a group.

REEMBODIMENT AND DISCOMFORT

The triumph of reason in modern Western culture has thus relied, among other complex operations, on the becoming metaphoric of the sensory. In the eighteenth century, the metaphorization of taste from the gustatory to the aesthetic and of tact from the musical to the social was one of the rhetorical tricks that allowed the Enlightenment to produce the universal Man by abstracting his body. Intangible (etymologically, inaccessible to touch), perched high above the vicissitudes of the particular and the social, and therefore better apt to serve as a figurative vessel for a new kind of transcendence, the abstractable body, as both subject and object of reason, became suitable to challenge the soul as the unquestionable justification of the political order. Metaphors were crucial in this process in that they provided the illusion that social bodies had been erased in favor of the abstract political body of the citizen. In reality, it was the actual bodies of various others that had been displaced by being banished from the City and confined to the recesses of the private sphere—or worse: categorized as objects to be studied, traded, exported, exploited, treated, policed, colonized, destroyed.

We also know, however, that the repressed has an annoying tendency to return. In fact, it is thanks to the repeated expulsion of the social others that are *made* repeatedly to threaten the boundaries of the system that said system perpetuates its existence. This is where the life and death of the system meet: what the system must imperatively do, in order to exist, triggers the possibility of its undoing, and it is by toying with the idea of its own end that the system survives. Nowhere is the simultaneous making and unraveling of a system's claim to universality more evident than in its compulsive need to expose its own limits and in the suicidal/murderous thrill it experiences in contemplating its own demise. "Islamists must be eradicated before they destroy Western civilization." "If we let Muslim girls wear headscarves in public schools, the Republic will be annihilated." "Should homosexuality become the norm, humanity would perish altogether." These are but a few of the patent, and eventually self-denying, absurdities that reason is capable of producing. Systems, it seems, get a kick out of flirting with the idea of self-destruction.

If this all gives the impression that "the system" is endowed with some sort of agency or volition, that's because it is. Or rather, the invention of a universal, autonomous subject allows agency and volition to be located in and relayed by the individual, giving the latter the illusion that such powers are his own. (I write "his" because the so-called universal subject is always a male position.) The individual, in other words, is a ventriloquist's dummy with a mind, a thinking mouthpiece of the system from which it stems and whose interests it had better serve if it is to survive. Whatever qualities the individual subject is endowed with were always present within the system from which it is an outcome. In Judith Butler's words: "Where there is an 'I' who utters or speaks and thereby produces an effect in discourse, there is first a discourse which precedes and enables that 'I' and forms in language the constraining trajectory of its will. Thus there is no 'I' that stands behind discourse and executes its volition or will through discourse." To put it differently, if an effect possesses certain qualities, it follows logically that these qualities were already present, if only as potentialities perhaps, in the cause from which the effect originates. Or: if, following Nietzsche, Derrida, and others, we understand that what makes a cause a cause is always retrospective in that it stems from the awareness of an effect as effect, then it is always already from the point of view and thanks to the characteristics of the effect (here the individual subject) that the cause (here the system) emerges as such. To return to the idea that the system is endowed with volition, or intentionality as Foucault has shown in his work on the question of power, one could make the following claim: what the system wants, it lacks, and what it lacks, it's had; therefore, what the system wants is what it has rejected in order to will itself into being: its own end—that is, both its own limit and its own demise.

If the universal citizen comes into existence thanks to his disembodiment, the bodies of others must then be simultaneously expelled and made visible, for it is their very visibility that subjects them to various regimes of control and modalities of expulsion. This explains the rise, in the nineteenth century, of biological-scientific discourses, whose Januslike status as both rational/abstract and empirical/concrete, true and real, allowed them to function as the interface (or border guards) between the universal and the particular, between the abstractable body of Man and the observable bodies of others. The biologization of gender, race, and sexuality thanks to the rational gaze of science was designed to define social others in terms of their visible, tangible bodies, thus disqualifying them by setting them radically apart from the intangible realm of the sort of citizenship defined by universal reason.

But it is impossible for science (or anything else, really) to be a buffer without also being a conduit. What separates connects. Modern medicine, for example, may not have sought to be a mediator between bodies but in the end it is, for once contact has been established, it matters little which side initiated it and for what purpose. Medicine's words may have been hurled at others, but, if you catch these words, and appropriate and resignify them to serve your needs, discourse may become dialogue and domination may turn into community. Caution is required here, however. As Butler insists, the reiteration of a norm does not automatically entail its subversion. But take AIDS politics. ACT UP's use of expert language provided AIDS people with the means to disrupt, if not fully solve, gay men's conundrum: having to entrust our lives to our sworn enemies. Doctors cannot touch us without being touched by us, the sick, the infectious, the dying.

Reason and truth, in other words, leave themselves open to the possibility of being affected and infected, that is to say, changed, from the very moment they conceive themselves as unchangeable, universal, and eternal in opposition to something else. Reason and truth, like the real bodies they have expelled, are vulnerable. They are going to bleed, get sick, and die, although they would have us (and themselves) believe otherwise. Reason and truth are subjected to the vicissitudes of life to the exact extent that life is where they have come from through the operation of metaphorization I talked about. They made only one mistake: they didn't realize that metaphors are modes of contact and that the sensory could never be safely othered. Or, rather, they denied it.

If Man, then, must come into regular contact (in touch, really) with expelled others, this raises a series of interrelated questions. What happens to the abstractable body when it touches actual bodies? How does this touch work to remind reason of its own denied and mourned corporeality? Do contacts give reason a palpable sense of its limits and finitude? If so, how is it possible for the universal to have a sense of its limits without experiencing the nagging yet thrilling suspicion that it may in fact not be universal at all? More generally, can the universal sense or experience without self-destructing? And is there something pleasurable about it? Given that the metaphorization of taste and tact sought to replace communities of bodies (bodies that ate together and made music together, respectively) with abstract communities in which actual relationality made way for an intangible sort of bond (the immanence of self-sameness), can the return of these bodies help us contemplate different or lost modes of collectivity?

When bodies return, they remind reason that it, too, has corporeality and that reason has never ceased to mourn its disappearance or, rather, its denial. Man, it appears, is not distinct from what he has defined and categorized as his own negation; each bleeds into the other, and this bleeding introduces interesting forms of discomfort that may disturb how we think.

REENTERING THE MOVIE THEATER

The modern dichotomization of subject and object—that is, the denial that they are effects of discourse—results from the metaphorical turn I just described and is a logical outcome of the mind–body dualism. If I may, though, I'll venture this: the collective enjoyment of bodies, our own bodies as well the bodies of others, and the social relations that stem from such an enjoyment constitute the lived and sometimes highly pleasurable experience of the untenability of strict Cartesian thought. My purpose, then, is to try to make life a little less still and nature a little less dead. And for that, we need to enter the dark recesses of movie theaters, where different kinds of viewership and social interactions take place, and where bodies do things together. I should warn you: it's not going to be pretty. That's the point.

To argue this point, I turn to three films taking place almost entirely within the confines of movie theaters where men go for sexual, but also *social*, encounters, demonstrating that the two need not be separated. One of them is a French movie from 2002, Jacques Nolot's *La chatte à deux têtes* (*Porn Theater* in its rather prosaic American title and a more suggestive *Glowing Eyes* on the international market). The story is set in a Parisian movie theater showing heterosexual pornographic films but teeming with sexual activity among men. The story, although one hesitates to call it that, since nothing happens in the traditional narrative sense, presents a collection of "characters" who remain unnamed. They are referred to in the closing credits as "the homeless man," "the naked man," "the man with the yellow dress," and so on. The three characters with whom we spend the most time are "the 50-year-old man," a gay man played by the film's writer and director himself; "the cashier," a middle-aged woman whose sexual identity may best be described as flexible—which means with no sexual identity; and "the projectionist," a young and candid heterosexual man fresh off the boat, or the train, from his native province. The fact that all the characters remain nameless is, no doubt, a reminder that the movie depicts what is often referred to as anonymous sex. But this also reflects the author's desire to emphasize contact over identifiable, subjective depth.

Throughout the movie, we encounter cross-dressers, hustlers, homeless men seeking a dark place to sleep, "regular" and probably married men, and eventually police officers. With the exception of the latter, these are the people HIV prevention has taught us to think of as "men who have sex with men," a fluid group defined by behavior rather than identity. As so many

French movies do, this one depicts several sexual encounters, along with smoking and a number of conversations about life and death in between. Finally, the cinema closes, and our three main characters leave the place together for what appears to be a three-way in the making. End of "story."

What sets this film apart is that it is the only Western one of the three, and, as such, it pertains to my point about Western culture more directly. The other two provide us with non-Western perspectives, although, to the extent that all three offer critiques of the globalization of sexual culture, we are bound to see some significant overlapping as well. One of these movies is Tsai Ming-Liang's *Bu san* (or *Goodbye, Dragon Inn* in its international, English-language title). From Taiwan in 2003, the "plot" (and there is even less of a plot than in the French film) unfolds in a giant Taipei movie palace, the Fuhe Grand Theater, on its very last night. (The actual theater used in the film had closed its doors for good not long before its fictional counterpart. Tsai looked for people who might be interested in preserving the grand old place but found no takers.) The movie being shown that night is the 1967 Taiwanese classic *wu xia pian*, or sword-fighting flick, *Long men ke zhen*, known internationally as *Dragon Gate Inn*. Our movie more or less follows a young, gay Japanese man who tries, without much success, to have sex with other men in the toilets or other discreet spaces of the nearly empty theater. Perhaps as a reflection of the young man's apparently limited ability to speak Chinese, perhaps as a desire to show nonverbal modes of social contacts, the movie contains almost no dialogue other than that of the old movie embedded in it. Tsai, whose films are known for being slow and contemplative, takes his long-take style to the extreme here, and the film is almost completely motionless.

At the end of *Bu san*, two of the actors of the original *Dragon Gate Inn*, Miao Tien and Shih Chun, here playing themselves decades later, meet outside as they are leaving the theater. Unbeknown to the other, they each had come to catch their old film one last time on the big screen. "No one goes to the movies anymore. And no one remembers us," says Miao to the older Shih, whom he calls *laoshi*, teacher. But the old man has his grandson in tow, and the sign in the window says "Temporarily closed." We know that Tsai's grandparents often took him to the movies when he was a little boy, and he saw *Dragon Gate Inn* as a kid in Malaysia where he grew up. Could this scene be a hint that the perpetuation of film rests in the hands of queer kids? Who knows what the future holds, right? This could be the final question that each of these movies asks of its audience.

My third example is Brillante Mendoza's *Serbis*, a 2008 film from the Philippines, depicting one day in the life of an extended family running, and living in, a squalid softcore porn theater in the city of Angeles. The theater, called "Family" (in English), is, we learn at some point, the last one the Pineda family still owns, and we understand that showing mild pornography, movies with titles like *Bedmates* and *Frolic in the Water*, is the only way for them to stay in business for as long as they possibly can and continue to serve not just their own interests but also those of the community around them—the community to which they also belong. (We hear street noises almost from beginning to end.) Clearly, the place used to exhibit more mainstream fare in the old, prosperous days. As in the other two movies, the theater is a place where men go to meet. Here we encounter all manners of them, some identifying as gay and some not, some flamboyantly effeminate and some very masculine, transsexuals, and young hustlers selling their services to older men. Prostitution is what the word *serbis* is referring to, although we soon realize that the notion of service is central to the movie's view of human relations as a complex web of interactions between people, places, and institutions, commercial or otherwise.

As Mendoza explains in the press kit: "In a broad sense, 'SERBIS' can mean 'SERVICE' of any kind: one's service to one's family; the family's service to its members; the cinema owner's service to their customers. Or the cinema's service to moviegoers and others; a citizen's service to society or country; society's or country's service to its citizens; men and women's service to humanity; humanity's service to man/woman; and so on and so forth." This may sound like a tall order, but what matters is that the film gives prostitution the same importance as any other servicing of human relations even though, in light of its defining corporeality, it could have been considered the basest.

In fact, the movie never allegorizes sex acts. It never, in other words, disembodies them in the name of some transcendent humanity or universal condition. With the trivial and the serious, the venal and the altruistic, all but impossible to disentangle, life in the theater unfolds as a series of vignettes, events both small and momentous, mixing family drama and social issues with very funny scenes. Nanay Flor, the matriarch, is suing her husband for bigamy; Merly is young, unmarried, and pregnant in a very Catholic country where abortion is illegal; a goat suddenly enters the dark theater and provides the movie with a slapstick chase scene at the end—a wink to the distant era of silent movies, to which *Bu san* also refers. Again, no story to speak of. Nanay Flor's ongoing lawsuit provides the closest thing to a sustained narrative thread and, tellingly, it ends in a loss for her. Another loss . . .

All three movies take place in a single day and although their styles are very different, each conveys in its own way a tender yet never maudlin affection for its characters. But more importantly, all three foreground the question of viewership by embedding it in the narrative. It is, in fact, their most salient feature, since the action hardly ever takes us outside the theaters at all. So here we are in a movie theater, watching a movie in which people are in a movie theater watching a movie. This sort of *mise en abyme* is a narrative device as old as the history of cinema itself. How could an art form so enamored of the narcissistic spectacle of its own mystique and technological prowess not be shamelessly self-referential from the get-go? But here the films within the films are, by dominant standards, specifically of the lowly kind, and with the exception of the French one, they are also shown in a large theater whose splendor and social status are now a thing of the past.

[From Tennessee Williams's "The Mysteries of the Joy Rio": "He did not go far and he always went in the same direction, across town toward the river where there was an old opera house, now converted into a third-rate cinema, which specialized in the showing of cowboy pictures and other films of the sort that have a special appeal to children and male adolescents."]

I find it quite striking that all three movies offer us love poems to genre cinema directed by three of the most sui generis directors I know. Pornography, *wu xia pian*, and cheesy erotica are formulaic genres centered on bodies. Because the pleasures they provide are based on repetition and adherence to patterns, what characterizes them is precisely that they lack the power to innovate that defines modernity, particularly aesthetic modernity. (I'm cheating a bit here, since the *Dragon Gate Inn* is widely considered a masterpiece today and its director, King Hu, a genuine auteur, but it nonetheless belongs to a highly codified commercial genre.) On the other hand, the films *we* are watching are meant to be considered art, and they were originally shown, at least in Western countries, in art houses. But what truly interests me in these movies, and what makes them particularly queer, I believe, is that they do not invent themselves as art by repelling, or aestheticizing, the lowly in a bourgeois way but, instead, by embracing it lock, stock, and barrel. And none does this more explicitly than *La chatte à deux têtes*.

For starters, the gay art film bears the same title as the straight porn flick being shown in it, suggesting that the two movies may not be so easily disentangled or ranked along a strict hierarchy of taste, with art on one side (up), pornography on the other (down). The fact that Nolot's film features its own scenes of graphic sex is thus crucial. But how does this work? How does the director make us accept his own film as art without transcending or sublimating the porn movie at the center of it, without producing good taste at the expense of bad taste? To put it differently, how does he create an art film without relying on the sort of exclusion that characterized the metaphorical turn of taste? The answer has to do with the audience.

From a social and demographic standpoint, "bad movies" have long been associated with minoritized communities, albeit in complex ways. It makes sense, of course, that most members of such communities would possess an aesthetic judgment at odds with dominant standards, since the upper classes have produced and maintained certain aesthetic values in order to serve their own interests. But minority groups also generate certain sets of values, and they do so for similar reasons. Objects discarded for being in poor taste may then be reappropriated and given a new valence according to the needs of a specific group. In the 1970s to early 1980s, for example, cheap kung fu movies (a redundancy, back then) were common fare in and around Times Square, where they overlapped with porn for a while until they disappeared almost completely. Kung fu flicks, churned out at a near-industrial pace in Hong Kong, found an audience among Western working-class men and, in the United States, among black working-class men especially, as the foreign genre soon converged seamlessly with a homegrown one, blaxploitation. Lower-class audiences were under no illusion that they were watching high-quality cinema, however. They knew full well what they were dealing with, but they also knew that discredited genres could be inhabited to their shared benefit thanks to repeated collective viewings. No political awareness necessary; just good clean fun.

But this relational dynamic works also at a deeper level. By embedding the act of viewing—the very act in which we, its viewers, are engaged—*La chatte à deux têtes* establishes what Ross Chambers has called a "'narratorial' (versus 'narrative') authority," thus making this form of art an "'art' of seduction"—the difference between the two kinds of authority being that the narratorial is engaged in "promoting a *relational*, not informational, concept of discourse." The embedding—or repetition—of the act of viewing reminds us that all *re*-presentation is a return (to and of a previous iteration) as much as it is a departure (from an original); or, in terms more redolent of modernity's founding aporia, to regress and to progress form distinct propositions only insofar as they come attached to a forward-looking ideological project. Progress is positively valued, and regression is its negative. But if we embrace the movie's relational concept of discourse, then it isn't just telling us that art isn't so different from trash after all but, more important politically, that the viewers of art are not radically different from the viewers of trash. Without a clear distinction between forward and backward, the lowly cannot be so easily relegated. This is how the movie avoids assuming a voyeuristic viewpoint: relationality always goes both ways.

From a normative perspective, such as the one represented by discourses of sexual pathology, voyeurism is a perversion, and specifically a perversion of the very faculty that endowed empirical science with power: the gaze. But we may embrace Foucault's idea that power and pleasure are so inextricably linked as to make "modern society . . . in actual fact, and directly, perverse," with power inventing perversions in order to derive pleasure from them and from its own exercise. In that case, the aesthetic distancing that distinguishes the viewer of art from the viewer of trash also creates a perverse, voyeuristic point of view, a form of visual slumming in a way, from which the spectator feels pleasure while exercising power. By giving both films—his own and the porn flick—the same title, then, Nolot manages *not* to produce such a dominating, exclusionary viewing perspective over his characters. The fact that Nolot chose to be on both sides of the camera only reinforces that impression. (*La chatte à deux têtes* is the second film in what is clearly an autobiographical series that, as of this writing, includes two more films, *Hinterland* [*L'arrière-pays*] and *Before I Forget* [*Avant que j'oublie*]).

I mentioned repetition, return, regression; these words bring out the question of time. The other pitfall the movie avoids is that of nostalgia. After all, *La chatte à deux têtes* depicts a "scene," in the social sense of the term, which hardly existed anymore at the time the movie was made. There are no diegetic or extradiegetic elements for the audience to date the story with any certainty, but we know that, with AIDS and the advent of home video (and now the Internet), pornographic theaters have pretty much gone the way of the nickelodeon, privatizing sex as never before. So we're guessing the late 1980s at the latest. In addition, the "50-year-old man" mentions the fact that he is HIV positive and that he is wearing the jacket of a friend of his who has died of AIDS, so that the departed may return to enjoy a place he used to like. This makes the theater haunted by the gay past but also prefigures the survivor's possible death of the same disease, reminding us that the epidemic isn't over at the time of the story and still not over at the time we are watching it. Will the jacket be passed to someone else? Is the director symbolically passing it on to us, the viewers, entrusting us to ensure that the narrator will in turn haunt theaters after he, too, goes? If indeed we cannot separate ourselves from the audience embedded in the movie, it is a plausible interpretation.

As for the other two movies, they too are about the end of something. *Bu san* shows us the very last night of its theater, not to mention, embedded in its story, a decades-old movie belonging to a mostly defunct genre in which all the action was performed by actual human bodies, not computer imagery, as in the global hit *Crouching Tiger, Hidden Dragon* by fellow Taiwanese director Ang Lee. Miao Tien sits alone in the audience, playing himself, as the phrase goes, and cries silently as he watches his old self on-screen. The encounter between what he is and what he no longer is (but keeps returning) uses the image of self-haunting to point toward a more generalizable haunting of the self. Miao Tien, who often plays fathers in Tsai's films, had "died" at the start of the previous one and reappeared as a ghost at the end. With this movie, Tsai was looking for a way to have the character return once more and initially imagined *Bu san* as "a film about a ghost that comes to a theater to watch a movie." Things didn't exactly turn out as planned, but a handsome and mysterious man does mention to the young Japanese visitor who comes on to him that the theater is indeed filled with ghosts, and, as he disappears, we have the nagging impression that he may have been one himself. In the movie's opening scene, we catch glimpses of a large audience that has mysteriously vanished in the story that follows. In fact, the theater appears completely full at first. It isn't until the young tourist takes shelter from the pouring rain, passes the deserted box office, and enters the theater proper that the place is revealed to have been nearly empty all along—a ghost ship in the eye of a storm. Who were all these people? The film's original 1967 audience? Were they ghosts of long-gone spectators and social interactions that no longer exist in a globalized world that has no more use for them? Or are they us, and the theater a mirror in which we see ourselves as the ghosts we are bound to become when our own practices of moviegoing have disappeared? Is the giant palace itself a ghost, haunting the city that surrounds it? This being a Tsai Ming-Liang movie, no clear answers ever come.

[From Tennessee Williams's "Hard Candy," a rewriting of "The Mysteries of the Joy Rio": "For the Joy Rio is by no means an ordinary theater. It is the ghost of a once elegant house where plays and operas were performed long ago. But the building does not exist within the geographic limits of that part of the city which is regarded as having an historical value. Its decline into squalor, its conversion into a third-rate cinema, has not been particularly annotated by a sentimental press or public."]

In *Serbis*, we know that the Pineda family may not be able to hold on much longer to their decrepit theater, the last relic of a once-thriving business. The name of the theater, "Family," can be read as an allusion to, all at once, the kind of clientele it used to serve, who runs it, and the traditional social structures being dismantled by globalization, of which the film industry is a representative. As the camera lingers on portraits of the characters' younger selves, there are also passing mentions of Nanay Flor's oldest son, Danny, now dead. We catch a glimpse of his diploma and his graduation portrait hanging on Flor's bedroom wall, but we have no explanation for what might have happened to him. What did Danny die of at such a young age, and why isn't anyone talking about it other than in oblique fashion? Could AIDS be haunting this theater as well? Given the goings-on and what we have been warned to associate with them, it is impossible not to think about it. And in this film, too, a piece of garment that once belonged to a dead man plays its part. This is a yellow polo shirt that Ronald and Alan, distant relatives whom Nanay Flor took in, fight over. Putting two and two together as best we can, we understand that it must have belonged to Danny. And before Alan leaves the Family (and the family) behind, in one very symbolic shot at the end of the movie in which he stands in the busy street with the theater and its name in the background, he decides not to take the shirt he seemed to value so much earlier that very same day. Danny, it seems, will remain a haunting presence in the theater. And beyond.

[From John Rechy's novel Numbers: *"The burlesque-movie theater. Occasionally, years ago, Johnny would go there when he'd be too tired from hustling but wanted to come back to the bars and the streets. He remembered the frantic activity in that theater—an activity of which he had not been an immediate part—being "strictly a hustler."*

Something incredible has happened to that theater, Johnny discovers when he enters. Every other seat has been removed. It's a decaying mouth, with teeth hideously missing. A giant, crystalline light glares down rudely on the men—several servicemen—scattered about, separated like naughty children. Evidently the City Authorities discovered What Went On—and they conquered. For now at least.

Where are the groping ghosts? Ghosts then, they're now ghosts . . . of ghosts.]

When I described the Pinedas as an extended family I also meant that it used to extend deep into the social fabric. Of course, this is what extended families always do: they stretch the social and the familial at the same time and keep the two from existing apart from each other. Mendoza's comment in the press kit maps out something like that. We don't know much about Alan's and Ronald's past, nor about their own relationship to each other, other than what Nanay Flor's son-in-law says when trying to break up their fight over Danny's old shirt: "You're both relatives of Zenaida." Since Zenaida is not a character in the movie and we hear no other mention of her after that, we can only conclude that she "appears" only as a name—a name that means "origin": "of Zeus." Everyone, then, is a relative of Zenaida.

Because these three films are about film, what they are telling us is that the experience of cinema is always a haunted one. The stars we watch up on screen are either already dead or will be dead one day, but their immaterial, spectral renditions will continue to return. This includes, of course, the ones we are watching in the three movies. But beyond the tender tributes to gay men's enduring love affair with the movies of the past, and of equal importance, is the impending disappearance of the social worlds, of the communities, that came alive in these theaters, both with sexual encounters and by the shared enjoyment of lowly genres. This is what the three movies are also about and could have constituted the object of nostalgia. But no. Or at least not exactly.

MOVING IN QUEER CIRCLES

The old cruisy theaters remain ingrained in the memories of those who have written books or made films about them as unique places brought about by social oppression but where, if only for an instant, it was possible to suspend that oppression and revel in pure desire, perhaps even love. Despite the complex mingling of memory and oblivion at play here, it would be easy to object that if these places and the ephemeral contacts they housed are so memorable, then they testify to the tenacity of the social structures that enable memory in the first place. The desire to seek interclass or interracial or intergenerational contacts remains indebted to the categories of class or race or age as *social constructs*. But this premise is an entryway. Once we have reached the bottom, the gutter, where nothing seems to taint our enjoyment of desire and love, we must also admit that desire and love are never purely themselves because they always bear the traces of their origin and that, for the same reason, we are never purely ourselves either in that process. Ephemeral contacts—oppositional forms of making do with constraints—are modes of disenclosure occurring in an enclosed space that is the space of sharing.

In his book *Times Square Red, Times Square Blue*, the novelist and scholar Samuel R. Delany mourns the demise of the old seedy universe of sex venues in the theater district of Manhattan, now replaced with more wholesome family entertainment, courtesy of Mayors David Dinkins and Rudolph Giuliani and the Walt Disney Company, who combined forces to make Times Square serve corporate rather than community interests. Clearly, the concept of family put forth by Disney is not of the same kind as in *Serbis*. Whereas the Filipino movie sees the family as embodying a do-it-yourself collective spirit of service that is equally embodied by the audience it serves, Disney proposes what we could call a we-do-it-for-you-and-instead-of-you corporate approach that, in a typical capitalist mode, alienates (in the Marxist sense) the audience and the very families it claims to champion. With the Times Square sex scene largely displaced by its new family orientation, so, Delany argues, is the kind of interracial, interclass, intergenerational socializing that took place in the old joints. The advent of AIDS provided the perfect excuse to eradicate undesirable social contact and to do so in the name of public health and safety. Tim Dean, with whom I share an admiration for Delany's work, notes:

It is terribly ironic that what made such institutions so vital to peaceable urban life—namely, that they facilitated the easy mixing of disparate races, ethnicities, sexualities, and classes—was exactly what made their destruction so readily marketable as a security measure. Since contact with those different from oneself, especially when they are strangers, tends to be regarded as risky (because unpredictable), institutions that sponsor such contact are easily perceived as hazardous, even when the opposite may be true.

What has vanished is what the novelist and essayist Bruce Benderson, also writing about Times Square, calls "the now old-fashioned urban value of contact," a phrase that, in a wonderfully compact way, encapsulates what to me matters about contact: it is out of sync with the future, it often pertains to city life, and it is worth something. What made the old Times Square crowd what I call a group, then, is its defining heterogeneity, whereas Disney's and Giuliani's corporate ethos is one of class, and its chief concern is to perpetuate a class system.

Delany tries to avoid nostalgia by describing a few ugly scenes of genuinely disturbing behaviors. (One may disagree on whether he succeeds or not.) In *La chatte à deux têtes*, Nolot makes no attempt to glamorize what's going on. The place looks filthy; the sex feels crude and unsexy; the men are not conventionally attractive overall. And in a manner at once disturbing and humorous, the patrons are shown checking the seats for fresh semen before they sit down and the front of their pants for the same thing before they exit. Bodily fluids are generously dispensed here, and this time the topic of AIDS explicitly broached. But it is less thanks to the introduction of graphic thematic elements that the director stays clear of nostalgia than to the proposal of a radical definition of time itself.

It would be naive of me to ignore the fact that the movies shown in the old Times Square and elsewhere could not be separated from capitalism and, in the case of pornography, sometimes tied to crime and human exploitation. So let's be clear: porn, kung fu, and the like were not primarily intended to serve the interests of certain disempowered audiences but to bring money to their makers. (*La chatte* and *Serbis* repeatedly show customers paying for their tickets, and, once inside, sex isn't always free either.) But in that sense, they are not wholly different from Disney cartoons and other family movies, so what *is* the difference? Size.

Discredited genres and movies made on the cheap are more likely to fall under the radar of society at large and to be appropriated by discredited groups. In that way, some corners of the entertainment industry may be tactically inhabited and transformed into a kind of entertainment bricolage. It isn't just that, in certain neighborhoods and certain theaters, the members of the audience, under cover of darkness, appear to flout the class system and other kinds of social barriers that prevail outside. Rather, the ingenuity, or making do, of the cheap movies that are up on the screen becomes fodder for the community of their viewers, regardless of how venal the original purpose was. Men who are not gay may have sex with other men. African American men may fashion their own masculinity by watching action movies made in Hong Kong and featuring Asian men, even though Western racial and sexual stereotypes have long placed each group at opposite ends of the spectrum of masculinity, excluding both in the process and thus unwittingly bringing them into contact. This kind of identification has become all but unthinkable with the multimillion-dollar nationalist epics now produced in mainland China, no matter how action-packed they are and how beautiful their stars. Big and expensive movies, unless they flop or tip over into absurdity under the weight of their own excess, may appeal to the nation or to the world; small genre movies, like failed and dysfunctional ones, are structurally diasporic and speak to scattered communities, allowing them to somehow connect with one another by sharing something largely regarded, like themselves, as having little or no value. The cheaper the work, the more it touches. (This is also, I believe, what explains the moving power of the 9/11 flyers on the streets of New York City, a power to appeal that no official celebration could ever approach.) But the sort of cross-community contact I am describing should not be mistaken for some utopian alliance of the marginalized. Contact, as I define it, may make daily life more pleasant, but its ephemeral nature probably forecloses larger political prospects for enduring social change.

There used to be, near the Barbès-Rochechouart metro station in Paris, a bustling movie theater—or should I call it a film palace?—named the Louxor. Annie Ernaux's young self must have seen it when she sought an abortion nearby. If you deduce from its name that this was one of those big 1920s orientalist pieces of kitsch you will be right, and if you have the nagging feeling that, with the passing of time, it acquired not patina but grime you will be right too. Did it used to play commercial American movies? Right. Did it then turn to other kinds of movies in order to cater to the neighborhood's North African and Indian immigrant population? Right again. Did it eventually close? Of course it did, and it even became a gay club for a while in the 1980s until its owner died of AIDS, before Ernaux's narrator returned to the neighborhood for her HIV test. The rest is just as predictable. Finally saved from destruction by the efforts of well-meaning neighborhood activists, the giant structure will be renovated and returned to its original vocation. Well, almost. Once gentrified—saved! but from what exactly and from whom?—the theater may become a commercial venue or a middlebrow art house, but either way it is unlikely to serve ever again as a haven for sexual outcasts from all walks of life and ethnicities as it did when it inspired Guy Hocquenghem, a French gay liberationist author, to wax lyrical about the fusion of cheap genre cinema and anonymous sex: "Hands jerk to the beat of antique oars whipping the ocean, just as they jerked to the accompaniment of karate grunts or Egyptian dances. Mouths suck with Greek cavalcades and western gunfights in the background."

If the so-called value of a film is enacted in and by its viewing (as François Truffaut once said, "A film that isn't seen doesn't exist"), then this value changes every time the film is seen and is an effect of situations and relations. And this, logically, applies to the kind of lowly, formulaic movie shown here within the art movies. If the formulaic movie changes with every viewing, then it is *not* a mere repetition of the same formula but a repetition of difference, as it were—that is, a repetition that is neither identical to an original nor to its future iterations. And inasmuch as the movie is "enacted" by its being viewed, this difference I speak of is that of, or within, the community of viewers. Save a little fading and scratching here and there and a little patina maybe, the film as physical object doesn't change, nor does the theater itself. Many of the patrons seem to be regulars, sometimes giving the porn theater in *La chatte* the feel of a typical Parisian *café du coin*, open for all day and available for anyone to pop in when the need or the occasion arises—often after work and before going home. And this turns the place into a narrow opening between the two structuring poles of capitalist culture and a temporary haven from alienation. In both the French and the Filipino films, the movies are shown in a loop, as they always are in such places, and customers care little about missing the beginning or the end. They come in and out according to *their* needs, not those of somebody else's story or somebody else's business. We're not sure about the Taiwanese film, but except for the aging actor the audience in it seems just as uninvolved as in the other two.

For Hocquenghem, the social function of the old theaters appears to be just as important as their sexual one. In fact, the two cannot be so easily separated, and desire without purpose allows for the perpetual reinvention of social relations as a series of seductive contacts with no future in mind:

> This is Arab-style cinema, not unlike Stendhal's Italian-style opera, in which the spectacle is neither a totality nor a mass but, rather, a kind of discontinuity cut up through and through with social relations, commentaries and conversations, and in which the staircase acts as an extension of the boxes' back row. A cinema with no beginning and no end, where the linear unfolding of the script is put through the mill and chopped as if by strobe lights by comings and goings and the fits and starts of pleasure. Oriental-style cinema, savored absently with one eye on reality, amidst the flirtatious fluttering of desire.

All this, of course, is happening alongside, in contact with, the larger city where the theater stands: "The neighborhood queens trade stories about the day's tricks, as they fix themselves up in front of spotty mirrors hemmed with flaky red paint, as if this was the latest salon."

I am reminded of a passage in David Leavitt's novel *The Lost Language of Cranes*, in which Philip, a shy, young gay man, hesitates to step into a porn theater in New York's East Village, circling and circling the place, as if enacting in space what is going on in time inside the theater—the circular world of homosexuality he is almost ready to embrace, for which the theater itself is a stand-in:

> The place he is going has no beginning or end. It runs on an endless loop. He actually called the theater a week earlier to see when the feature started and the woman on the other end of the line laughed at him. The circle he is walking includes the crucial block of St. Mark's Place, with its haircutting salons and clothes shop; the Indian ghetto on Sixth Street; Third, Second, and First Avenues. He knows every inch of this territory by now. He has been walking for an hour.

The metonymy (the trope of contact) that opens the passage—it isn't literally the place that "has no beginning or end" but the sort of film viewing occurring in it—signals that contiguity, or nearness, is key. The woman's laughter has to do with the incongruous meeting of two different modes of time and two different social worlds: one temporality is linear and structures the open world; the other, circular, runs the darker recesses of marginal sexuality. "On the other end of the line," it seems, there is no line. The two corresponding sets of circles, one in urban space and the other in time, indicate that this "place" the young man is about to enter—really homosexuality—follows different rules. And there is little doubt that the sexual and the social cannot be disentangled any more than the theater and the city at large.

We're inside at last. An older man wearing a cap makes a move for Philip. Sitting in front of him, the man reaches back with his arm, making more and more circles whose center gets unexpectedly . . . decentered: "The hand strokes Philip's thigh, back and forth, gently, and the capped head does not turn around. The hand goes in circles, larger and larger, over his lap, landing on his groin, but not resting there. Instead—to Philip's surprise— the hand reaches for his own hand, and coils around his thumb." The faceless older man's actions seem to be attributed to his body alone, not to the volition of an autonomous self: "the hand," "the capped head" are the subjects of the verbs in the passage. Of course, this reflects the viewpoint of our protagonist and gives us a sense of what the pursuit of anonymous sex in a dark space feels like to him, but the final gesture—a hand grabbing another's hand—brings bodies and selves together in a way that is simultaneously sexual and social, yet still anonymous. In a dark movie theater, people have no faces. Well, stars have faces—or rather *had* faces, as Norma Desmond remembers well. But that was before movies got chatty.

Loops, circles, and formulas notwithstanding, the community of viewers, a socially dynamic group rather than a static class, does change with each viewing. Yet it never adds up to anything. Nothing is ever gained with each successive viewing. The "meaning" of the movies doesn't become any clearer nor its spectators more enlightened. In fact, I hesitate to call this process "successive" because it is as if with each viewing and each random sexual encounter the world gets reinvented anew, with no memory of the previous viewings or the previous encounters on which to build anything resembling a narrative succession. And without memory there is no possible nostalgia and, therefore, no stable object to sentimentalize or feel nostalgic about. This is no *Cinema paradiso*, in other words, but, with its concentric circles, more like *Cinema inferno*. In the end, that's what the embedding, or repetition, of the act of viewing does: it proposes a vision of time that isn't linear, as is that of Western modernity, in that it leaves nothing—and *no one*—behind in the name of progress; but this isn't a cyclical model of time either, because the same thing never recurs identically. The films may then offer a critique of modernity's linear, forward-looking temporality and embrace a nonmodern, even archaic, form of sociality, without falling into the trap of nostalgia for clandestine homosexuality. They do not represent a return *to* pre-Enlightenment collectivities but *of* them. This, in a nutshell, is the difference between nostalgia and haunting.

SPACES, PEOPLE, AND ACTIONS (I)

Another way in which these three movies figure alternatives to modern, exclusionary modes of viewership is by diffusing their focus onto the entire theaters. Modern viewership, inherited from the Renaissance, claims to result from the perspective of the individual viewer when, in reality, it produces the liberal concept of the autonomous individual as if it had always been there—a naturalness effect, in a way. In our three movies, however, the aesthetic experience is inscribed within specific sets of material conditions, means of production, and social relations. The title of the earlier section, "Reentering the Movie Theater," sought to be a transparent allusion to Roland Barthes's essay "Leaving the Movie Theater." In his essay, Barthes considers film as a whole moviegoing experience in which art is touched or affected by what and who surrounds it and isn't maintained at an awe-inducing distance. The erotic charge of the place as a tangible site where acts of viewing occur restores a degree of corporeality to cinema, an art form often described as disembodied.

It is true that there is a physicality, a tangibility, present at the movies that, paradoxically, no longer exists as much at the theater or the opera even though actual human beings are onstage. I confess that my views on the matter are largely intuitive, and my intuition, based on personal experience, is that the elevation of certain forms of spectacle to the level of high art has produced another set of acceptable behaviors. There does remain a space between quiet reverence and codified outbursts, however, and to transit through it—like all in-betweenness it isn't strictly speaking inhabitable, or at least not comfortably so—often brings the recognizable tingles and thrills of transgression. Indeed, it's always great fun to spot fellow queers at the opera, and you may even pick up someone there, but, like most homosexual practices, this largely happens below the radar of our straight friends. Moreover, the film audience, freed by the absence and deferral that define images as opposed to live performances, may turn to the place itself and to other spectators, deflecting the gaze away from the disembodied kind of aesthetic experience and toward a more social, embodied one. I am not implying that none of this ever happens during high-art performances. There is something to be said for enjoying great art in a gorgeous venue in the company of beautiful people. I am only proposing that such a turn to the materiality of things and corporeality of people occurs more often when the object of our gaze is of a lesser value in the hierarchy of taste, its aesthetic rewards less enlightening or less distracting from other matters at hand, so to speak. Screaming, laughing, even talking may be acceptable while watching junk at the multiplex surrounded by a bunch of high-school kids, but try doing this at your local art house (if you have one), and you'll get shushed by indignant patrons, usually of the white, middle-class persuasion. Traditionally, art is meant to be enjoyed with our minds, not our bodies. In fact, that's how we know it's art. Gay men love going to the theater and the opera, it's true, but they don't have sex there. Because of its role in the construction of a hetero-sexual class system, high art, in other words, is less homosexual than trash. But there are ways—ways, when the need arises, to shun disembodied aes-thetics and restore the full sensory and communitarian dimension that the ancient Greek concept of *aesthesis* seems to have lost in the modern shuffle. One of homosexuality's most enduring characteristics is, after all, the ability to make do; another is drawing on our continuing relation with the past as a living entity whose stubborn resilience mirrors our own.

THE RETURN OF TOSCA (ENTR'ACTE)

Several gay friends with whom I talked about seeing a stage performance of *Tosca* told me some version of the same story, and I have the strong suspicion that it has made the rounds for a while. It goes something like this: in the famous final scene, Tosca jumps to her death from the prison castle's walls, and, naturally, there isn't a dry gay eye in the house. In this given performance—in some cases, the friend heard it from a friend, in another the friend was actually there—a trampoline was strategically placed behind the wall to cushion the singer's fall. Yes, a trampoline. So there's only one way for this story to go, really—up. Sure enough, a mere second after the poor singer takes her fall—in one version of the story it is none other than Montserrat Caballé—she bounces back into view, turning the audience's tears into roars of laughter.

This story stretches credibility in so many ways and is much too good to be true. How many people who tell it actually believe it? Probably very few. Yet it appears to be going around in gay circles, so to speak. When the friend who claims to have witnessed the incident told me the story, I never once thought of calling him on it. On the one hand, this is another example of how a minority community uses storytelling to form and maintain itself, and it matters little that the story isn't actually true so long as it is shared. It is sharing that makes communities, not truth. Truth alone can sometimes unmake them. (In his famous 1882 discourse "What Is a Nation?" Ernest Renan argues that countries may have much to gain by selectively forgetting certain unappealing facts about their history.) In Western cultures, these stories may take the form of grand myths that one is expected to believe or else, and they tend to be written, often in books, sometimes in stone. But in the case of communities whose members are aware that they have been relegated to the margins on the basis of lies in the first place, the stories tend to be oral, face-to-face, and smaller in scale (as in gossip), widely understood to be apocryphal (as in our story or in the case of fabled pitch-perfect repartees), or about lies (as in conspiracy theories). Sometimes, debating the veracity of the stories is how they become shared. In any case, smaller, subcultural myths often inhabit larger ones, just as subcultures themselves inhabit dominant ones—in oppositional ways, making do in subtle ways with processes of inferiorization.

On the other hand, there may be something specifically campy about the strange tale of the bouncing soprano, something perhaps about the desire to trash things up and cut art down to size. ("But Puccini *is* trash!" Ross exclaimed, and he knows a thing or two about opera. "Not true!" later countered Helmut. "Well, *Madama Butterfly* yes, that really is trash, but certainly not *Tosca*.") If you've seen Gus Van Sant's film *Milk*, about the career and death of Harvey Milk, you know that *Tosca* figures in the movie as a marker that punctuates moments in the life of the openly gay San Francisco supervisor. Piling tragedy upon tragedy, the end of the film brings together Tosca's suicide and the murder of Harvey Milk. The theme, writer, and director of the film may be gay, but its style isn't. And that, I believe, accounts for the unanimous praise it received. What we have in our little story is far more irreverent in its genre-bending mixture of tragedy and comedy and, quite literally, high and low. Rather than a Marxist "second time as farce," I want to see this as a principle of camp physics: what goes down must come up. And I'm reminded of Oscar Wilde's aphorism: "All of us are lying in the gutter, but some of us are looking at the stars."

End of entr'acte.

SPACES, PEOPLE, AND ACTIONS (II)

All three examples devote considerable screen time to squalor and poverty, to lobbies and restrooms, to cashiers and janitors and projectionists, providing a sort of peripheral vision that doesn't redundantly emphasize the characters' social marginality so much as inscribe their (sex) lives in the thick of social existence. Spaces, people, and actions keep intersecting in mutually defining fashion, undoing the limits that seek to keep them apart conceptually. But the characters use the various spaces that constitute the movie theaters in funny ways. In *Serbis*, the grand staircase serves as a red carpet for a transsexual cheered on by hustlers, and the lobby provides a place for gossiping, catching up, or talking shop and trading stories about sexual customers. In *Bu san*, men stand at urinals without urinating. In *La chatte à deux têtes*, the restroom becomes the dressing room in which an overweight man turns himself into a woman before entering the theater not as a patron but as a star, the man's transformation into a fabulous creature entailing the similar transformation of the place, although neither is particularly pleasant to look at—that's the point.

[*From Tennessee Williams's "The Mysteries of the Joy Rio": "The angel of such a place is a fat silver angel of sixty-three years in a shiny dark-blue alpaca jacket, with short, fat fingers that leave a damp mark where they touch, that sweat and tremble as they caress between whispers, an angel of such a kind as would be kicked out of heaven and laughed out of hell and admitted to earth only by grace of its habitual slyness, its gift for making itself a counterfeit being, and the connivance of those that a quarter tip and an old yellow smile can corrupt."*]

Faking and pretending—acting, in other words—is at work on and off the screen, which is why, in addition to the darkness they provided, old movie theaters made such great places for public sex. Public sex, in that it occurs in spaces designed for other purposes and may be frequented by "legitimate" users, not to mention cops and gay bashers, requires of its participants the ability to emit and decipher opposite bodily messages—"I'm really here to watch the movie but I'm not really here to watch the movie. What about you?"—and to do so simultaneously. In the specific venue that is the movie theater, this form of acting—always an unstable hybrid of desire and corruption, an adulteration—further blurs the contours of the audience as audience and contributes to redefining the place's social purpose and the relationships that take place in it.

[*From John Rechy's* Numbers:*"Lights scurrying like electrified mice, a bright movie marquee proclaims that the theater is:*

* O *

* P *

* E *

* N *

ALL NIGHT *** ALL NIGHT *** ALL NIGHT ***
Two Technicolor Hits. And Smoking. In The Balcony.
It's open all night, and there's a balcony. Johnny knows—just as anyone who has hung out in gay bars knows—what that means. The hunting shadows in the dark . . . the frantic moving in and out of the toilet."

And later: "A man sitting smoking idly in the lounge stares at Johnny as he walks by. Another man is making—probably only pretending to make—a call in the phone booth; he also looks at Johnny.

In the restroom, Johnny stands before the urinal; but he can't pee.

Even before he hears footsteps, he knows that one of the two men—or both— will soon be here. And here's one: standing only one urinal away from him. In his anxiety the man has even forgotten to pretend he's standing there for any purpose other than to see Johnny's prick; he hasn't even opened his fly in the charade of pissing."

And later: "Along the stairs several men, smoking or pretending to smoke, watch Johnny, perhaps trying to determine what purpose he's down here for. Johnny pegs them right away as sexhunters."

Later still: "Another one pretending to wash his hands, comb his hair— actually staring in the mirror at the reflection of the others' backs. Johnny picks up immediately on what all this would mean."

Looking in mirror at someone else in the hope, acknowledged or not, that the other will catch you doing it, is a common gay trope for plural identification. It is found, for example, in André Gide's The Immoralist *and Jean Genet's* Querelle de Brest.]

And, of course, in all three movies sex occurs where it isn't "supposed" to. The theaters, commercial spaces in their normal usage, become redefined by their users to serve their own social and sexual needs. As Mendoza explained, the title of the Filipino movie refers to prostitution, but it can also be read as an allusion to the larger social role the space plays in the community, beyond and including male prostitution. Throughout his film, the near-constant noise of the city in the background reminds us that the Family, with its motley assemblage of misfits, does not stand in a vacuum but in the heart of a bustling urban neighborhood, partaking in life beyond its crumbling walls.

Even the work of exhibiting movies is presented from unexpected angles. In *Serbis*, the restrooms have an annoying tendency to become flooded, and the guy in charge of cleaning up the mess is none other than Alan, the one who paints the large, garish reproductions of sexy movie posters. Painting and mopping up shit go hand in hand. (I don't know if this is intentional, but it reminded me of the time Jean-Luc Godard famously criticized Truffaut for mythifying cinema in the latter's film *Day for Night* [*La nuit américaine*]. Instead of the more glamorous and artistic film professions, Godard suggested, Truffaut should have focused on the guys painting giant tits on porn theater marquees. Godard is a lot like Barbra Streisand that way; he just *loves* the little people.) So what we have here is a notion of taste as an effect—or as a series of effects—of material, economic, and social conditions and, therefore, a notion that isn't premised on the abstraction and exclusion of the body.

Indeed, bodies are extremely present in these films. Not just people—bodies. Alan, the cute painter-cum-janitor, also has a hot butt, with a giant boil on it, and in a later scene sports a visible hard-on. So does Ronald, the projectionist, who likes to jerk off in the booth and cums in a Coca-Cola bottle. Take that, corporate scum! (In the 1960s Godard and Nagasi Oshima, his sort of Japanese counterpart, often used Coca-Cola to signify US imperialism, which they criticized for pervading and alienating youth culture.) If *Bu san* prefers to show us the silent, delicate dance of men circling each other, pretending to piss next to each other, but with no visible sexual outcome, *La chatte à deux têtes* and *Serbis* give us far more graphic images. They depict fucking and sucking involving drag queens (and you'd be surprised to see who's doing what and to whom), hustlers, men of all ages, social classes, looks, body types, as well as sexual and gender identities and men of various ethnicities. In all three films, the bodies we are shown are far from perfect. They are neither ugly nor beautiful. Sometimes, they are dysfunctional. Because of the painful boil on his ass, for example, Alan keeps limping around the place. And so does the manager in *Bu san*, as her gait provides a ticking clocklike rhythm to several shots of large spaces that time has inexorably emptied. When a distraught Nanay Flor bathes after her loss in court, the nakedness we see is the unadorned one of an old woman. Here, bodies, like the spaces they occupy, are aging, breaking, growing, transitioning, wasting, dying; they are engaged side by side in the process of life. The dynamic difference of community is made visible, tangible almost, in these movies.

But it isn't just bodies that we see. Again, movies have a long history of showing us bodies. In fact, that's what movies are for—the good ones, I mean. What matters more here is what these bodies do and don't do together and where. And what they don't do very much is watch the movies to which tickets were bought. Rather, people both provide and enjoy the show that they make up themselves. As we say in French, *Le spectacle est dans la salle.* Just as with other diners sitting around the table, the supposed object of their attention—the film, the food—is but a pretext, albeit also a necessary condition, and although it must be consumed, it is also a reason for the equally indispensable social interactions, not between subject and object, but among people who are brought into collective life by the things they do with their bodies, such as fucking or eating.

In the theaters, darkness is intended to figure and enforce (in this case there is no difference between the two because it is a work of policing) the primacy of sight and disembodied aesthetics by literally leaving the body in the dark, unknowing. What the patrons do is reincorporate bodies that get to know one another thanks to the reconnection of all senses. This operation is made possible by the lower value of the object of vision, a low aesthetic value that reflects the low social value of the patrons themselves. Thanks to the physicality of the whole moviegoing experience as *aesthesis,* Man gets his body back. Or rather, Western modernity's abstract concept of the self makes way again for the multiplicity of actual people, whose inner sense of self doesn't disappear of course but is felt through the ephemeral touch of surfaces—contact, tangibility, contingency in their full etymological kinship. Whereas the politics of disclosure seeks to fabricate a sense of subjective interiority to sabotage unruly communities, inside the theaters, enclosure becomes invested with an outward-looking form of desire.

Reflecting on what he calls "claustrophilia," Cary Howie, a scholar of the Middle Ages, outlines the ontological potential of such a move: "To touch is to experience a limit and open a connection. Whether this touch is figured visually, hermeneutically, or sexually, it traces the outline of a community of embodied lovers expropriatively given over to bodies, texts, and buildings sensibly intensified by this gift." And he adds that "such an ontology is committed to the *intensification* of these materialities in their very mystery and withdrawal, the multiple and proliferating enclosed spaces upon which we inevitably, extensively touch." To experience oneself in this way is to understand that all selves are relational by definition and are made possible not by any inherent and permanent quality but by what's outside them in specific situations: the bodies of others. With the return of the body into the political–aesthetic equation, the strict separation or policing of categories gives way, allowing once more for multiple and unruly modes of contact. Intimacy, yes; privacy, no. This could be the motto of public sex.

AGAIN, WHERE ARE THE POLICE?

A scene in *La chatte à deux têtes* depicts a raid, and a rather routine one, I might add, judging by the police's obvious lack of enthusiasm and the patrons' matter-of-fact reaction to it. Three cops enter the theater with flashlights and—not a big surprise if you've ever heard stories about the French police—start checking the papers of men of color, looking for undocumented immigrants, the *clandestins*. Sure enough, they arrest a few North Africans. They also chase people from the restrooms and wake up a presumably homeless man with "This isn't a hotel!" As they leave, a cop tells his colleague, "I don't know what these fags are doing here. They should go see gay movies. I never got that." We have the sense that the question has been lingering on his mind for a while ("I *never* got that") and that it is meant to linger in ours as well. How do we understand what is going on in the theater? How does it somehow upset our sense of identity—not just our own but identity in general? Are we in any way complicit with the policing work that takes place here?

In two minutes, the scene demonstrates most of what I have been discussing. The process that, following Rancière, I have called "policing" is figured by actual police officers. Their role, real and symbolic, is to enforce the strict delineation of social and spatial categories, delineations that had been redrawn by the theater's patrons' engagement of them. For the police, sex should take place in private, restrooms are for pissing and shitting, a movie theater is not the same thing as a hotel, homosexuals shouldn't watch heterosexual pornography, and Arabs don't belong here. Checking identity papers is an especially significant narrative device in this passage. For one thing, it is a symbolic stand-in for the enforcement of the modern concept of identity. But more profoundly, it also disrupts the sort of separation of the figural and the actual that was the basis for the metaphorical turn of taste. Within the movie's fictional world, the "actual" police embody the symbolic work of policing at the core of Western modernity, interpellating people in both senses of the word. (In *May '68 and Its Afterlives*, Kristin Ross shows how the two are one and the same. To this I would just add that it wasn't until the nineteenth century that the primary mission of the police shifted from political to social regulation.) And as one symbol stands for another symbol, moving farther and farther away from any original, reality is shown to be an aesthetic effect—and so, logically, is the social system that rests on the supposed naturalness of reality and on the reality of nature.

As for the cop's weary bafflement as to why homosexuals should come to a heterosexual porn theater, it recalls Foucault's observation about the inherent perversity of modern society. Why indeed would a cop want to "get it"? Cops are not supposed to understand, only to repress. But here, one has the impression that the cop in question, unsuccessful as he may be time and time again, is trying to put himself in the place of those he is expected either to discipline back into social normality or, more likely, to exclude to a radical exteriority. How can this be done by putting oneself in the place of the other? Can one "get it" and not "be it" somehow? Our young police officer, it seems, would like to be some kind of expert, both inside and outside his field of investigation, dominating it but also deriving pleasure from it, from his complicity with it, from his desire for it. The French verb *comprendre* used in the original dialogue functions here in its full acceptation of "taking together"—and that includes the cop himself, who is not only contemptuous of the sociality he sees and fails to get but also frustrated by his own exclusion from it. In a sense, he is there to apprehend these people: to grasp them both physically and mentally. The police, as enforcers of social norms, are by definition in a liminal position. Their role may be to keep the normal and the abnormal safely separated, but they also inevitably bring them together. The police, too, enter the dark recesses of the movie theater. They see the reprobates and interact with them. They have to touch the untouchable. But because their mission is twofold—they protect us and/as they repress them—they are also touching us and bringing the two sides into contact. Jean Genet understood very well this defining ambivalence and, in his novels, endowed the cops with the same erotic charge as he did the thieves, exposing the former to the corrupting power of the latter, and vice versa until all that is left is the inexorable corrosion of all social order at the exact point of its articulation. As for Pier Paolo Pasolini, his provocative praise of the working-class riot police who repressed protesters in May '68 reminds us that cops (like gay bashers) are often equally despised by those they crush and those they serve. They get their hands dirty, they are unclean, and that can make them sexually interesting.

Desire is inherent in contact. It may not arise in every instance, and when it does it may become sublimated or repressed, perhaps even turned into violence. But desire is always there as a possibility as soon as contact occurs, and so is corruption. If women have long been used as the caregivers of choice (nurses, nuns, for example), this may have less to do with alleged maternal instincts than with the fact that they are largely perceived as disposable. Cops, but also doctors, teachers, or priests, as well as more literal gay bashers, are especially vulnerable to this, whether as objects or subjects of desire, because, as border guards, they are the very vectors of contact. They simultaneously separate and combine an abstract body of law and the concrete bodies of those they police, treat, educate, and so on. The contact person isn't inherently erotic, however. It is the process of coming into contact that carries the erotic charge, as well as its counterpart, corruption, and distributes both with great generosity to everyone and everything involved. And this process applies as well to contacts between the abstract and the concrete, the intangible and the corporeal, reason and unreason, as though each side of these foundational divides longed, in a sort of Platonic erotics, for what it once had but lost and has mourned ever since—longed for and feared, since contact inevitably brings corruption to the system that rests on these separations. Conventional forms of tact are a way to solve this paradox thanks to an operation of disembodiment that specifically seeks to replace the tactile dimension of human relations with a set of normalizing principles.

The police, of course, are never as efficient as when their work is taken on, internalized even, by civilians. Gay people have not been exempt from this, far from it in fact, as political demands have increasingly focused on assimilating and normalizing. In his novel *The Beauty of Men*, Andrew Holleran brings out the link between sight, aesthetics, and social exclusion, as he puts these thoughts in the mind of his narrator cruising in a park during the day:

> What he does fear is not the reputation the place has for policemen, but something more frightening: chicken. . . . The young can stand daylight. The old cannot. That is why, he thinks as he crosses the deck of the reception area, the Boy Bar opened in New York in the early eighties with brightly lighted rooms. The point was obvious. And that other bar on Second Avenue that looked like an art gallery—a bare room, blazing with light, behind a big plate-glass window. Both bars pushed back to the dim margins, like a vampire reeling from a crucifix, anyone who could not stand the glare.

And Christopher Coe's *Such Times* sheds more direct light, as it were, on what this is also about: AIDS. Here, we are talking about sex clubs where patrons are expected to be naked, save for their socks and shoes. This time, the context is San Francisco: "One reason nakedness was required, apart from any lubricity that might inhere to it, was, I now believe, that unless he had them on his feet, which has been known to happen, no man could hide any markings, Kaposi's lesions, that he may have had on his skin." Forced disclosure is a central task of the police, which is why they are so prone to use physical coercion on people, and as much as we would like to dissociate them, brutality and the political fight for rights have that in common. Liberal civil societies may be anchored to the concept of privacy, but they leave you no place to hide. You must speak up and fess up.

So let's return to the confused young cop, who may also be missing even more than he thinks—in multiple senses of the term: lacking, misunderstanding, and regretting. If the abstraction of the body is the Enlightenment's precondition for citizenship, it is also very telling that the cops, bringing light into the dark theater, should zero in on possible noncitizens. The world they literally enlighten with their flashlights isn't just a dark space; it also figures a sort of dark ages, a cave even, in which the modern categories of race, class, gender, and sexual orientation—to name the most obvious ones—do not function as stable and separate entities according to which citizenship may or may not be granted. The modes of sociality that gay normalization, AIDS, and home-based communication technologies have made obsolete thus stand in for even older ones, sending us back to a past far more distant than the pre-Internet, pre-AIDS, or even pre-Stonewall years—a past in which Man didn't exist but people did, and people had bodies.

[From Tennessee Williams's "The Mysteries of the Joy Rio": "According to Emil Kroger, who is our only authority on these mysteries which share his remoteness in time, one lived up there, in the upper reaches of the Joy Rio, an almost sightless existence where the other senses, the senses of smell and touch and hearing, had to develop a preternatural keenness."]

There is something archaic, and perhaps less than human, about darkness; that metaphor is hardly new. The anthropologist Michael Taussig puts it beautifully: "For if the visual settled in with a nice sense of distance between self-enclosed subjects and other-enclosed objects, this distancing was annulled with nasal perception, such as the senses ran riotously into one another as much as into the Other, as with the dog, man's best friend, loyal to a fault, never happier than when its nose is up the Other's rear end." The collectivities of contact figured in La chatte à deux têtes do evoke a kind of archaic, pre-Cartesian, premodern age, but the movie asks us to identify with it—or rather dis-identify with it. By refuting the separation of subject and object of the gaze and the dualism of body and mind, the embedded audience in the movie is also, in a way, staring back at us, the actual audience, as if telling us, "You know, it is quite possible to socialize in the dark. And it can be fun, too."

In all three, as an echo of the nonlinear and noncyclical temporality they figure, the absence of a central storyline brings out the constant crisscrossing of minor stories with no other narrative center than the movie theater itself, a place with no inherent value, that comes to life only when people use it for no real purpose other than being together. The refusal of bourgeois narrative development echoes in the movies' form the critique of urban redevelopment implicit in these movies' themes. If bourgeois art is concerned with producing individual viewing subjects, what matters *in* our movie is the collectivity formed by the audience, a collectivity as devoid of center and purpose as these multiple stories. (This is precisely what the cop doesn't "get" but wishes he did: like the "stories" themselves, no one is going anywhere.) Here, however, the separation that bourgeois notions of taste effect between viewers of art and viewers of trash no longer holds. In the end, the actual movie that *we* are watching creates a movement of simultaneous self-presentation and self-erasure, leaving us with questions about the relationality of our own moviegoing experience: we too are watching a movie together with other people. After all, these cruisy theaters hardly exist anymore, but *we* do. And the movie functions as a distorted mirror in which we are made to face the need to reembody our own aesthetic experience if we want to oppose the forces that seek to police us, our behaviors, and our relations with whomever we want to have relations with. And by "we" I do mean gay men. But not only. Let's make this clear: the film genres we are asked to embrace, centered on bodies and considered in poor taste, represent homosexuality itself, that is, a form of taste despised as lowly, mechanical, pointless, and incapable of transcending its corporeality and reaching the higher, abstract plane of true love. We fags are stuck in the cave and we like it. But just as the circles in Leavitt's novel encompassed the city over which they ripple, gay men are only the beginning, a mere entry point from where a larger critique may originate and thanks to which a reembodied, or reincorporated, *aesthesis* becomes a way of being in the world.

One could argue, though, that if Man gets replaced by men, even gay men, then this hardly constitutes a progressive gesture. Exclusions would appear to be only slightly displaced, with their principle left intact. Even though the sort of pointless circularity of group dynamics I have been describing does evoke Hocquenghem's ideas on the political potential of homosexual desire, these movies are no more revolutionary than the characters in them. And the old Times Square was the product of a culture of exploitation, not a utopian undoing of it. At best, Times Square offered some people a place to live (and fuck) within the system. Similarly, the collectivities represented in the three movies, mourned and longed for, are semiclandestine. They function in the dark recesses of modern Western culture but neither outside it nor against it. The men who check that there are no semen stains on their pants as they return to the world outside just want to make sure that no telltale trace remains of the world inside. An oppressive social reality can be "exposed" as a discursive effect; it is no less real and oppressive for it. The abstraction of Man's body through the becoming metaphoric of taste was intended to have very concrete effects on those whose bodies were said not to be capable of a similar abstraction. People were and continue to be subjected to actual bodily harm, such as rape, torture, unaffordable health care, or extermination.

Still, in their stealthy, tactical way of appropriating and resignifying public spaces, our movies present us with a critique of the entire modern system of identification and categorization. The inside of the theaters may be all or mostly male, for narrative purposes and because, in these cases, the critique is coming from gay men. You have to start somewhere, and universality is not a somewhere. It is an everywhere, and therefore a "nowhere." Bodies, however, are particular by definition. The bodies of men are as "valid" as any in that respect and do not in themselves signify phallocentrism. *La chatte à deux têtes* ends with a heterogeneous group leaving the theater, as the middle-aged, gay, HIV-positive protagonist, the young straight male projectionist, and the omnisexual foreign woman who sells the tickets all walk out together in broad daylight. She, of course, is not a border guard, nor is she a caregiver exactly, but, as her multidirectional desires suggest, more like some sort of queer matchmaker. There is even an unseen fourth character in that closing scene: the ghost of the friend who died of AIDS and whose jacket Nolot's character is wearing. The heterogeneity of the group, this one but also the concept of group that it stands for, is what allows me to bring into contact movies from different cultural traditions, mindful of their differences, naturally, but as unconcerned as they themselves are about any kind of supposed cultural integrity.

Furthermore, the "presence" of the ghosts alongside the living doesn't merely return the unseen to sites, cultures, and forms of knowledge defined by the visual. Or rather, it does so by giving us the sense that contact isn't limited to the spatial, the social, or the cultural, but that it establishes a poetics of nearness among different times as well, or what Howie calls "the fundamentally erotic approximations of anachronism." What could be more appropriate for the misfits of the time-space collusion that is modernity! As the art historian John Paul Ricco reminds us in *The Logic of the Lure*, "One is attracted to the dark to the extent that one cannot be put in one's place there." Darkness, then, becomes "a way of moving beyond oneself, is a becoming-disappeared through what we might refer to as a *spatialized ascesis*. This spatial unworking renders identity, subjectivity, and sociability unbecoming." If cruisy movie theaters make up especially poignant sites of AIDS haunting, it isn't for the simple reason that undisciplined sexual mingling allegedly provides efficient avenues for HIV transmission but because they eroticize our relation to the disappeared. (And in the political context of the epidemic, I understand the latter term in its *desaparecidos* sense, meaning those who, as in the case of Argentine or Chilean dictatorships, were disappeared violently by the forces of power.)

In nearly all his films, Tsai Ming-Liang shows an uncanny deftness at conveying in visual terms the sensual contact between different times as a loving and elusive caress that allows people to connect no matter how far apart they may be from each other in time and space. If time, the most unbridgeable of gaps, may in fact be bridged, then so can all other, more tangible forms of separations. Old men are watching their younger selves onscreen, as vanished sexual worlds ask to reestablish contact with us. Did the crowd filling the theater at the start of *Bu san* represent the one that flocked to showings of *Dragon Gate Inn* when it first came out? Is the Pineda family of *Serbis* and its queer extension to the whole neighborhood a thing of the past? Can the reincorporation of our senses serve as a way to be in touch with archaic notions of the body? Ripples, it seems, run along the surface of time as well as space. All this, the movies, the characters, and the ghosts, challenges us to make life a little less still, nature a little less dead when we leave the theater and walk down the streets.

Tact

MY CONTACT IN THE UNDERGROUND

With its endless corridors and steep flights of stairs the Paris metro has little mercy on the weak. My father was in his early eighties then, and he was becoming very frail, as he had been for a while. It was clear that our urban strolls were taking an increasing toll on him and would soon be a thing of the past. That day, at the same time as my father and I were making our way up from a station at an excruciatingly slow pace, his left hand on the banister, my left hand under his right arm, a young man no older than seventeen was rushing down the stairs toward us. We came face-to-face. He stopped. His body and expression stiffened in defiance, as if to indicate that there was no way in hell he was going to yield to us, or anyone else for that matter. In a flash, before I even had time to become angry or register astonishment, he seemed to come to his senses. He gave me an almost imperceptible nod and walked around us. He was fast and we were slow. He was strong and we were weak. Yet he surrendered graciously and without a word, and his physical avoidance of us was in fact an odd mark of small social recognition. The encounter, the simple fact of coming across each other, had turned into a contact. The whole scene lasted no more than a few seconds, but I haven't been able to get it out of my mind. Only later did I understand why, and it took a lover.

It took a lover who washed his hands too often and too long, who recoiled from intersections and crossings, who drove around and around in circles because he'd convinced himself that he had run over someone and just had to drive and check, again and again and again, in a spiral of ever-increasing, whirling madness. When that happened, there was nothing I could do but wait and, once it became clear that these occurrences were not going to stop ever, learn to be patient when my day suddenly came to a standstill. To walk with the slow is to be as slow as they are, if only for a brief time. If you want to be with them, it has to be on their terms, not yours, and you must accept being at a competitive disadvantage in a world where speed is all and destinations matter less than how fast you reach them. In fact, you might as well drop out of the race altogether. And because it is often out of love that one gladly accepts to be held back and restrict one's own freedom, or what passes for it, this tells us much about the nature of that emotion. Love is a loss, not a gain, and our most unforgettable lovers are often the ones who drag us down to where there is nothing left to distract us from the matter at hand—love itself.

The other reason why the episode in the metro stayed with me is its structural resemblance to tactfulness, a question that had been on my mind for some time. While the encounter that took place that day cannot be said to be a manifestation of tact exactly, the two have a lot in common. There was, first of all, an encounter between two people whose statuses, within the parameters of the encounter, were unequal. (And I say "two" because at that moment I was one with my father rather than a separate, third player.) When such encounters occur there are many ways to deal with them. Tact is one of the nicer ways, at least on the surface. Others include oppression, exploitation, all kinds of violence, and other means of reinforcing inequality in ostensible ways. Tact may very well do the same thing but, by definition, not in an ostensible way.

The other element that pertained to something like tact was the young man's ability to read the situation in an instant and react to it in the least amount of time possible. In no more than two seconds maybe, he examined what was going on, gauged how power was distributed among the various participants, came up with a rundown of the options open to him, decided on one, and acted. Naturally, people may react swiftly in situations where tact is not the issue, as when they are in imminent danger, for example. But the young man's reflex was neither fight nor flight. Nor was it both of them at the same time. It was something else. He didn't force us to get out of his way in order to continue with his trajectory as planned, and he didn't retreat and run back up the stairs to where he came from. Instead he took a detour. He temporarily altered his course of action by acknowledging our otherness to him.

I never loved my father more than when he was weak and he needed me. The young man's fleeting hostility—or what I perceived as his hostility—exacerbated my instinctive protectiveness toward my father and my sudden twinge of anger at his "attacker." It felt like a rush of indignation. But the fact that my feelings against the kid could turn to respect so fast, as fast really as it took him to realize how misguided his initial reaction had been, testifies to tact's power to affect social interactions and to do so with tremendous swiftness. At that instant, and for that instant, he willingly suspended his power over us, opting to behave as if he didn't have that power. This sort of leveling down, or *nivellement par le bas* in French, is what I call contact—a meeting with the other that sidesteps all thought of growth or improvement, momentarily circumvents the dynamics of power, and restores equality downward, as if power differences, and thus power itself, did not exist.

So was that what it was, then? The comedy of powerlessness? Like the master in a comedy, who dons his valet's clothes but only for a short while, before reasserting social order and his own power position at the end? To be sure, what happened didn't change the fact that my father was old and frail and the young man strong and vibrant and therefore at a great advantage in many avenues of life where such things matter. But if this was all a comedy, where was the audience? Where was the laughter? Nowhere in sight. I suppose I could count as the audience here. The kid did look at me right before he walked around, and, as fast as the whole thing went, there was a kind of mutual acknowledgment going on. But he didn't come back for a curtain call. He never benefited from his good action in any way, other than with a sense of self-satisfaction for having behaved with grace perhaps, but in that case he would stand as his own audience. As I said, however, his tactful gesture was not directed at me but at my father, who, as far as I could tell, never even realized what had happened because he was too busy looking down at the steps, trying not to fall. (Or was he being tactful by pretending he hadn't seen the young man's initially shameful behavior? My father was the kind of person who felt embarrassed by other people's mistakes.)

Finally, what reminded me of tact in all this was the fact that the scene and whatever happened in it had no existence outside itself. Its pure randomness means that it had no past and the fact that we would never see that kid again, no future. Contact has no temporality as such. It exists only when it exists, so to speak. And the same can be said about the form of contact that is tact. You can only react tactfully, that is, in relation to a specific context that will never recur in exactly identical terms. The context, by definition dynamic as the prefix *con* indicates, is always at work within the tactful gesture (or statement, or silence—more on this later) and makes it impossible to import an old occurrence of tact in a new context as is, as if it were a separate, autonomous object. Simply said, even if you were to find yourself in a situation that does resemble one you've experienced before, you'd still have to read all the elements at play in it before making your decision as to whether it may be a good idea to act tactfully and how. You may draw on a past experience of tact, of course, but in the end you only become better at starting from scratch, which, I guess, could represent a form of accretion. This is why the suspension of power that may occur in tact—a kind of *faire avec*—is just that, a suspension. It doesn't carry over, doesn't have a direct political resonance in the world that exists outside the encounter.

Unless one is moved by a feeling of love, perhaps, and wants to experience it again. Anything you gain you can lose, but love, because it is a form of loss to begin with, is free to take its time and linger long after its object has vanished. Loss is its own afterlife, and the same may be said of love. In both, feeling and event cannot be disentangled.

HOSTILE BODIES (AND THE PEOPLE WHO LOVE THEM)

To liken oneself to a very old person was once a common trope in AIDS writing. Hervé Guibert often described the feeling that his illness had erased the gap between him and his nonagenarian great-aunt, while Gilles Barbedette, another French writer who died of the disease, titled one of his books *Mémoires d'un jeune homme devenu vieux*, the memoirs of a young man who became an old man. But in light of what I've just said, it is a passage in another book that came to my mind, Oscar Moore's collection of his newspaper columns, *PWA: Looking AIDS in the Face*. ("PWA," you may recall, stands for "Person with AIDS"—or rather *stood* for it; it isn't used very much anymore.) Here Moore talks about stepping out on the busy streets of London after overestimating his strength and, as he comes to realize, refusing until then to acknowledge the full reality of his illness:

> I could not walk. I could walk but no faster than an infirm ninety-year-old. I felt as light and fragile as a piece of cracked Meissen. I crept, one foot gingerly placed after the other, down Charlotte Street but was almost swept away in the rip tides of Oxford Street. I suddenly felt totally helpless, knowing that if one person walked into me I was finished. I would probably sprawl back into another who would push me away and I would be bounced between hostile bodies until I fell. I crept along, clinging to the wall, emaciated, etiolated, wrapped up in jackets and scarves and hat, and feeling very conspicuously a PWA.

In the social context in which this book appeared (1996, soon after the author died), most people, if you asked them out of the blue, would probably understand the danger involved in encounters with people with AIDS as one of contamination of the healthy by the sick, of the strong by the weak. People with AIDS are dangerous and they place others at risk. Moore, of course, sees it as the opposite. The "hostile bodies" are the healthy ones.

What this apparent disconnection indicates, however, is a shared feeling of vulnerability. I don't mean to imply that the strong are just as vulnerable as the weak, obviously, but that the strong are always liable to lose their strength and the uninfected to become infected, and that may explain why, even though the danger may not be real, the perception of it is. Whites feeling under attack by blacks, men by feminists, and straights by gays, even though the political reality points to the opposite, are examples of that phenomenon; to cultivate a sense of victimization among the strong is intended to legitimize violence against the weak as self-defense and therefore morally acceptable. The Nazis did it; Serb nationalists did it.

But when Moore writes, "if one person walked into me I was finished," I am tempted to extend the meaning of "finished" into that of "finite." The French language, having only one word for the two meanings, would make this less of a jump, perhaps. Still, the image of two people walking into each other, even if they are in unequal positions, one strong, one weak, raises the possibility of there being contact (and an awareness of mutual constituency) rather than a simple encounter. "Walking into" doesn't quite mean the same thing as "coming across," and it opens up certain relational possibilities— albeit risky ones. If Moore is contemplating his finitude when thinking of physical encounters with the bodies of others, he is expressing an awareness of his limits, those of his life ("finished" means dead or just about, death ineluctable and near) but also the limits of his body. And when these limits come into contact with the bodies of others, each body involved experiences the sensation of its corporeal finitude (if only at a physical level and to the extent that an experience may be said to be strictly physical).

To transform this physical sensation into a contact would involve not just the feeling of one's limits but also of one's limitations, that is, not just the objective limits of the body but those, subjective, of the self that comes with that body, the self without which it is impossible to utter the phrase "This is my body." Indeed, in the words "my body," the possessive "my" pertains as much to the subject as to the object, and the words side by side acknowledge the split between the two and bring them together at the same time. (This is in the nature of touch.) It is thus impossible to say "my body" without, at the very least, questioning the separation of subject and object, mind and body. And since no first person may conceive, let alone express, itself without a second, one cannot say "my body" without indexing "your body." For the strong and healthy, then, the risk of contact isn't one of contamination ("You can't get AIDS from 'casual' contact," remember?) but one of loss of integrity—the abstract integrity of the self made manifest by the tangible integrity of the body.

Etymologically, "manifest" means what can be seized by hand, while both "tangible" and "integrity" come, like "tact," from the Latin *tangere*, to touch. I have much more to say about this connection in the pages that follow, but for now I want to venture this: I may have an *idea* of the self only by disembodying it, but I can protect it only by thinking of it in corporeal terms, that is, by conceptually reembodying it. I hope to protect my subjective integrity by avoiding the touch of bodies I consider not only infected but infested (from the Latin *infestus*, hostile, that must not be touched). The contact at play here is one between bodies and between selves but, at a deeper level, between body and self. Once again, contact occurs when one agrees to let oneself be contaminated by the other's weakness and shortcomings. Agree to it with pleasure and you may call it love.

SHARING: FROM DISCLOSURE TO TACT

Aaron Shurin's slim volume *Unbound: A Book of AIDS*, published in 1997, is a collection of short pieces, written in different genres over several very bad years. In a passage from 1988, Shurin, a gay man who lives in San Francisco and, in contrast to so many of his friends and acquaintances, is HIV negative, brings together several of the strands I too am trying to weave in these pages, but unlike me, I fear, does it with the graceful economy of the poet.

Disclosure, he posits, pervades so many exchanges among gay friends at the time as to make the act of sharing an inevitable factor in group maintenance: "We have conversations in various forms whose essence is *disclosure*. One is sero-positive or negative, another has just been diagnosed. The build-up to announcement along a route of suspense: Sit down, I have some bad news, X got . . . , or Did you hear about. . . ." And later: "His news precedes him: scent on the wind. (I'd heard about S but I hadn't seen him yet. When I did see him I asked him, 'How are you feeling?' He looked at me—about to disclose his diagnosis—tilted his head quizzically—then realized because I'd asked not How *are* you but How are you *feeling*, that I already knew.)" Part news and part gossip and often viral in the ways that it spreads and acquires a life of its own, disclosure, however helpful it may be in and for a group of friends, is bound to share some features with its external, more malevolent manifestations. Even inside the group (given the fact that insidedness is a situational effect rather than a quality inherent to its members), one is not, indeed cannot be, immune to the exclusionary power of disclosure to the exact extent that disclosure's power consists precisely in delineating an inside and an outside:

> Sometimes we know things about each other we didn't want each
> other to know—whispers and hand-me-down disclosures—and
> we are even *friends*—but we know that vocabulary in the hands of
> others creates stigma, grows in the social body as the body grows in
> the physical. "Positive" and "negative" become signs not just for our
> physiological trials but for civil restrictions, and in these matters
> we are rarely wrong in trusting our deepest paranoias. (On our first
> date, W—handsome, warm, mature, sexy—told me he had mild
> symptoms of ARC [AIDS-related complex]. My desire was confounded, cauterized at the source. He left feeling embarrassed and
> somehow guilty; I left embarrassed, guilty, and ashamed.)

Shame: the feeling of being judged by our peers for failing to abide by the standards of the group. Yet shame: the feeling of discomfort signaling that outer boundaries have come into mutual contact and threaten to come down.

"Eric was my good friend T's sometime lover"; Shurin goes on, "hence in proximity to my daily life if not exactly in it." This proximity, understood as nearness and distance at the same time, allows Shurin to perceive how Eric, while gravely ill, has now repurposed his irrepressible power of seduction to fuel group friendship instead, one assumes, of erotic pursuits no longer possible: "His desire to charm outpointed his powerful adversary. A small army of friends were his defenders, scheduling precisely his daily meetings, meals, sheet-changes, medicines, and 'dish' sessions. Eric's dying was a site of empowerment. The server and the served were connected by the line of interdependence that constitutes a meaningful act. As Eric got sicker, T tried to draw me into this nexus of exchange." This last phrase, the "'dish' sessions," and "the line of interdependence" underscore the dynamic of sharing at the core of the group. Recognizing T's own needs, rather than Eric's, Shurin decides to join: "It was for *him* I did it, as if he were the one in need of care (as, of course, he was)." But ultimately, it is Eric's tactfulness that brings to the surface the fact that the ethics of sharing propels not just the group of friends but everyday life—"the serious business of being casual"—making the group something like a testing ground, perhaps even a model, for something much larger: life itself: "I was nervous, hadn't yet confronted anyone head-on who owned the disease, wanted to be correct, polite, less fearful than I was, more comfortable than I anticipated being. First we tended to functional details, then Eric and I got to the serious business of being casual." This is when something like a reversal takes place:

> Almost immediately, he showed me the way. "You know," he said,
> "one of the nice things about being sick is that I get to see people I
> like, but wouldn't ordinarily spend time with." With a swift lunge
> of graciousness he'd assumed the position of caregiver by putting
> *me* at ease, making *me* feel good. By turning the occasion away from
> illness and towards sociability, he located himself as a giver as well
> as a taker—a liver instead of a dier. Eric was *living of* AIDS.

This "lunge of graciousness," phrased itself as a disclosure of sorts, figures the generous movement of one's body toward another's body: tact as contact as sharing.

TACT AND DELICACY (I)

It is worth noting that the English "tact" is often used where French speakers would use "*délicatesse.*" I noticed this often in translated texts, for example. But what are the differences and similarities between the two? "Tact" is also a French word. Delicacy implies fragility and precariousness, much as in the English phrase "a delicate balance," something that threatens to come undone at the slightest touch. As for the expression "a delicate situation," it gives the sense of something socially complex that needs to be handled with care. Whether it refers to fragility or complexity, delicacy does share unmistakable attributes with tact, a kind of delicate touch and careful handling allowed both by an accurate evaluation of the facts at hand, so to speak, and by a reasonable prediction of possible consequences of such or such external action in relation to these facts.

Another element of delicacy, and one that I find particularly fruitful when thinking about tact, is that it doesn't define the sole object but may also apply to the person who interacts with that object. When a delicate object or situation is handled delicately, it transmits its fragility—its weakness—to whoever has the power to threaten it, and such transmission has the potential to make power itself as precarious as that to which it may be applied.

TACTLESSNESS

"How can you of all people be writing a book about tact?" a friend once laughed. "You're the most tactless person I know!" I chose to ignore the fact that the remark wasn't exactly tactful either and retorted instead that, by definition, one doesn't research something one already knows. The truth, though, is that tactlessness may provide a way to throw a wrench in the system, to lay bare the hypocrisy of it all and unveil the mechanics of exclusion. Like a well-placed profanity, it can also be loads of fun. But to be tactless just right is probably as delicate a matter as to be tactful and may require skills no different in nature.

TACTFUL ENCOUNTERS

To feel as sincerely as I have that my personal experience of testing positive for HIV and living with the virus couldn't be separated from the events of 9/11 and the wars that followed doesn't mean that it was easy for me to put these feelings in writing in the hope that someone would read them and see pertinent connections. Have I crossed a line I shouldn't have when I likened some of what I've been through to torture? Are some parts of this book, in other words, tactless and in poor taste? These are legitimate concerns, and now that tact has become my main, and final, focus I think the time has come to address them more directly than I have so far and to try to answer some uneasy questions. For example, if bearing witness to traumatic events, both personal and historical, is an act of bricolage that makes use of other events, does this necessarily entail that these other events merely become instrumentalized, perhaps even exploited? Can tact provide us with a way to avoid this risk and promote a different, nonexploitative kind of contiguity between the otherness of others and our own? What happens to the self, including the writing self, in such situations? To answer these questions, it may be best to start where they hurt the most.

Many historical instances of mass death have been compared to others, but few comparisons have inspired as much anger as the one that brings together AIDS and the Holocaust. We may be tempted to dismiss this hostility. It may emanate from defenders of the absolute uniqueness of the Nazi genocide. Perhaps it is spouted by homophobes or racists who won't acknowledge that the early association of the disease with marginalized groups prevented governments and societies from reacting in a timely fashion. Dismissals may be warranted at times, but they fail to account for what I believe is a more subtle feeling that runs through such vehemence—a fundamental fear of contact, not just between specific people and histories but contact as a mode of being with others in the world. To be sure, a frightening disease transmitted by a virus lends itself easily to the embodiment of certain cultural fears. This is especially so when, as was the case with AIDS, the epidemic was initially identified with people with whom contact was already shunned and who were perceived to be themselves defined by modes of contact (homosexuality, prostitution, immigration . . .) often feared as illegitimate or pathogenic in the first place. In that context, advocating any kind of sharing may sound too much like sexual promiscuity, global migration, and junkie etiquette not to give certain people pause. But we are, after all, talking about rhetorical and not actual contact here, so why the fear? Beyond the traumatic experience itself, what is it about certain modes of writing or speaking about it in a comparative mode that prompts hostility and rejection?

When Guibert compared his AIDS-ravaged body to that of an inmate of Auschwitz, or when he likened a physician to a Nazi in a war movie, he was not the first witness to turn to the Holocaust in an attempt to make sense of the pandemic and of his own experience of it. Another French writer, Alain Emmanuel Dreuilhe, had already systematized the trope for matters of personal as well as collective survival, positing AIDS as a historical turning point in gay history and relying on the cultural memory of the Holocaust to help shape the relationship between disaster, community formation, and political legitimacy. In the United States, where the political culture is much more pragmatic and less timorous in its rhetoric if the goals are deemed both worthwhile and urgent, the trope raised fewer eyebrows. This may be due to the fact that, whereas French culture in general puts a greater premium on a single, unified, and unifying national memory, Americans tend to accept more readily the idea that their country has been shaped in part by the crisscrossing, often diverging, but ultimately shared memories of different communities. From this vantage point, no fundamental contradiction exists between the fact that certain memories belong to certain communities and the idea that they are also shared across the nation these communities make up.

To compare AIDS to the Holocaust—or rather, to bring out their structural similarities—served some communities well in the first decade or so of the pandemic. It wasn't long before the trope escaped the confines of literary testimonials and was summoned to politicize the AIDS crisis and energize activists fighting for their lives. Drawing from a well-known historical legacy of societal indifference and government complicity allowed AIDS activist groups, in particular ACT UP, to denounce inaction in the face of mass death striking specific communities. They even called for trials that they compared to the Nuremberg trials. In some quarters, the reaction was fierce, especially in France, where ACT UP–Paris's combative rhetoric was often denounced by the mainstream press and some intellectuals as apocalyptic and no different in essence from that used by the extreme Right, especially by the Front National. Just like members of the Front National, AIDS activists were accused by some of undermining the basic principles of contractual citizenship in favor of divisive identity politics. Once again, two incompatible concepts of the national community came into conflict and, as was the case with the Jews at the time of the Dreyfus affair, a minoritized group found itself at the heart of it all.

Certain visual tropes, however, never had to face the same level of hostility as rhetorical ones did. To draw parallels between emaciated patients and concentration camp inmates generated little mainstream outrage, and the media relied heavily on these tropes in the 1980s, even if they left the viewer in charge of making the connection. As the atrocities committed in Bosnia in the 1990s would soon demonstrate once more, certain bodies automatically reawaken images of the Holocaust in Western minds. But why such disparities in public reactions between words and pictures? As Douglas Crimp shows in his reading of an early exhibition of photographs of people with AIDS, portraits purporting to bring out the supposed universality of human suffering ended up erasing the political and social dimensions of the epidemic and producing images so abstract and so removed from the vicissitudes of daily human lives that they paradoxically impeded all possibility of empathizing with their subjects. In short, comparing AIDS to the Holocaust appeared acceptable inasmuch as it constructed a seemingly immediate image of AIDS sufferers as politically passive, essentially other, and soon to be dead; it did not when it underscored, as the argumentative dynamics of words can easily do, the realities of social exclusion and raised uncomfortable questions about its actual workings. Universal humanism didn't produce a palpable sense of contiguity with AIDS sufferers. Rather, it resulted in the reinforcement of distance. Images of the Nazi death camps sometimes had the same effect, making their attendant claim never to let such atrocities happen again little more than a piety—as AIDS or the war in Yugoslavia demonstrated so nakedly.

The condemnations of activist rhetoric often concerned the trivialization of the Holocaust, said to be the inevitable outcome of comparisons. The political success of these comparisons, however, depended on their ability to respect, not dilute, the power of the Holocaust to evoke exceptionality— and to do so precisely by latching another historical event onto it. But how can this seemingly contradictory connection occur? I believe that tact, when understood as a relational play of differences, can work by acknowledging proximity and distance at the same time. In other words, it can represent a form of deconstructive contact whose status as mediation does not rely on, and indeed undoes, the self-enclosed sameness of who and what it connects. Acknowledgment without knowledge (*reconnaître sans connaître*) is, I think, how tact offers us clues to grasp the dynamics of community at play in the act of bearing witness. Mediation makes such dynamics possible because it acts both as a community's contours and as its interface, suggesting the community's inherent vulnerability to difference—its alterability. I've already described—in the context of movie houses—how the police, their corporeality restored, may unwittingly serve as mediators, connecting what they separate. Tact, a mode of indirection in language, may also function as just this sort of mediation. And it too has been initially entrusted with a policing mission.

When used as empathy, tact is concerned with relationality. And so is witnessing that, like tact—and with tact—relies on a kind of effacement of the writing or speaking self (its unmaking into words) in order to leave room for others and make community. The indirection of tact is what allows AIDS and the Holocaust to be brought into proximity, if of an uneasy sort, and form something like a community of the traumatic. But such a community is itself a traumatic community in that its founding commonality is always mediated by difference—the wordless shattering of the self—and not reassuringly fused in sameness. In that sense, to rely on the shared, cultural memory of the Holocaust, as so many AIDS activists and witnesses did, served more than the communal interests of those directly affected; it was also intended to produce a larger view of community as difference against the hierarchical and exclusionary distinctions—the politics of enclosure— that were responsible for the spread of the disease to begin with. In other words, the AIDS–Holocaust trope often sought to convey the idea that the pandemic was not caused by dangerous contact but, on the contrary, by the dangerous fear of it, by the refusal to envision certain bodies as anything other than hostile.

In a world of reason, where discernment and synthesis are everything, contact can be understood only as leading to a switch in positions or as dissolution-fusion. Thoughts of HIV, for example, remain largely structured by a polarized discourse of normality and pathologization—you have it or you don't, you're sick or you're not—that makes it impossible for many to understand being HIV positive as having a disease but without being ill. Contact is thus felt as seroconversion, and seroconversion can lead only to death—even if only of the social kind these days. This also explains why people often express their hostility to the AIDS–Holocaust and other tropes with a dismissive "They're not the same thing." This common reaction betrays, first and foremost, a misunderstanding of how tropes work, but it also reveals that, between radical difference and radical sameness, nothing appears even conceivable. Tropes, however, are modes and conveyors of contact. They are a process of alteration and transition that goes nowhere. The point of origin is indexed but no longer recoverable; the destination remains out of reach. With contact, dynamic in-betweenness is all there is. In practical terms, this intermediate space is where my lover and I shared HIV and OCD and, as I described in another book, my father and I shared Jewishness and queerness.

I would thus like to argue for tact as a trope for a form of relationality bringing nearness and distance together—which, naturally, is what all tropes do, since one does not substitute a thing for itself but for something different. As Ross Chambers tells us, what cannot be compared cannot be known, because it cannot be recognized. This is the apparent paradox of troping as a way to acquire knowledge: to know a thing, another thing must be substituted for it—or at least, such substitution must be possible. In other words, the only way to know what something is, is to put it in contact with something it isn't. This other "thing" that the original object is not may very well be language itself, the words without whose mediation no knowledge is conceivable but that inevitably expose concepts to a perpetual process of alteration, to their alienation from pure reason. This inherent differentiality, or relationality, is what prevents knowledge from congealing into Cartesian categorization or, worse, Nazism, the absolute negation of the relationality of all things and all people.

With the 1985 release of Claude Lanzmann's documentary *Shoah*, which paradoxically did not focus on France at all, the specificity of Jewish history during the Vichy years attained an unprecedented degree of recognition in a political culture long averse to so-called communitarian assertions. At the same time, the AIDS pandemic was reaching catastrophic levels and ravaging the gay community. The overlapping of these two different histories of mass death may have been an accidental encounter, but the fact that the memory of the Holocaust, with its role in rethinking the place of Jews as Jews in the nation, should have provided a model for gays was not. The memory of one collective disaster was soon enrolled in the fight against another, ongoing one. And things didn't stop there. This rhetorical borrowing may have served tactical purposes, but it also uncovered something else, namely, that Jewish history and gay history had in fact long been entangled. In the wake of the gay community's newly acquired political legitimacy, the focus soon turned to the fight for the official recognition of homosexual deportations under Nazi rule. That, too, created discomfort within the French Republic, and it did so in two ways: it put different histories in uneasy contact with one another, as demonstrated by the violently homophobic reactions of some camp survivors against attempts to include wreaths with a pink triangle in official commemorations; and it also shed a light on the disturbing kinship between supposedly incompatible strategies for erasing differences.

There exist two main tendencies to homogenize. One, universal reason, disembodies just as it reembodies through discourses of science or pseudoscience. The other, right-wing totalitarianism, reembodies in order to disembody by way of murder. If knowledge is to resist both, it can only take the unstable form of approximations or nearness, which necessarily leaves stones unturned and particularities respected. But the particularities of others—their otherness—can be respected only by being touched: acknowledged if not fully known. One may, as many AIDS sufferers have done, invoke the memory of the Holocaust to help make sense of other historical catastrophes befalling other human communities as communities; but one must do it with tact, for tact brings into thought and social relations the simultaneous dynamic of touch and distance that characterizes all tropes. And because AIDS, the Holocaust, and other catastrophes are not confined to the pages of books written by people now long gone, tact may serve as a general model for a poetic form of remembering history in the present, reading the social and dealing with others—a form of contact with people one fails fully to comprehend. In that sense, tact's phatic function underscores its focus on contact rather than on the expression of accurate statements. Moving beyond the informational, the interpersonal, and the allegorical, the trope of tact may become a model of reading (with) others that brings different historical "events" into a neighborly relation without erasing their difference—indeed by understanding difference as that which makes community possible—or, to use a musical metaphor: as a kind of disaccord. The cultural memory of the Holocaust, then, is not denied but perpetuated in AIDS testimonies that, by appealing to past events, let themselves be haunted by them and bear witness to them. This could allow us to read history neither as a linear succession nor as a cyclical repetition of finished entities but as a dynamic of nearness and concurrence: something that, like all encounters, only exists when shared.

TACT AND DELICACY (II)

There is a wonderful moment in François Truffaut's film *Stolen Kisses* (*Baisers volés*). In the course of the story, a young Antoine Doinel falls under the charm of Fabienne Tabard, a fabulous older woman played by the no less fabulous Delphine Seyrig. Fabienne is not only phenomenally desirable, she also happens to be married to Antoine's employer, a racist, sexist, paranoid prick. The Tabards are rich too, while Antoine, a working-class kid, tries to make ends meet, one menial job after the other. One day Antoine is invited for lunch at the Tabards' elegant bourgeois apartment. After the meal and with the husband out of the way on an errand, Fabienne pours the coffee and sets out to play a record. In a low, smoky voice reminiscent of Marlene Dietrich's androgyny, she asks the nervous young man, "Do you like music, Antoine?"; to which Antoine replies in a high-pitched voice, "Yes, sir." Overcome with embarrassment and gender confusion, he drops his cup and, literally running out of the apartment, he exits the *scène*, both the scene and the stage. After wandering the streets for a while, he eventually returns home to find a small gift waiting for him by the door. Of course, it is from Fabienne. On the note attached, she has written a little fable, and as Antoine reads it, it is her seductive voice-over that we hear. Her extended presence–absence beyond the boundaries of the earlier scene blurs the distinction between the written word and the spoken one and brings to her tactful reaching out to Antoine more than a hint of sexy physicality. If the young man's overwhelming desire for Fabienne was the source of the embarrassing scene, the sensual reading of the note indicates that the embarrassment has in no way disrupted that desire, quite the contrary.

So here's the story Fabienne tells Antoine:

> When I was in middle school, my teacher was explaining the difference between tact and politeness. A gentleman caller mistakenly opens a bathroom door and discovers a lady stark naked. He withdraws immediately, closes the door, and says: "Oh! pardon me, madam." That is politeness. The same gentleman, opening the same door, discovering the same lady stark naked, and telling her, "Oh! pardon me, sir," *that* is tact.

I return to this passage—the story and the scene that precedes it—quite a bit in what follows; it is so rich. But first I would like to comment briefly on the gender issues at play in it.

In his 1977–78 lectures on what he called the neutral, Roland Barthes devotes a couple of sessions to tact, or as he actually calls it in the original French, *délicatesse*. At one point, he explains how tact may be socially frowned upon because of its association with effeminacy. This rejection of tact not only applies to its more obvious social dimension but also to its association with certain modes of cognition. Barthes thus notes—and the choppy style is due to the fact that the book is a posthumously published transcription of the lectures:

> Tied to language, founded by it, tact: falls under the prohibition of preciosity.
>   1. The bottom of this prohibition: the protestation of virility: *Delicatus* = effeminate; virile condemnation of the delicate, of the precious one, of the "deliquescent," of the "decadent"; this combined with a virile representation of empiricity: the useless, the futile are feminine . . .
>   2. Principle of tact: contiguous with a kind of social errancy, takes upon itself excessive marginality . . . Principle of tact: . . . a kind of social obscene (the unclassifiable).

Gender mishaps pervade Fabienne's story, both in its tenor and because of the incident that triggered its (re)telling. Antoine mishandled gender propriety twice in that scene: he called a woman "Sir" and, by contrast, feminized himself. There is no hint of homosexuality here, however; Truffaut is as straight as they come, I'm afraid, and so is Antoine Doinel, his fictionalized counterpart in the series of somewhat autobiographical films to which *Stolen Kisses* belongs. The feminized role that Antoine inadvertently assumes merely registers, thanks to the eroticism that pervades the scene, as a displacement of class inequality and age difference into the realm of gender. Feeling at once socially inferior to Fabienne and filled with sexual desire for her, he unconsciously sees her as a man and himself, given the unambiguous heteroerotics of the episode, as a woman or a girl. But if Barthes is right, Fabienne's story does not seek to restore the "proper" distribution of gender roles or the inequality that rests on it. By emphasizing Antoine's tact, she feminizes him again and redefines his social inferiority and his incongruous presence in the Tabards' apartment as "social errancy," a far more complex political proposition.

As for the cognitive dimension of tact, the way it approaches reality to make sense of it, it too has a relation to gender, as Barthes explains. Not only is Fabienne fabulous, that is, unreal and an effect of storytelling, she also tells a fable, a mode of transmitting meaning that is as indirect as tact itself. No information is bluntly conveyed here and no reality empirically described. The story's purpose is primarily phatic and gives Fabienne an opportunity to make contact with Antoine despite the social barriers that separate the two. Yet the barriers have not fallen. As her voice-over hints, she is, just like the desirability and the tactfulness she embodies, at once near and distant. In that respect, the story goes nowhere; politically, it is "useless" and it is "futile." It is feminine and it is sweet. Indeed, Barthes goes on to liken *délicatesse* to *douceur*, which the English translation of the book renders as "sweetness" rather than the more accurate "gentleness." This word choice, however, has the unfortunate effect of neglecting the other meaning of the French original: softness *of* touch and *to* the touch, a quality also shared by subject and object on both sides of the interaction, like delicacy. As for the sharing of the story, it allows both participants to partake in and of its qualities themselves as well and to do so behind the back of the revolting Mr. Tabard, the epitome of bourgeois power.

In this particular section of *The Neutral*, Barthes expands on a small fragment of an earlier book of his, *Sade, Fourier, Loyola*. In it, he had reflected on a letter Sade wrote to his wife, and in a later lecture, Barthes quotes it again. Sade's wife had asked her husband, who was imprisoned at the time, for permission to collect his dirty laundry, presumably to wash it. But Sade pretends to misunderstand what she means and chooses to uncover a sexual meaning behind his wife's request. He goes on to explain in jest that, as she knows full well, he is not one to judge other people's sexual tastes, no matter how peculiar. The implication, if I understand the letter well, is that she longs for him sexually, just as he does for her. He calls her alleged cageyness about it—she would be masquerading the sexual desire supposedly at the source of the request but also redirecting that desire away from her husband's body to the garments that were in contact with it—"complete tact" ("une délicatesse achevée"). Ultimately, Sade's feigned misunderstanding is itself a playful and tactful gesture—a loving wink at his wife and a recognition of the feelings they have for each other. In an exquisite double-take on tact, Sade, for whom matters of the body are famously not unspeakable and not so easily disentangled from matters of the mind, pretends to see sex where there may not be any.

To describe the avoidance of conflict, Barthes uses the French phrase *prendre la tangente*, translated as "dodging" in the English text. Again, the translation doesn't render the semantic richness of the original. The French expression does convey the meaning of dodging, it's true, but a tangent is more than that. In a stricter sense, both mathematical and etymological, the tangential implies a kind of touch, a form of contact that delicately brushes against the surface of another entity, leaning and diverging at the same time—contact reduced to its smallest possible form, a single point that consists of nothing other than contact itself. And not only does this moment pertain to tact, in the letter, but it also describes the kind of fetishistic displacement its author pretends to understand, investing with the desire, not the body of the other, but what was once contiguous to it. *Prendre la tangente* brings all these meanings together and, underscoring their kinship, allows us to envisage fetishism as the most tactful form of sexual contact.

And Sade adds that "the most singular and bizarre of them [tastes and fantasies], when well analyzed, always depends on a principle of tact ['un principe de délicatesse']." I wish that Barthes had included in his quotation what Sade immediately adds in his letter, namely, that he, Sade, can prove this at any time because "vous savez que personne n'analyse les choses comme moi." What makes this sentence so lovely is that we may understand it in two ways: you know that nobody analyses things *as well as I do*—the most obvious meaning here; and, you know that nobody analyses things *the way I do*. This sort of analysis, as Barthes concludes nonetheless, is of a radically different kind from the more traditional, empirical version because, for Sade, it is suffused with corporeality and pleasure:

> Sade's very utterance exposes what the principle of tact is: a pleasure [*jouissance*] in analysis, a verbal operation that frustrates expectation (the laundry is dirty in order to be washed) and intimates that tact is a perversion that plays with the useless (nonfunctional) detail . . . and it's this cutting and rerouting that is the source of pleasure→one could say: pleasure in the "futile" . . . In short, tact: analysis . . . when aimless [l'analyse qui ne sert à rien].

This aimless analysis, the subtle understanding of a situation with no discernible consequences for the future, is all at once one of the more intriguing possibilities opened up by tact and one of its most politically frustrating. Not unlike dysclosure, such analysis seems to have no existence beyond the playful, pleasurable mess it makes in the present moment, and Fabienne's story may have originated in a classroom: it isn't exactly what people, of late, have been calling a "teachable moment."

THE SHOWER SCENE

Tact always teeters on the brink of its undoing. An excess of it can be just as devastating as the lack of it. There I was, alone in the gym's shower room, showering, when a line of people, men of course, all of them fully dressed, began to walk right by me on their way to the pool in what I gathered was some sort of business tour of the facilities. Two? Five? Ten? How many more of them were there? Now, I'm really not bashful about being naked in a locker room, but this endless parade, reminiscent of two dozen clowns stepping out of a Volkswagen Beetle, was a bit too much even for me. As these clothed men passed by little naked me one after the other, trying their best to appear suddenly fascinated by their loafers or staring in the opposite direction, at nothing, I grabbed my towel and covered myself clumsily while childhood nightmares about going to school without clothes on seemed to have come uncannily to life. The embarrassment was palpable on both sides.

Is it possible, I now wonder, to be tactful as a group, or even in a group? Is there such a thing as collective tact, or does it remain the province of the sole individual? The answer will have to do with how one defines the individual and tact itself, of course. If tact is a social convention pertaining to class systems, cultural norms, and other forms of power distribution, then it is always collective. Even if it appears to come from the unaltered will of an autonomous self, it has to be measured against an external set of criteria. Furthermore, if the individual is an effect of social relations and not a precondition for their existence—if, in other words, there is no such thing as an autonomous self—one reaches the same conclusion, only using a different route. Tact, it appears, can only be a collective thing. The sense of measure or perfect balance between extremes is what has made it such a perfect bourgeois value. It mirrors the defining quality of the social class that claims it as its own. This ideal quality, however, does not inhere in tact, as if it were natural and outside the realm of the social, waiting, like land, to be reunited with its rightful owners and to legitimate them. Tact was historically elaborated from within a given social class to serve the particular interests of that class. This also means, though, that others may reappropriate it as well.

TACT AND DELICACY (III)

For all its power to articulate social relations and maintain power structures, tact often appears tainted by its gendered association with the delicate. Does tactful persons' reliance on intuition and immediate, that is, nonanalytic, apprehension of human relations mark them as feminine somehow? And to pose the question bluntly and narrow it a bit, is there something queer about tactful men? Jung, Freud's student and rival, seemed to think so. In his essay on the mother-complex (where else), he notes:

> Thus a man with a mother-complex may have a finely differentiated Eros instead of, or in addition to, homosexuality. (Something of this sort is suggested in Plato's *Symposium*.) . . . He may have good taste and an aesthetic sense which are fostered by the presence of a feminine streak. Then he may be supremely gifted as a teacher because of his almost feminine insight and tact. He is likely to have a feeling for history, and to be conservative in the best sense and cherish the values of the past.

I won't even attempt to unpack everything that is wrong, yet somehow endearing and unwittingly provocative, about these remarks. Let's just note very briefly the association of taste and tact, and focus instead on what it is that could make tact appear feminine to some.

Freud, who mentions tact in passing here and there, did see it as a possibly useful quality for an analyst to possess, or rather to exercise, for example, when discussing sexual subjects with female patients. But more important and beyond simple matters of propriety, tact is for him what allows the analyst not to feel needlessly constrained by a straitjacket of technique and rules. Tactfulness, in short, defines the good analyst. In 1928, Freud wrote in a letter to Sándor Ferenczi: "The 'Recommendations on Technique' I wrote long ago were essentially of a negative nature. I considered the most important thing was to emphasize what one should *not* do. . . . Almost everything positive that one *should* do I have left to 'tact.'" This, then, seems to associate tact with the dominant and perforce masculine side of the doctor–patient relationship and, I would like to argue, with Freud himself, to the extent that what he "left to 'tact'" was itself left tactfully unspoken so perhaps that his readers may exercise this very quality when reading the master and thus demonstrate their professional merit.

For this reason or simply for lack of interest, Freud never bothered to define with great precision what he meant by *Takt* other than to say that one should not think of it as undefinable. In his 1910 essay "'Wild' Psycho-Analysis," he made a point of explaining that "medical tact" was not to be "looked upon as some special gift," an idea he expanded on in the letter to Ferenczi when discussing the latter's definition of tact as "the capacity for empathy":

> All those who have no tact will see in what you write a justifica-tion for arbitrariness, i.e. subjectivity, i.e. the influence of their own unmastered complexes. What we encounter in reality is a delicate balancing—for the most part on the preconscious level—of the var-ious reactions we expect from our interventions. The issue depends above all on a quantitative estimate of the dynamic factors in the situation. One naturally cannot give rules for measuring this; the experience and the normality of the analyst have to form a decision. But with beginners one therefore has to rob the idea of "tact" of its mystical character.

Where to begin? For starters, Freud reasserts that tact is a masculine trait and that whoever lacks it also lacks self-mastery and the ability to keep unmoored subjectivity in check. Somewhat paradoxically, however, even though any professional understanding of the "situation" at hand is quan-titative in nature, there can be no "rules for measuring this" other than the analyst's parallel qualities of "experience" and "normalcy." But what to make of tact's "mystical character" then, and why would it spell danger for the inexperienced who, logically, may not be quite normal yet? This, I believe, is where Freud cannot completely shake off tact's association with the fem-inine and leads Jung to mark it as a potentially homosexual character trait. The "delicate balancing" Freud mentions is located "for the most part on the preconscious level" and therefore beyond the scope of normal heterosexual-ity, which establishes itself only with maturation. Tact's "mystical character" would thus hark back all at once to the premodern, to the pre-oedipal, and to women's propensity to fall under the sway of magic and superstition rath-er than science and reason. The link between tact and "feminine insight" as backward looking may then find its logical extension in homosexual men's loving remembrance of things past and search for lost time in that homo-sexuality itself represents a form of developmental and social archaism.

TACT, POWER, AND THE POLICE (I)

"Tact," Benjamin Disraeli is said to have said, "is the intelligence of the heart." In our modern era, tact, not unlike grace and taste (another one of its etymological kin), is often defined as a natural elegance of the mind, unteachable and elusive. You either possess it or you don't. The teacher in Fabienne's story does not teach what tact is and never actually defines it. Instead, he or she uses a fable and relies on one trope to define another. Fabienne does the same thing in her own story, so does Truffaut in the movie, and so do I in these pages. The endless chain of substitutions illustrates how "tact," the signifier, points toward a transcendent, forever deferred signified and thus eludes all possibility for the idea to receive the clear contours that would make it possible for all to grasp and use it. The idea of tact spreads in the culture but remains available only to those capable of deciphering the tropes and producing their own in due course. Tact, without its own contours, nevertheless provides the outline of a linguistic community of sophisticated readers and allusive storytellers.

One thing that makes tact attractive, perhaps charming even, desirable in any case, is how it brings together improvisation and the expert command of rules that accompanies privilege, forming the sort of know-how that, like dilettantism, remains out of the reach of those who have to work for a living—hence, I believe, the disruptive potential of tact when appropriated to serve the interests of those who have been socially devalued by it and its distancing usage.

Because it requires the ability to gauge social situations and discern their dynamics instantly, tact appears effortless. It gives the impression that it does not require thought and that, therefore, it isn't a skill one could work to acquire like politeness or etiquette, the stuff of manuals. If politeness provides us with a set of rules and instructions on when to apply them, tact is a way to deal with the unexpected and it appears to require more intelligence, in both senses of the term. This, in essence, is what accounts for tact's superiority to politeness in the story. In reality, of course, tact has long been a construct and a mode of social policing linked to shame and embarrassment. It is often required to respond to situations—slips, mishaps, and a variety of failures and shortcomings—that isolate a person from the social. But if it is a measure of group membership, and therefore not available to all, then tact is really designed to establish social hierarchies and enforce something like class privilege—reframing social proximity as distance. Think of k***, for example. Remember him? His rejection of me may have stemmed less from my being HIV positive than from my inability to pick up on his subtle avoidance of the topic. However, as a policing device, concerned with establishing and surveilling social boundaries, tact inevitably, if unwittingly, facilitates forms of symbolic contacts across difference, thus allowing those it polices to oppose it and repurpose it in order to enact more egalitarian relations between people. But first, there is policing.

Tact indicates that, in our modern culture of truth telling, transparency may not be the obvious proposition we make it out to be. As with mandatory (self-)disclosure, principles and practices of tact play out modalities of power by policing speech. Power positions, however, do not get distributed simply according to the opposition between truth and nontruth, the former speakable and the latter not; nor do they emerge from the separation of two kinds of truths—those that must be told and those that may, or even ought to, remain unexpressed. To the extent that policing society means policing actual people, the truth-value of a given statement is largely arbitrary in the end. What matters most in the process, I contend, is the difference between who, not what, may remain silent and who must speak up. Here silence (or the possibility to opt for it, whether partially or totally) is a sign of power, not oppression.

It is thus possible to discern a certain degree of continuity between the classical culture of discretion that characterized the seventeenth century and the modern reliance on confession and self-disclosure. Foucault admits that much:

> It may indeed be true that a whole rhetoric of allusion and metaphor was codified [in the seventeenth century]. Without question, new rules of propriety screened out some words: there was a policing of statements. A control over enunciation as well: when and where it was not possible to talk about such things became more strictly defined; in which circumstances, among which speakers, and within which social relationships. Areas were just established, if not of utter silence, at least of tact and discretion.

As for Theodor Adorno, he sees an explicit link between tact's appearance as a social value during the Enlightenment and the concurrent consolidation of bourgeois power. Both, he says, are premised on emancipating the individual:

For tact, we now know, has its precise historical hour. It was the hour when the bourgeois individual rid himself of absolutist compulsion. Free and solitary, he answers for himself, while the forms of hierarchical respect and consideration developed by absolutism, divested of their economic basis and their menacing power, are still just sufficiently present to make living together within privileged groups bearable.... The demise of the ceremonial moment seems at first to benefit tact. Emancipated from all that was heteronomous and harmfully external, tactful behaviour would seem one guided solely by the specific nature of each human situation.

But to deny that tact does in fact rely on convention—how else could one determine that tactful behavior is required if not against some sort of deviation?—makes the complete emancipation of the self politically problematic, to say the least. All human interaction rests on conventions that make it possible, and to pretend that it doesn't negates human relationality in general. For Adorno,

> when emancipated, [tact] confronts the individual as an absolute, without anything universal from which to be differentiated, it fails to engage the individual and finally wrongs him.... Beneath the demand that the individual be confronted as such, without preamble, absolutely as befits him, lies a covetous eagerness to "place" him ... in the ever more rigid hierarchy that encompasses everyone. The nominalism of tact helps what is most universal, naked external power, to triumph even in the most intimate constellations. To write off convention as an outdated, useless and extraneous ornament is only to confirm the most extraneous of all things, a life of direct domination.

What makes the idea of the absolutism of the individual so disturbing to contemplate isn't just the idea that tact may in fact be an oppressive form of civility, but that it brings the age of reason into proximity with its most radical opponent.

In *Anti-Semite and Jew* (*Réflexions sur la question juive*), Jean-Paul Sartre observes that tact appears to fall outside the realm of reason the better to outline, and reinforce, a community's boundaries:

> To act with tact is to appreciate a situation at a glance, to embrace it as a whole, to feel it rather than to analyze it, but it is at the same

time to direct one's conduct by reference to a multitude of indistinct principles, of which some concern vital values and others express ceremonies and traditions of politeness that are altogether irrational. Thus to act "with tact" implies that the doer of the act has adopted a certain conception of the world, one that is traditional, ritual, and synthetic; one for which *he can give no reason.. . . .* it takes on its whole meaning only in a strictly defined community with common ideas, mores, and customs.

It makes sense to conclude that this social mastery over others is available only to members of the classes that have the power to define what social values are and how to transmit them. Although tact seemingly escapes reason and thus cannot be taught, like taste and grace it must be learned—and learned from proximity. But if tact delineates social groups, proximity can occur only within the same class. Indeed, that is the primary purpose of tact as a tool of social policing. What matters most is that people capable of exercising tact may be able to recognize each other and do so at the expense of the person in need of tactful treatment. "Tactors" are people who not only understand how the social works and do so wholly and instantaneously but also exercise mastery over society. In addition, the mutual recognition of fellow tactors must be tacit to be effective. Should this recognition be expressed in words, tact would run the risk of being, like politeness, encoded in ways that make it accessible to whoever learns the code. If that happened, tact would cease to unify a specific class and keep others at bay. The perception of tact's unteachability and elusiveness seeks to naturalize a certain social system, discipline people, and perpetuate the allegedly undisputable superiority of one group.

Yet if tactfulness—the practice of tact—may bring cohesion to a certain class thanks to wordless mutual recognition, it can work only thanks to physical nearness. Tact-as-policing seeks to enact the silent ritual that disembodies community by performing two tasks: keeping bodies that allegedly do not belong together at a safe distance from each other, and keeping the body away from thought. But since its metaphorical turn, tact, like taste, has been haunted by the body it has expelled and repressed. Tact as a form of social ritual is felt to be imperative as soon as the repressed body threatens to return. (Embarrassment is the emotion that signals this return.) The expulsion, however, must never be completed for that would constitute a suicidal move, erasing tactee and tactor all at once. This is a basic difference between fascist self-annihilation and bourgeois resilience, and it explains why tact pertains to the latter: bourgeois capitalism is cynical. What, then, does this tell us about the operation of disembodiment that made tact shift from the sensorial to the social in the first place? How can tact be intangible if it can never sever its ties to the body?

In Western modernity, tact pertains to the bourgeois ideal of discretion as propriety. Indeed, the word acquired its current meaning in the decades preceding the French Revolution. Forms of tact can be found in other social classes, of course, such as lower-class men, among whom a certain type of delicacy may (paradoxically or not) be required to preserve masculinity. In some cases, looking away allows someone else to "save face," preserving the sense of self that face (re)presents to the world. But just like taste (again tact's probable etymological kin), the dominant, normative form of tact belongs to the class that is itself in the dominant position. In any case, it is no surprise that the body (and the contiguous notions of sex–gender, race–ethnicity, sexuality–illness) should play an essential part in all this. Tact is often required to avoid attracting attention to certain bodily functions, for example. It may appear polite to use phrases such as "Bless you" and "Bon appétit," but doing so has nothing to do with tact. And recall Annie Ernaux's shame when her mother appears at the doorstep with urine stains on her nightgown. But the concealment of bodily functions or sexuality or race—their privatization, in the modern context—cannot be separated from the body itself and the actual people it belongs to. After all, if the art of tact is transmitted by contiguity within the same class, bodies cannot just be wished away altogether. The bodies of the dominant class must be concealed because their power rests on their access to abstraction, the bodies of the dominated must be made spectacularly visible to disqualify their owners. Bourgeois propriety and property, it seems, are germane, and what connects them is a division: that of the public and the private where bodies are said to belong. You inadvertently open a bathroom door, you breach a boundary, and embarrassment ensues.

Because tact brings together bodies and the class system, distributing the former according to the categories of the latter, it has served as a tool for social inclusion and exclusion, while its unteachability ensures that class boundaries are not breached inappropriately. (As Jean Cocteau once revealingly put it, underlining tact's connection with all sorts of limits: "Tact consists in knowing how far to go too far.") The supposed tactlessness of the Jews, for example, which triggers Sartre's observations, has worked as a way to assign them a specific place in bourgeois society—the place of the misfit. In the meantime, non-Jewish bourgeois may recognize and appreciate each other's mastery of tact, confirming that they naturally belong together and have power over others. For Sartre, to allege that Jews are tactless is a ploy to keep them at the margins of a community cemented by a mystical, magical bond unattainable by individual conscience—or what Jean-Luc Nancy called a community of fusion. One can think of Barresian nationalism or, as Sartre reminds us, of the right-wing writer Charles Maurras's contention that Jews will never be able to understand—that is, to absorb all at once as if by magic—Racine's line: "Dans l'Orient désert, quel devint mon ennui." (I won't attempt to translate Racine; the words *Orient*, *désert*, and *ennui* make this clear enough.) But if tact functions as a tool of bourgeois power, it follows that the contractual, rationalist concept of the nation, premised on separating the public and the private, also contains an element of magic and irrationality designed to forestall the unraveling of the community from its margins. A group's sense of social distinction and ability to be discriminating produces just that: distinction and discrimination, or in more technical terms, essentialized identities and social exclusion.

The specific stereotype of the tactless Jew seems to have appeared with the Emancipation. It represents a form of exclusion that relies on Enlightenment notions of taste and suggests that, no matter what the law says, Jews will never truly belong to the community because to belong is to possess certain inalienable qualities. Here tact is seen as the externalization of this internal trait into the realm of social relations, which simultaneously opens up the undoing of its policing power. To begin with, tact historically pertains to the Enlightenment and reason, but is understood to stand outside the rational and against the very idea of the community as a contract freely entered into by equal and autonomous subjects. In other words, tact is a product of reason that undoes reason. It is also supposed to be an inherent quality that binds the "natural" members of the community and keeps the riff-raff out—or rather, at the margins. This can only imply, however, the existence of a semi-external object, or intimate other, defined as lacking tact but with whom tact must be exercised. (The Nazi project of extermination can be seen as the most radical attempt to do away with this intimate proximity.) As Sartre's phrasing suggests, if one must act with tact, then tact doesn't inhere in the subject but is as exterior to it as the person it applies to. The feeling that tact is an interior quality is thus produced *with* the outside—an outside–in dynamic as much as an inside–out one. Furthermore, because the tactor cannot be reminded of that fact without losing face, the tactee can exercise tact as well and refrain from mentioning that the emperor is naked. In short, the contractual community based on reason becomes undone by its unstated belief in purity and magic, while magical tact becomes undone by the denied relationality at its core, making protofascists like Barrès and Maurras much closer than they think to the philosophy they repudiate. And vice versa, I'm afraid. No matter how we see it, we can never disentangle tact from the question of community. Its ineffability is a way to cover up the material conditions that make power and inequality possible. To put it differently, tact reveals how modern reason could claim to ground a new, democratic ideal while operating little more than a simple rearrangement of power.

TACT, POWER, AND THE POLICE (II)

In general, one needs to exercise tact when one's interlocutor is, in one way or another, vulnerable, when that person has failed at something and is feeling touchy about it. To feel embarrassed or ashamed is a way to acknowledge our failure and to have it confirmed by others around us. As the sociologist Erving Goffman notes, "To appear flustered, in our society at least, is considered evidence of weakness, inferiority, low status, moral guilt, defeat, and other unenviable attributes." A person in need of tactful treatment is, in a sense, broken—not intact. His or her integrity as an individual (that which cannot be divided or broken down) has come into question insofar as feeling embarrassed presupposes the ability to judge oneself, standing on both sides at once at the doorstep of shame. The avowed purpose of tactfulness is to mask the individual's failure to remain undivided, metaphorically covering his or her nakedness, if you will, and pretend that nothing happened.

Oftentimes, however, tact singles *out* what it purports to ignore. That's the point. But to expel inevitably means to bring boundaries into stark relief. Elaine Scarry, for one, understands torture as a spectacle of power that makes the private visible. Like mandatory disclosure, it "makes people talk" in order to silence them. Tact, as a form of policing, finds itself caught in a similar double dynamic. On the one hand, it outlines discrete categories, and, on the other, it betrays a synthetic view of a world in which the tactee is a kind of resident outsider, so to speak, providing in full view of the world the repellent spectacle of outsidedness. Visibility is thus central. The tactee must be seen, as if on a stage where a private drama unfolds for all to see. The tactor's tactfulness, to be legitimated as such, must be witnessed by potential fellow tactors. The act of concealing, then, increases visibility, and with this come certain risks that must be addressed. If a person isn't intact, presumably because he or she is delicate, the rupture extends beyond the boundaries of the individual into the small worlds that people make when they come together.

Reflecting on tact and embarrassment, Goffman notes:

> During interaction the individual is expected to possess certain attributes, capacities, and information which, taken together, fit together into a self that is at once coherently unified and appropriate for the occasion. Through the expressive implications of this stream . . . the individual effectively projects the acceptable self into the interaction. . . . At the same time he must accept and honor

the selves projected by the other participants. The elements of a social interaction, then, consist of effectively projected claims to an acceptable self and the confirmation of like claims on the part of the others. . . . When an event throws doubt upon or discredits the claims, then the encounter finds itself lodged in assumptions that no longer hold. The responses the parties have made ready are now out of place and must be choked back, and the interaction must be reconstructed.

The sociologist Anthony Giddens, who sees tact as central to Goffman's thought, adds, "Thus people routinely shore up or 'repair' the moral fabric of interaction, by displaying tact in what they say and do, by engaging in 'remedial practices,' and helping others to save face. . . . If day-to-day social life is a game . . . , it is a game into which all are thrust and in which collaboration is essential."

That's one way to look at it. What Goffman and Giddens recognize, even though neither one phrases it quite this way, is that tact has a normalizing function. Something is broken. It may be a person's sense of self or it may be social cohesion, that is to say, the coming together of selves in a mutually agreeable manner. Either way, or both, things must be repaired. I see little to dispute here. But the idea that tact's primary purpose is to restore the kind of interaction in which all selves are recognized as equally acceptable and honored, to use Goffman's terms, seems much more problematic. How can tact normalize social relations without, at the same time, producing the very rupture it claims to mend? Or to rephrase the same question with the self in mind rather than the social, how can one have a sense of what a functioning self is without contrasting it to a dysfunctional one that must be rejected for the contrast to operate? If tact's purpose is to normalize social relations, then it really expels who it pretends to integrate. Discretion, in all its senses, is something one exercises like power, and tact as a mode of policing ironically erases others by bringing out their singularity. It seeks to define its relation to others as distinction—an essentializing move that links the discreet and the discrete. Indeed, the tactor's discernment is a multipurpose quality pertaining as much to tact as it does to taste and that relies on all the semantic possibilities of the word: the ability to identify, distinguish, separate, discriminate, judge. Collaboration may occur in this process, it's true, but I fail to see how it can be a matter of common and equal interest.

The distribution of power, however, is not clear-cut. If the tactee's embarrassment is an experience of alienation and self-policing—envisioning oneself as a judging other—social embarrassment is also highly transmissible. By using tact as a way to bond with one's own kind and keep the weak at a safe distance, the tactor may be looking to self-protect from the same shattering results and avoid experiencing the fragility of his or her power. Goffman was well aware of that, which is why he sees the undoing of the self as a risk that extends to the world around it. To begin with, embarrassment automatically affects the person who makes the other one feel embarrassed, and both are "sharing this sentiment just when they have reason to feel apart." And he adds,

> By the standards of the wider society, perhaps only the discredited individual ought to feel ashamed; but by the standards of the little social system maintained through the interaction, the discreditor is just as guilty as the person he discredits—sometimes more so, for if he has been posing as a tactful man, in destroying another's image he destroys his own.

In Fabienne's story, for example, who was embarrassed exactly? The woman who failed to lock the door and whose body was exposed, or the man who failed to knock and saw the naked body? Both I imagine. And both go through a comparable process of doubling and experience of alienation that temporarily dislocates them. The fact that tactor and tactee may *share* this dislocating feeling of failure opens up the possibility of understanding tact in certain situations not as distinction but as empathetic difference. If embarrassment is contagious, so then are the solutions to it. The powerless, too, may behave with tact. That the tactor may also be treated with tact is what I meant by the nakedness of the emperor. Or the empress. Ultimately, if tactor and tactee may share a degree of embarrassment as well as an appreciation of tactfulness, another community may emerge in which difference becomes embraced rather than rejected.

Fabienne Tabard is a wealthy woman of exquisite tastes, whose maturity and social superiority contribute much to the charm she exudes. Antoine's palpable discomfort inside his boss's elegant bourgeois home owes in equal measure to sexual desire and social out-of-placeness in an intimate space that isn't his own. Perceiving both at once thanks to a well-tuned sense of discernment, Fabienne symbolically turns the table on Antoine. She is so tactful in fact that she tells Antoine a story that makes it look as though he were the tactful one and she the one who had said or done something wrong—seducing and intimidating him, presumably. In the end, however, determining who has truly committed a faux pas and who has truly exercised tact is of no relevance. What matters is that the story has momentarily equalized the relationship between the two participants, or interlocutors, at the expense of the racist, sexist—and absent—husband. The success of the parable, or fable, is premised on Antoine's ability to understand Fabienne's indirect use of language and, therefore, on her assumption that the young, working-class man may possess a sense of discernment equal to hers in sophistication. The subject of the fable may have been ostensibly about inequality and power, but its object was in fact equality, an equality grounded—in this case—in desire. In a different context, Rancière writes:

> Behind the fable's moral, which illustrated the inequality of functions in the social body, lay quite a different moral, one inherent in the very act of composing a fable. This act of composition was on the assumption that it was necessary to speak and that this speaking would be heard; the assumption of a pre-existing equality between a wish to speak and a wish to hear. Above all, it put this presupposition into practice.... The moral of the very act of fabulation was thus the equality of intelligences. And this equality shapes and defines a community, though it must be remembered that this community has no material substance. It is born at each and every moment by someone for someone else—for a potential infinity of others. It occurs but it has no place.

Through her fable, which presupposes, if not Antoine's wish to understand maybe, at least his ability to do so, Fabienne restores, or retrieves, a foundational equality. The use of fabulation may suggest that the power relations it fabulates are constructs, that inequality is a fiction; it does not, however, effect any kind of social revolution. Fabienne's tactful gesture posits equality as a premise, a moment that precedes the current distribution of power: the tactee can be touched by the tactor, thus evoking a corporeal proximity whose denial forms the basis of social and political inequality. This is, after all, a story of bodies and desire. But it doesn't, in turn, replace one fiction with another, nor does it try to give the false impression that social equality will ensue. Fabienne Tabard was and remains in a position of superiority in relation to Antoine Doinel, but both are, for different reasons, socially inferior to Mr. Tabard. Unstated in the fable itself, Antoine's and Fabienne's equality was an effect of utterance and must be effected anew each time, for it never outlives the moment of its utterance. Yet, when the young man looks at himself in the mirror—a common visual trope for processes of self-identification in the movies—and repeats his own name several times until he replaces it with hers, we are glimpsing the dizzying realization that all selves are relational, all individuals divided.

Here we begin to see how tact-as-policing may not be so easily separated from tact-as-contact. All borders connect and disconnect at the same time, and since they have no tangible existence in themselves, it is whoever guards them that embodies this dual status. As we saw with the cops in the movie theater, the police always bring together what they separate. And because the role of the police isn't simply to police individuals but, through them, all society, the repercussions are inevitable. Goffman once more:

> But of course the trouble does not stop with the guilty pair or with
> those who have identified themselves sympathetically with them.
> Having no settled and legitimate object to which to play out their
> own unity, the others find themselves unfixed and discomfited.
> This is why embarrassment seems to be contagious, spreading, once
> started, in ever widening circles of discomfiture.

With this last image in mind, think again of the anxious young gay man in *The Lost Language of Cranes*, circling the porno theater he's afraid to enter and, in the process, spreading his anxiety to the rest of the city around it. The transmissibility of tact through contact, which produced the class cohesion of one side at the expense of the others, is also what signals the possibility of undoing its policing power. When Sade sexualized tact he made it subversive—which is Barthes's point: "Sadian tact is not a class product, an attribute of civilization, a style of culture. It is a power of analysis and a means of *jouissance*: analysis and *jouissance* join together to produce an exaltation that is unknown in our societies and which constitutes therefore the most formidable of utopias." Contact, as I define it here, is of the metaphorical kind, of course, but it is not by accident that I chose sexual encounters to figure the social. Being an operation of disembodiment, tact always undoes itself, and with this ultimate failure comes that of the entire system of thought that rests on the strict division of body and mind.

TACT AND CONTAMINATION

Were the Nazis tactful? The question is a little disconcerting, perhaps even disturbing, but so is the novel that made me think of it, Jonathan Littell's *Kindly Ones* [*Les bienveillantes*], a long and absorbing book about the Holocaust as told from the perspective of its Nazi narrator. I am not trying to find out whether Nazis were capable of exercising tact—or showing a lack of it—in normal social situations, that is, in those situations similar to the ones where we too might be called on to exercise tact; I couldn't care less and I don't see why they wouldn't be anyway, since they came out, by and large, of the same cultural mold as other Europeans at the time. What intrigues me is whether the notion of tact may prove pertinent in the context of what Nazis did as Nazis, of what defined them as Nazis—the extermination of the Jews. Can tactfulness and tactlessness, in other words, be invoked as part of a political project that negates the very culture whence tact came?

We know that high-ranking Nazi officials in charge of organizing the "final solution," chief among them Heinrich Himmler, went to great lengths to avoid nearly all direct mention of what they were doing. Some people involved in the "evacuation" of the Jews (die Judenevakuierung), for example, were referred to as "bearers of secrets" (Geheimnistrager). Was the systematic use of euphemisms, this indirection in and of language, a form of tact in that it sought to avoid discomfort and unease among interlocutors and functioned structurally in the way that tact does? Conversely, would it have been tactless, in some circles, to describe in explicit terms what was occurring in remote corners of the eastern front?

In two speeches, now famous but secret then, Himmler did just that as he addressed a selected audience of Nazi officials in Posen, in occupied Poland, on October 4 and 6, 1943. Instructing his listeners never to share with anyone else any of what he is about to tell them about the killing of the Jews, he goes on to discuss the topic bluntly, going as far, in the second speech, as to evoke—and justify—the killings of women and children. This is the speech the narrator of *The Kindly Ones* happens to attend. Although he is himself a bearer of secrets and has been directly involved in the extermination, Himmler's frank speech takes him by surprise: "I found it, considering the secrecy rules we were bound to, truly shocking, almost indecent, and at the beginning, it made me very ill at ease, and I was certainly not the only one, I could see the Gauleiters sigh and mop their foreheads or necks." Himmler, the narrator continues, insisted that, yes, we were indeed killing the women and the children too, so as not to leave any ambiguity linger, and that's precisely what was so uncomfortable, that total absence, for once, of ambiguity, and it was as if he were violating an unwritten rule, even stronger than his own rules he decreed for his subordinates, his *Sprachregelungen* already absolutely strict, the rule of tact perhaps, that tact he spoke of in his first speech.

In that speech, two days earlier, Himmler indeed called "tact" the silence that surrounded the so-called Night of the Long Knives, the 1934 liquidation of the SA leadership by the SS, and that he now urges with regard to the extermination of the Jews: "That was, thank God, a kind of tact natural to us, the self evidence of tact, that we have never conversed about it amongst ourselves, never spoken about it" (Das war so eine Gottseidank in uns wohnende Takt, Selbstverständlichkeit des Taktes, daß wir uns untereinander nie darüber unterhalten haben, nie darüber sprachen). The notion that tactfulness precludes the mention of bodies is taken here to its extreme.

To shroud in silence murders committed collectively is not an unusual phenomenon when both murders and silence bring about and sustain a given community, protecting it like a wall or a barrier, to which silence is often compared, against the intrusion of dangerous foreign bodies. Nazi Germany may represent only the most dramatic occurrence of this. Most of us would balk at the idea of calling tactful the hushing of mass murder and the use of impersonal administrative lingo, but I understand why Nazis would prefer to do so. As Himmler describes it in his speech, tact is supposed to be a quality natural to Germans as a collective entity, and *Selbstverständlichkeit*—what goes without saying—turns out to be both what defines tact and what it covers up. Moreover, as he goes on to describe Jews, using the usual Nazi metaphors of disease (I'll spare you that part), he indirectly affirms tact's function as a safeguard against contamination. It is thus particularly cunning of him, as the narrator surmises, to use tactlessness to propagate another sort of metaphorical contamination—that of guilt and complicity—as the kind of community that is Nazi Germany begins to unravel in the aftermath of Stalingrad and as a result of intensified Allied bombings of cities:

> But perhaps it was also a matter of something other than the question of tact and of those rules, and that's when I began to understand, I think, the profound reason for these declarations, and

also why the dignitaries sighed and sweated so much, for they too, like me, were beginning to understand that it wasn't by chance that the Reichsführer, in the beginning of the fifth year of the war, was thus referring to the destruction of the Jews before them, without euphemisms, without winks, with simple and brutal words like *kill*.

The realization that Himmler's words could not have been uttered without Hitler's knowledge or against his wishes leads the narrator to this inevitable conclusion:

> There could only have been one reason, hence the perceptible emotion of the listeners, who grasped this reason very well; it was so that none of them could, later on, say that he didn't know, couldn't try to make people think, in case of defeat, that he was innocent of the worst, couldn't think he might someday be able to get off scot-free; it was in order to *drag them in* [pour les *mouiller*], and they understood it very well, hence their distress.

The French verb *mouiller*, meaning "to implicate" here but literally "to wet" or "to get (something or someone) wet," constitutes a metaphorical continuation of the very real sweat that runs down the listener's faces and necks. The mutual contamination of the figural by the literal—which is, at bottom, tactlessness's most elemental affair—represents *en abyme* that of the listeners being compromised in the crimes, tainted and altered because they could not keep their distance from these crimes. Himmler's tactlessness, his direct mention of bodies and what is being done to them as he speaks and his audience listens, joins together by soiling them the members of a community that can no longer look the other way and pretend to believe in its own purity.

It is true that if tactlessness brings into contact what tact tells us must be separated—the ideal and the corporeal, the abstract and the tangible—its occurrence produces social discomfort, perhaps even disorder in one form or another. But if it emanates from on high, and thus carries the normative weight of power and the organizing function that is usually tact's purview, tactlessness may also work as tact's mirror image rather than its disruption, thus fulfilling the same purpose while appearing to do the reverse—to keep the riff-raff in, to build a community of the unclean.

TACT AND SILENCE

Whereas tactlessness means saying the wrong thing, one is tactful when saying the right thing means saying the wrong thing on purpose and saying it right. Sometimes, though, it means saying nothing at all, and silence too may be a form of social policing. If the phrase "It isn't done" signals politeness, what defines tact is more like "It isn't said." In both cases, though, the passive voice leaves the agent conveniently unspoken, giving the impression that proper behaviors are in fact justified by some sort of unquestionable transcendent authority rather than by social conventions. But the link between tact and silence often appears as elusive as silence itself. First of all, for silence to be tactful it mustn't in fact create an effect of amplification, a sort of echo chamber or emptiness in which embarrassment may expand unchecked and make matters worse for everyone. To stare dumbstruck at someone else's mishap is not tactful. Clearly, not all silences are made of the same stuff. Distinguishing between *tacere* and *silere*, for example, Barthes brings out the crucial difference between, on the one hand, what is deliberately unspoken and thus verbal in essence and, on the other, the absence of sound or noise: "*Tacere* thus, as silence of speech, is opposed to *silere*, as silence of nature or of divinity." Tact, in that it always indexes something that remains implicit, pertains to the first case, to what Barthes calls "worldly tactic":

> In such a "semiology" of worldly morality, silence has in fact a
> "speakerly" or "speechly" ["parolière" ou "parolante"] substance: it is
> always at the level of the implicit. When in the field of worldliness,
> of strong sociality (and what else is it but an excessively social,
> worldly language?), the implicit (and the silence that works as its
> "index") takes part in the worldly combat: It is a polyvalent weapon.

Silence, then, may have a direct relation with power in one way or another: "In fact, in every 'totalitarian' or 'totalizing' society, the implicit is a crime, because the implicit is a thought that escapes power." One may be "'imprisoned by reason of implicitness'—or better, 'condemned by reason of silence.'" Himmler's initial, euphemistic silence about the reality of the "final solution," which in turn gestures toward the bystanders' *tacit* approval of it, indicates that some kinds of silence may not be tolerated in liberal democratic societies either, at least in principle, if they violate certain basic values. The nondisclosure of one's HIV-positive status isn't criminalized in totalitarian regimes only, as we know; but to force people to speak is totalitarian by nature, regardless of what kind of society in which this coercion takes place. In fact, it isn't too far-fetched to consider the forced display of the yellow star as the ultimate mandatory disclosure.

The issue of power remains a blind spot in Eviatar Zerubavel's sociological study of silence and denial, *The Elephant in the Room*. Noting as a starting point the discrepancy "between the private act of noticing and the public act of acknowledging," he goes on to add:

> And the difference between what we actually notice and what we publicly acknowledge having noticed is at the very heart of what it means to be tactful. . . . As when we forgive someone or pretend to have forgotten the promise he once made to us but never kept, being tactful involves at least outwardly treating things we actually do notice as if they are somehow irrelevant and, as such, can be practically ignored.

The mistake in this description consists in positing the "private" as no different from the "individual." (The book starts off with "The Emperor's New Clothes," by Hans Christian Andersen. Everyone can see that the emperor is naked, but no one says a word to anyone else.) This conflation, when applied to tact, cannot account for the role of tact in class formation and maintenance. If a class is closed to outsiders, it cannot be said to be public in the strict sense of the term, but that class is nevertheless a key player in establishing a political system that extends beyond the boundaries of the class in question. And, clearly, class isn't an individual matter either.

Zerubavel's stated purpose is to "examine institutionalized prohibitions against looking, listening, and speaking that, whether in the form of strict taboos or more subtle rules of tact, help keep certain matters off-limits." The problem is that tact doesn't only keep matters off-limits, but also people—especially people. Nothing prohibits members of the tactful class from talking about the hapless tactee in any way they want to so long as the latter isn't around to hear it. And they may discuss among themselves certain subject matters they will avoid with others in the name of tact. As some people are fond of saying, even the queen goes to the loo. And, I would add, she can talk about it too, as long as it's with the appropriate people. Whatever behavior is met with tact doesn't need to be unspeakable (nothing is) but simply unspoken in certain situations. The different situations in which something may or may not be spoken do not exist in separate societies, just in different compartments of the same society. If tact does "keep certain matters off-limits," it does so in order to produce these very limits.

Later on, when bringing the question of denial into the mix, Zerubavel makes what I think is his next, related mistake. Assuming that silence about the elephant in the room cannot be discussed either, he adds, "In other words, the very act of avoiding the elephant is itself an elephant! Not only do we avoid it, we do so without acknowledging that we are actually doing so, thereby denying our denial." But to acknowledge denial would essentially end it. To deny that there is denial is always part of the process of denial, not an additional layer of silence upon silence. And unlike what Zerubavel thinks, tact is not a form of denial anyway. If fellow tactors sometimes do not speak to each other about what just happened, it isn't because they can't but because they don't need to. The closeness among members of the same class is such that no words are necessary for there to be understanding between them. The complicit may remain implicit or tacit.

What then is the untold function of the tactors' silence if it isn't a matter of denial? What is it that they have to be discreet about? The answer is power itself and the fact that some people share it at the expense of others. The tacitness of tact among tactors is due simply to the fact that a quality shared need not be expressed. But it also gives the impression that what needn't be spoken really cannot, placing such a quality beyond the purview of discussion and, with it, the power of the class that shares it. As Jacques Rancière remarks: "The very principle of superiority collapses if it has to be explained to inferiors why they are inferior. This discourse assumes that it will be apprehended on its own terms, but the fact is that it portrays a community, governed by equality, which is quite different from the one that it promotes." This is why tact essentially pertains to democratic societies and appeared as an important social value at the same time as they did. Only when power is supposed to be shared does its unequal distribution need to be concealed. In that respect, a sovereign's magnanimity has nothing to do with tact, for example. Tactful silence, in other words, indexes the secret sharing of a social bond among the powerful. Not only do we not need to say anything to recognize each other as being "in the know," but social discretion may in fact be a manifestation of political discretion. To be discreet or tactful about being rich, for instance, is a way to protect the power that comes with wealth. Those in power cannot reveal how much power they really have or how it works for fear of losing it or worse, sharing it. Power is indeed the opposite of sharing (whence my distinction, earlier in this book, on disclosure as confession and disclosure as sharing).

Applied to others, silence is intended to pass as respect, the better to hide the fact that the very same silence, shared "among us," means something else altogether. The Latin *cernere* gave us the words "secret," "discretion," "discrimination," and "discernment," among others. It also gave us the French verb *cerner*, which means to surround and to comprehend and brings the two together around the idea of enclosure. All these are central to tact. The sense of social discernment that allows a person to determine if a given situation requires tactful handling and of what kind is inseparable from a more global discernment of the inner workings of society in general. Discretion, like discreteness, is intended to keep such knowledge a secret and set up strict boundaries between classes.

The alleged tactlessness of the Jews and tastelessness of the nouveaux riches are telling phenomena. Think of the insistence, in some circles, on former French president Nicolas Sarkozy's supposed vulgarity. Although I assume that few dared to make explicit mentions of his Jewish and immigrant origins in that context, he soon earned the racially tinged nickname of "President Bling-Bling." The man's ostentatious tastes, his fascination with money and social status, his predilection for rubbing elbows with showbiz celebrities, all were interpreted as evidence that, even though he has been elected president, he was not and never would be quite "one of us."

TACT AND FAILURE

For something defined by what it doesn't say, it is amazing how many forms tact may actually take: euphemisms and understatements, parables and fabulation, silences, even deflecting speech by speaking to a third party rather than directly to the intended recipient of the tactful gesture; tact's obliqueness, circumventing or sidestepping its object, is what makes it difficult to define and imitate. But I am focusing here on the sort described in *Stolen Kisses*. Within Fabienne's fable, tact is itself a mode of failure—a willing failure of language ("Pardon me, sir" for "Pardon me, madam") that rewrites Antoine's unwilled lapse ("Yes, sir" for "Yes, madam"). In this case, tact is not located in the actual statement but in the conditions of its utterance. We can find another, far more tragic example in Charlotte Delbo's *Measure of Our Days*. In this scene, Charlotte and two comrades say good-bye to a dying friend in Auschwitz. Sylviane can no longer speak, and words seem all but pointless in the situation. Carmen tries: "Comment vas-tu, ma petite Sylviane? demanda Carmen, et cette question qui était fausse sonnait juste." An English approximation would be something like, "How are you, dear little Sylviane" asked Carmen, and this question, which was false, sounded right." I prefer to quote the original French text rather than the published English translation because the last segment is rather difficult to render. "Fausse" suggests falsity but also hypocrisy—the hypocrisy of tact—and "juste" implies not just accuracy but justice and fairness. "Fausse" and "juste" also evoke music, especially when used near the verb *sonner*. Carmen's question may be *fausse*, but the contact it establishes with the dying friend is *juste*. The community at work here represents a form of disaccord.

The "false statement" that is Carmen's query, because it is also right, conveys some kind of truth. The question is, what kind of truth? Truth here—or perhaps rightness: rightness of feeling, of care, of support; "The tenderness in Carmen's voice was true"—doesn't occur despite the statement's falsity but thanks to it. Had Carmen addressed the reality of Sylviane's situation bluntly, she would not have been able to convey with accuracy the friendship of the group. But rightness that may not be separated from falsehood cannot be grounded in the sort of reason premised on the objective separation of the two. Yet in the context of the concentration camp, that is to say, in the face of an experience in which the self no longer exists as such, it would be equally inaccurate to describe the rightness of the scene as subjective or even, despite my use of the word *feeling*, as affective. I prefer to think of it as rightness in and as relation, emerging neither from a purely objective source nor from a subjective one. This sort of rightness is thus in and of the moment. Not unlike dysclosure, it changes with each utterance without being any less right for it. In this specific scene, the rightness is *about* Sylviane but it is also, and more importantly, *for* Sylviane. It is the rightness of friendship.

TACT AND UNREASON

The fear of contact is both a fear of death and a fear of life. To be touched is to acquire more than a sense of one's corporeal limits; it gives a sense of one's finitude and end—the stuff of life. To be touched is to begin a process of undoing close to putrefaction. Indeed, the Spanish word *tocado* is synonymous with "blemished" and "spoiled." Goffman, as we know, used this last word to describe what happens to identity as a result of stigma. But there is more. "Touched" may mean crazy as well, and this second meaning is also conveyed by the French *toqué*. When reason is touched it unravels. Not only does it cease to be universal from the moment it experiences its limit, but to touch reason is to undo its separation from the corporeal and the material, a separation on which its very existence rests. To shun contact is an attempt to maintain the other's body at a safe distance from mine but also to keep the body away from the mind.

THE KINDNESS OF STRANGERS

Sometimes, strange things happen when you open a door or you forget to close it. A gentleman caller may inadvertently catch a glimpse of a naked woman, for example. For Blanche DuBois and her young husband the consequences were just terrible. "There was something different about the boy, a nervousness, a softness and tenderness which wasn't like a man's, although he wasn't the least bit effeminate-looking—still—that thing was there." Poor Blanche couldn't figure out what that "thing" was, "and all I knew was that I'd failed him in some mysterious way and wasn't able to give the help he needed but couldn't speak of!" Until, one day, someone forgot to lock a door. "Then I found out. In the worst of all possible ways. By coming suddenly into a room that I thought was empty—which wasn't empty, but had two people in it." What to do? "Afterward we pretended that nothing had been discovered. Yes, the three of us drove to Moon Lake Casino, very drunk and laughing all the way." There, Blanche finally let it all out, screamed at her young husband, "I saw! I know! You disgust me . . . ," and "the boy" shot himself in the mouth with a revolver—perhaps one of the queerest demises in Western theater since Edward II's impalement.

Silence in *A Streetcar Named Desire* is not of the tactful kind but stems instead from the inability of its characters to put homosexuality into words or to decipher its codes when disclosed obliquely. Yet tact—the delicate balance of touch and distance—is all that Blanche seems to be asking from others, including the audience. "Handle me with care, I'm so delicate," she tells us in essence. "Treat me with the kindness I should have given the boy but didn't." Is it then to atone for her lack of tact that she ended up absorbing the very qualities of her dead husband—vulnerability, softness, tenderness, even nervousness?

That the character of Blanche DuBois should be read as a homosexual man—or rather as the transfer of unspeakable homosexuality onto the visible body of a woman—is not a new idea, especially to generations of gay men for whom this has never been even an "idea," really, but a no-brainer and a lifeline. By that I mean a form of vital if fragile contact not just with the character of Blanche but, through her, among gay men themselves. As was the case with those three films about film, a collective dynamic may emerge at the periphery of society by embracing the discarded. By reencoding herself as a homosexual man Blanche encodes within the text a meaning that, at the time, it was safer not to state too explicitly, namely, that the "desire" of the title is (also) a homosexual one and that it deserves the kindness of the strangers who see or read the play. That this simple message should be embodied by a madwoman who gets taken away to a lunatic asylum at the end of the story may now sound understandably dated and depressing to some. Be that as it may, I prefer to see it as recognition that, once contact has been made, analytic reason fails to account for it. Blanche may be delirious and delusional, but the truth she speaks will not be denied. As a Southern belle, she epitomizes propriety, yet she is also shockingly improper in many ways. In her madness, she externalizes for all to see the mess that rests inside her mind—she embodies it in her words, manners, and actions. What makes the rest of us look sane in comparison is not that our minds aren't messy— they are—but that we have enough sense not to show it. We keep our doors safely locked. But as we do so, we shut ourselves off from the kindness of strangers.

SUNDAY IN THE PARK WITH . . . ?

The small, wooded section of New York's Central Park known as the Rambles is a notorious cruising spot and has been so for a very long time. This is where Andrew Holleran first met O. on a beautiful Sunday afternoon in the 1970s. In 1985, O. has AIDS, and the city has become a very different place. Andrew is back in town and calls on O. How, Andrew wonders, can he properly express his friendship for O.?

> I wondered as we sat talking if I should, or could, tell O. how much I admired and liked him—but to do this seemed artificial and awkward. So I wondered if he knew without my saying so. And I began to think of Proust's aunts. In *Remembrance of Things Past*, the narrator's two aunts are so horrified at the idea of thanking Swann for the wine he brings them one day—thanking him in an obvious way, that is—that they ignore it altogether, until, shortly before Swann leaves, they slip in a reference to the gift so subtle that only the narrator realizes they are acknowledging the wine, so oblique that Swann leaves oblivious of their gratitude. I sat there thinking O. had given me wine, too—in this very room—a lot of wine, a lot of laughter, a lot of wit, conversation, happiness. But I could no more refer to it than Proust's aunts could draw attention to Swann's present. Even worse, I didn't want to thank O. for giving me anything; I wanted to thank him for being. . . . And there was certainly no way I could phrase that. So I left. I left O. twenty minutes before his own departure to visit a doctor.

There is such a thing as too much attention, when caring for someone turns into its opposite. Andrew leaves "thinking, *There is no need to stay. That would be too solicitous.*"

Charlotte Delbo: "What can one say to a twenty-year old girl who's dying?"

Andrew Holleran: "I left O.'s block refusing to think this might be our last conversation—who could? And what if? There was *still* nothing to say."

Christopher Davis: ". . . and then without speaking he pulled off his shirt and pushed his pants down to his knees and showed me the dark purple marks on his still-beautiful body. I gasped and shut my eyes and I did not know what to tell him: What do you tell a beautiful young man who thinks life is the proverbial banquet with no end in sight and who finds out he has been condemned to death? Even now I cannot answer that question."

Roland Barthes: "The courage of discretion / It is courageous not to be courageous."

The impossibility to express certain things with words doesn't mean, however, that, confronted with extreme horror and injustice, one can only be stunned into silence. There exist other ways, as Carmen found out. As for Andrew, he starts heading for the park, "the sites of those strolls, those springs, those conversations whose jokes now seemed to have occurred in another language." The sun doesn't shine as brightly as it did that day in the seventies when Andrew first met O., but still, a man follows him and the familiar dance begins anew: "I looked back, and we began to circle." The wordless encounter that follows doesn't exactly go without saying. Earlier in *Ground Zero*, Holleran had described how gay interaction in the city had been transformed by AIDS: "His friends were dying; my friends were dying; and New York was merely a place where one went to funerals and avoided the eyes of other men on the street—at least, in our generation." Yet life must go on in the city, gay life must go on, contact must be made, and sex with strangers must happen. In this case, "we said nothing; I unbuttoned his shirt and ran my hands on his body; he turned away moments later and ejaculated into the air; zipped up, walked off, and disappeared from the park—without saying a word. All the way home the city seemed pervaded by silence." To turn away and ejaculate safely registers here as a sign of care for the other but also as a reminder of times when contacts were more direct, more involved perhaps. As for the silence that extends from the encounter in the park to the rest of the city, it doesn't deny reality but, on the contrary, acknowledges with tact the ravages of the epidemic—if not for the anonymous man then, at least, for the narrator and the readers. In this scene, silence is not empty, it is filled with death and mourning. It tells something about the truth of AIDS and does so with great eloquence.

THE YELLOW STAR

The yellow star may very well be the most violent form of disclosure ever designed. When, in the early years of the AIDS crisis, the right-wing author William F. Buckley (first) proposed that HIV-positive gay men be forced by law to have their serostatus tattooed on their buttocks, the parallel with Nazi anti-Semitism wasn't lost on activists. It should come as no surprise, then, that once again I look a few decades back for ways to make do and for pointers on how to move from distress and anger to more subtle ways of engaging the world around me.

Hélène Berr was a musician and a student of English literature at the Sorbonne during the Occupation. She was also Jewish. Between 1942 and 1944, she kept a diary that was published in France in 2008 and translated into English that same year. Arrested, deported, Berr was murdered in Bergen-Belsen. Like all diaries with tremendous literary value, hers is at once ordinary and extraordinary. I focus here on a few brief scenes that directly evoke the impact, on herself and on those around her, of the yellow star the Nazis forced her to wear—a shock that makes the extraordinary intrude on the ordinary and redraws the contours of the speakable.

At first, Hélène wears the star with defiance, the only way she knows how to gather up the courage to go out in public. She stares at people; they look away, or not at all:

> I was very courageous all day long. I held my head high, and I stared at other people so hard that it made them avert their eyes. But it's difficult.
>
> In any case, most people don't even look. The awkwardest thing is to meet other people wearing it. This morning I went out with Maman. In the street two boys pointed at us [nous ont montrées du doigt] and said: "Eh? You seen that? Jew." Otherwise things went normally. . . . I went back to place de l'Etoile on the métro on my own. At Etoile I went back to the *Artisanat* to get my blouse, then I went to catch the 92. At the stop there was a young man and woman in the line, and I saw the girl point me out to her companion. Then they exchanged some remarks.

Everything seems redefined, and encounters once seamlessly woven into the familiar fabric of everyday life now signify exclusion from it: the sight of other Jews, the impropriety of children, the complicity of young couples.

And although no mention is made of this, even the word *Etoile* (star) conveys how tainted Parisian life has become in its very cityscape. A word that would have gone unnoticed not long before startles us now.

The following day, Hélène meets Molinié, a fellow student, at the Sorbonne. He behaves as if nothing were wrong and talks about normal student business. Recognizing his friend's touchiness about her predicament, Molinié decides not to touch on the subject of the star at all. This is without a doubt a gesture of sympathy and a kind of contact in its own right, but that's just it: what would have been an ordinary conversation in regular circumstances and would not, in all likelihood, have made its way into a diary has become a meaningful gesture that denies the casualness it flaunts. The ostensible absence of gesture is the gesture. The ordinary, once unspoken as such if it is to retain its ordinariness, must now be underlined to oppose the extraordinary that is the yellow star; the extraordinary, once the source of endless speech (gloss, interpretation, conjectures . . .) must now remain unspoken:

> I got to the main courtyard of the Sorbonne on the stroke of 2:00. I thought I saw Molinié in the crowd, but as I wasn't sure it was him I went into the hall at the library. It was him; he came over to me. He spoke very kindly, but his eyes drifted away from my star. When he looked at me, he looked up [au-dessus de ce niveau], and our eyes seemed to be saying: "Don't take any notice." He'd just sat his second philosophy paper.

The moral high ground (*au-dessus de ce niveau*) that Hélène and Molinié take by means of silence (or: the high ground that each one may take thanks to the other's tact) is compromised from the outset. What their eyes are saying is that what goes ostensibly unnoticed is noticed. The same goes with other students: "We talked about the exam, but I could feel that all their thoughts were on this badge [insigne]." The word *insigne*, we know, implies remarkability.

Language use thus becomes displaced. As is often the case, what it states and what it conveys do not coincide, and the studied casualness of a conversation simultaneously veils and unveils something phatic: the purpose is to make contact in the face of a political order that prohibits it:

> My confidence got a boost at the Department. Obviously I created a stir when I came in, but as everyone there knows . . . no one was

embarrassed. Monique Ducret, who is so sweet, was there, and she talked with me at length, deliberately—I know how she thinks; then the boy called Ibalin turned around . . . and gave a start when he saw, but made a show of coming over [il s'est approché ostensiblement] and joining the conversation (we were talking about music). It didn't matter what the subject was; the main thing was to display[de faire comprendre] the unspoken friendship that connects us.

One could argue that the topic does matter in this case, for the silent bond that ties these young people together, their "unspoken friendship," their tact, constitutes a form of social music making. More on this soon.

Later in the diary—the year is now 1943—Hélène confronts a fundamental dilemma touching on the limits of tact as contact. Sometimes, one must tell. But can one tell without individualizing what is by definition a collective experience, without denying the experience in the process of representing it? At the university again, Hélène faces this question with another student:

Yesterday at the Sorbonne I had a talk with one of my very nice classmates, Mme Gibelin. There was an abyss of ignorance between us. However, I believe that if she knew, she would feel the same anguish as I do. That's why I was terribly wrong not to make a real effort to tell her everything, to shock her, to make her understand. . . . It's just that that brings you up against a serious problem: human nature is such that people only understand if you present immediate evidence, evidence which concerns *you*; they aren't upset by stories of other people, only about *your* personal fate. You only succeed in creating a little understanding by describing the misfortunes that have befallen you yourself. And then? I realize with disgust that I have become the center of interest, while the only thing that matters is the torture others are experiencing; it's a question of principle, it's the thousands of individual cases that make up this question; horrified, I see that the person I am talking to pities me (pity is much easier to get than understanding, for that requires the gift of one's whole being and a complete reconsideration of oneself [une adhésion de tout son être, une révision totale de lui-même]).

Here Hélène is bringing out the fundamental difference between autobiography, a form of individualizing and distancing, and bearing witness, a mode of relating and remaking the world that inscribes the self within the collective and the collective within the self. With this particular classmate, the community of tact—what I call contact—is not working because it does not entail a rethinking of the self as inherently plural.

"How to escape this dilemma?" asks Hélène. "There are very few souls sufficiently generous and noble to face the issue itself [la question en soi], without seeing the person telling the tale as an individual case, and to see through that person the suffering of others." The phrase "la question en soi" implies a depersonalization of the Holocaust and, therefore, the recognition of its collective dimension. Can we read it as "the question in oneself"? There is no indication that Berr intended to suggest this other meaning so directly, but she does evoke the fact that an ideal listener must possess the ability to imagine himself or herself as other:

> Souls like that must be endowed with great intelligence, and also
> great *sensitivity*, because seeing is not sufficient; you have to be able
> to feel, you have to feel the anguish of a mother whose children
> have been taken away from her, the torture of a wife separated from
> her husband, the huge stock of courage that every deportee is going
> to need every day, and the physical suffering and misfortunes that
> he must endure.

Whereas Mme Gibelin "reads" Hélène naively, not perceiving the enormity of the situation, the ideal interlocutor seems to have an elusive sense of discernment and intelligence. This ability resembles reading because it presupposes figuration and the understanding that the part—the individual—stands for a much larger whole. If a sympathetic but literal reading can be a form of denying ("seeing is not sufficient"), to recognize that there is a metonymy at work pluralizes the individual case by connecting it to others. The empathetic feeling Berr describes signals that contact has been established and that the awareness of internal pluralism, or self-otherness, has been transmitted to the interlocutor via the act of bearing witness. The blend of "intelligence" and "sensitivity" that combines the intellectual and affective meanings of "understanding" is precisely what links witnessing and tact. Far from excluding Hélène as a token other—a Jew who stands for other Jews but would still stand apart from non-Jews—empathy places otherness within the self, pluralizing the individual *en soi*.

Sartre recalls how people who were once forced to wear a yellow star in public often felt harmed by other people's marks of sympathy, charitable gestures that looked suspiciously self-serving and only made matters worse by objectifying them as Jews. Acknowledging that embarrassment goes both ways and speaking in the name of those Gentiles who recognized the paradox of ostensible sympathy, Sartre writes:

> In the end we came to understand all this so well that we turned our eyes away when we met a Jew wearing a star. We were ill at ease, embarrassed by our own glance, which, if it fell upon him, made him a Jew in spite of himself and in spite of ourselves. The supreme expression of sympathy and of friendship lay here in appearing to ignore, for whatever effort we made to reach to the *person*, it was always the *Jew* whom we encountered.

And the body reappears, for this Jew is the one produced by racial anti-Semitism, whose strategy was to make emancipated Jews visible again in order to make them radically invisible by way of extermination. The yellow star is the mark of this reembodiment. This definition of Jews as radical others is what Sartre seeks to reject here, yet his use of the first-person plural seems at odds with his stated goal. Who is this "we" he speaks of in "we came to understand all this so well"? The community it outlines and that, by definition, does not include star-wearing Jews, seems endowed with, indeed defined by, a binding sense of discernment. But because it stems from embarrassment, this kind of understanding is not analytic but affective in nature. Sartre seems unaware that what he is describing here is the kind of magical tact he denounces a few pages later and that his "we" bears a disturbing resemblance to the one fantasized by anti-Semites. Obviously, this cannot be what he had in mind.

Tactful silence is another kind of statement—*un silence qui en dit long*, a silence that says a lot. I explained how tactful silence is often used for policing purposes. However, one of the things silence is saying in the situation Sartre describes is this: The tactor's glance, the glance by which one is able to feel the situation as a whole and exercise power, is itself altered, or redirected, by the other's embarrassment. What was intended to bring a feeling of naturalness and belonging becomes instead a source of discomfort, alienation, and discordance; or rather, it is revealed to have always been so. The key lay not in ignoring the situation but in "appearing to ignore" it, since to know when to look away presupposes that one has already seen and understood. True friendship may come at that price: embracing artifice, in this case, experiencing oneself as other—a form of distance from reality that may feel (or sound) false but is an effect of figuration.

Tact, whether as statement or absence of statement, is an experience of alienation by means of trope—less a figure of speech than a figure of thought perhaps, but based on figuration all the same: what it conveys does not coincide with what it states. If we understand Fabienne's note as a parable, then it doesn't just tell a story of tact, it is a tactful story. This, in short, is why tact isn't natural but cultural: like irony, it is an utterance effect and, therefore, occurs only in what Goffman would call a situation of copresence. It may not be, however, a rhetorical tool of persuasion; that would imply reducing the possibility of noise or interpretive errors. To make sure that one's tactful statement or act is "properly" understood as such would be, well, tactless. To recognize that a statement is tactful implies that we can contrast it with at least another, tactless statement. Fabienne's story, by opposing tact to mere politeness, makes this explicit. In other words, in every tactful utterance, tactlessness is indexed and there somehow, if only as a trace, as soon as one recognizes that it is a tactful utterance.

Ideally, tact should be understood as a poetic trope whose readability leaves room for multiple interpretations and maintains the tactee's agency and freedom not to see the tactor as tactful. In short, empathetic tact must contain the possibility of the tactor's own tactical erasure. (Tact and tactics are not etymologically related, by the way, and that's really too bad.) A Gentile tactfully pretending not to notice a yellow star on the chest of a Jew runs the risk of being misread as indifferent or worse (assuming that in this context "indifferent" and "worse" are not the same thing). But that is the price to pay—except for the fact that tact-as-its-own-erasure falls precisely outside any dynamic of exchange. It is a present that is never present but that one cannot refuse without acknowledging it. While always situational, tact can never present itself as tact without self-destructing. (In that sense, it evokes the gift that ceases to be a gift the moment it creates an obligation, as Derrida has shown.) "True" tact, because it must remain unacknowledged, is thus purely relational. It does not even produce identities, which, like selves, emerge only from mutual recognition. In the absence of any stable object of knowledge, then, all that remains is empathy itself, that is, the pure play of relationality between the people involved—what I called acknowledgment. Tact-as-policing, however, seeks to silence others under the pretext of respecting their privacy. In that case, if saying the right thing still means saying the wrong thing, enforcement of class privilege is the "right thing" and social exclusion the "wrong thing,"

TACT AS SOCIAL MUSIC MAKING

Here's another example, from Hervé Guibert's AIDS memoir, *The Compassion Protocol* (*Le protocole compassionnel*). One day, the narrator enters a neighborhood café where he has been a regular customer for ten years, often having a cup of coffee at the counter, even though the waiters have always seemed hostile to him, presumably out of homophobia. Hervé, ill and extremely frail, trips on the doorstep and falls to his knees, unable to muster enough strength to get back up on his feet. The other customers are staring at him: he has committed a literal faux pas and feels like a burn the social death of the fallen. He finds himself in an uncomfortable position—again, literally—and is making onlookers uncomfortable as well, this time metaphorically. Contamination is the source of discomfort, and this includes the contamination of the literal by the figural.

Something happens then that Hervé did not expect:

> Not a single word was uttered, and there was no need for me to ask for help, for one of the two waiters I had always thought to be an enemy came up to me, took me in his arms and put me on my feet again [me remettre sur pied] *as if it were the most natural thing in the world*. I avoided the other customers' eyes, and the man behind the counter simply asked: "Coffee, sir?" I feel deeply grateful towards those two waiters I'd never liked and who I thought detested me, for having reacted so spontaneously and with such tact [délicatesse], without a single unnecessary word.

Notice that Hervé is the one looking away. As was the case with Berr, it is difficult—and probably unnecessary—to determine whether he is trying to shield himself from the gazes of others or treating their own discomfort with tact. Regarding the waiter's gesture, when Guibert writes "as if it were the most natural thing," he underscores a fundamental aspect of tact-as-policing: that it is not natural but must appear so in order to stay out of reach of those it singles out for exclusion. But in this particular scene, the waiters' tact testifies to their professionalism. Whether they actually hate Hervé doesn't matter. What does matter is that their professionalism allows the two men neither to enforce nor to erase their power over Hervé, but only to deflect it without singling him out. By doing so, they maintain their difference from him—they are waiters; he is a customer—but it is a difference that rests on the codependency of the two social positions.

(I don't know what the German translation of the text looks like, but the verb *aufheben*, all at once, to pick up, to abolish and to keep, would fit nicely.) So when the first waiter proceeded to *ease* Hervé back up, he may have wished to conjure away the latter's *dis-ease* and the customers' *malaise*, but Hervé perceived his professional distance as an act of community occurring within the delicate, ephemeral parameters of a specific situation.

When Hervé realizes that he cannot get back up on his feet, the verb used in the original French is *relever*. (*Relève*, incidentally, is the French translation of the Hegelian *Aufhebung*.) And *relever* is what the waiter eventually does to Hervé. The word offers interesting possibilities. Its English cognate, "to relieve," reminds us that the verb means "to alleviate suffering," which is what both waiters do with regard to his body as well as to his feelings. Indeed, the expression *remettre sur pied* may mean "to be back up on one's feet," but its more idiomatic sense suggests restoring someone's well-being, be it physical or psychological. Furthermore, *relever* almost means "to notice," a dual meaning that may also be found, conveniently enough, in the English "to pick up"—as in "to pick something up" and "to pick up on something," something that is presumably *relevant*. That too is what the waiters do: they pick up on what what's happening and one of them picks Hervé up. With their professional casualness, they bring him *relief* by treating the whole incident as ultimately *irrelevant*. This doesn't mean, obviously, that AIDS is irrelevant, or Hervé's suffering, but that what happened to him does not pertain (*ne relève pas*) to any essential inferiority. If the policing mission of tact is to make certain people irrelevant, in some cases it is the police itself that is no longer relevant.

Throughout the book, Hervé also praises the professionalism of some doctors and nurses and often does so by emphasizing their linguistic restraint. By contrast, he fires the well-meaning doctor who tells him, "I understand," a tactless statement in this French middle-class context because it is read as condescending. He soon replaces him with one "who never utters one word more or less than is necessary." The professional distance of the second doctor appears more beneficial to Hervé than the sincere but misguided sympathy of the first.

The corporeal nature of medical relationships reminds us that tact is touch and the tactful tactile. Soon after telling us how the waiter took him in his arms, Hervé describes a similar, albeit more expected, gesture from his masseur: "I'm so knocked out after each session that my muscles no longer respond, and I always have to put my arms around the masseur's neck."

After describing their sessions as a shared struggle, he adds: "That was the contract we embarked upon every Wednesday afternoon, between three and six, again without uttering one unnecessary word [un mot de trop]." The masseur's professionalism, as that of the waiters, links the studied withdrawal of language to a physical embrace, embodying the etymological link between the two and suggesting that tact, a sign of social dexterity, may also be contact, the tactful tactual. What was made to appear intangible (what cannot be touched) is in fact contingent (contextual, sometimes fortuitous, and a matter of contact and physical proximity). We thus begin to glimpse a form of relationality established by means of touch. Tactful community, it appears, rests on what in French is called *doigté* (the ability to handle delicate situations), whereas tact as a tool of social exclusion is a way to *montrer du doigt* (to point a finger).

The use of the word *tact* to describe social discernment and quick judgment starts to appear in the eighteenth century in the writings of Voltaire, Montesquieu, Diderot, and other Enlightenment philosophers. Until then, one of its dominant meanings, along with the older sense of "touch," was that of the German *Takt*, meaning beat or pulse, a musical term that referred to the organizing beat that the master of music would bang on the floor with a stick—what is known as "marking time." At the same time as taste (whose probable etymological kinship with tact, via a frequentative form of *tangere*, is still seen in *tâter* and the improvisational, bricolage-type version of analytic reason known as *tâtonner*, to grope, as if in darkness) saw its meaning shift from the strictly gustatory to encompass aesthetic judgment, tact went through a similar metaphorical turn.

An anecdote that Goethe recounts in his *Travels to Italy* seems to dramatize (in hindsight, of course) the transition from one meaning to the other. The year is 1786 and the poet finds himself in Venice. He makes his way to the Church of the Mendicanti, which houses the city's conservatory. There he attends a concert in which women sing an oratorio behind the church's grating. The event is almost perfect, save for one irritating detail— the clash between two meanings of the word *tact*:

> The performance would have been a source of great enjoyment, if
> the accursed *Maestro di Capella* had not beaten time [den Takt],
> with a roll of music, against the grating, as conspicuously as if
> he had to do with schoolboys whom he was instructing. As the
> girls had rehearsed the piece often enough, his noise was quite

unnecessary, and destroyed all impression, as much as he would, who, in order to make a beautiful statue intelligible to us, should stick scarlet patches on the joints. The foreign sound [Der fremde Schall] destroys all harmony. Now, this man is a musician, and yet he seems not to be sensible of this; or, more properly speaking, he chooses to let his presence be known by an impropriety [unschicklichkeit], when it would have been much better to allow his value to be perceived by the perfection of the execution.

By refusing to efface himself graciously in favor of an indirect, more subtle perception of the music—and of his own talent—the hapless conductor condescends to the singers as well as to the audience and commits an act of tactlessness. The sound he makes by beating time is "foreign" to the music and constitutes an "impropriety," and these two words suggest that he doesn't belong, somehow, to either of the two groups—the singers and the audience—whom he is mediating. Clearly, the harmony the poor man is destroying is social and historical as well as musical. He is supposed to be marking time but, by emphasizing musical tact the way one would have in the old days, he contravenes the new social tact. He may very well be beating the rhythm perfectly, but it matters very little in the end. He is simply out of sync with the times, an embarrassingly obsolete creature at a moment of great historical upheaval. Our master of music is all but deaf to what is happening around him, both socially and historically. What he does is out of place, what he is, is out of time. Naturally, I find him endearing.

In his memoirs, Hector Berlioz recounts a similar episode taking place in the 1830s during a concert at the Teatro San Carlo in Naples. After offering his somewhat condescending praise for the orchestra, the French composer notes how "supremely" irritated he felt at what he judged to be the *maestro di capella*'s lack of delicacy in the way he loudly beat time on the music stand ["le bruit souverainement désagréable de son archet dont il frappe un peu rudement son pupitre"]. Being told that without such heavy-handedness, the musicians would have a difficult time following the beat, he goes on to blame Italy's lack of sophistication in relation to its neighbors, "for in a country where instrumental music is more or less unknown, orchestras the like of which are found in Berlin, Dresden and Paris would be too much to expect." Italy, it would seem, had remained stuck in its old musical ways, which Berlioz experienced as a lack of manners.

Moving from the corporeal to the subjective, this shift in the meaning of tact during the period pertains to the larger disembodiment and abstraction of Enlightenment's Man occurring in the period. Forms of togetherness involving sensing bodies that did things together (eating, playing music) moved away from contingent copresence and made way for disembodied classes based on transcendent, universal reason. One can, however, lure tact away from its police duties, as I have been doing, and reclaim it for a radical undoing of the Cartesian mind—body dualism that underlies the metaphorical turns I describe. Those that tact excluded for their supposed inability to transcend and abstract their own bodies would have much to gain from this operation. The idea, of course, is not to reclaim reason in the name of the powerless but to reembody the abstract, to touch reason and remind it of its denied corporeality.

This, I believe, is what we see in the writings of Delbo, Berr, and Guibert. There was, remember, Delbo's dissonant question to a dying comrade, and Hélène and her friends talking about music to oppose the yellow star. With more levity, there was Fabienne's question: "Do you like music, Antoine?" There is also the following remark of Guibert's, encompassing nearly all the issues at stake. After having initially gone through a particularly painful fibroscopic exam, which he compared to torture, the narrator describes a second procedure in very different terms: "The alveolar lavage, unlike the first nightmarish fibroscopy, and despite the barbarity of the act itself, became, thanks to the delicacy and lightness of touch [grâce au doigté et à la délicatesse] of a young woman doctor and two nurses, almost a medical string quartet in which I was the fourth instrument playing in complicity with the other three." The barbarity he speaks of lies in the violent treatment by a person in authority of a human being reduced to being a body. Ernaux's hospital experience after the abortion was of the same nature. In the contexts of catastrophic illness and genocide, this reduction of humans to their bodies *is* the barbarity from which all others stem, but it is one that finds its source in the rise of disembodied reason as the basis for citizenship. Guibert uses words like *doigté* and *délicatesse* in such a way that it is impossible to determine whether we should understand them as literal or metaphorical, hence the difficulty of translating them. But that's the whole point. Being a homosexual dying of AIDS in the face of political indifference, not unlike being marked for racial extermination, makes it impossible to escape one's own embodiment. What we read in this passage is an assertion of community as a form of social music making in the context of mass death. This is not, however, like the band of the *Titanic*, playing on as the ship sinks, or the orchestras established in the Nazi camps, and it cannot be confused with the abstracting kind of aesthetic gesture either, since that would require the expulsion of the body. Quite the contrary, the manifestations of friendship we read here are glimpsed thanks to the reembodiment of tact as con-tact, that is, a recognition that failures, shortcomings, and vulnerability are everyone's lot.

The incongruous spectacle of a young man unable to get back on his feet showcases his failure as much as his vulnerability. That was the late 1980s. Back then, however, doctors and scientists, unable to solve the riddle of AIDS and to come up with effective treatments, were failures too, alienated from their own mission. If the notion of "patients' rights," which began to appear in the 1970s, is commonplace today, one should never forget that few had heard of it until AIDS activists finally imposed it, for the benefit of all, on a medical establishment that was forced to confront its own powerlessness so that the doctor–patient relationship became more like a matter of cooperation. Paradoxically, patients gained much from medicine's shortcomings, as the recognition of shared powerlessness allowed for a more egalitarian redefinition of doctor–patient relations—a community based on difference—and, in turn, made medical progress possible.

The Compassion Protocol, Guibert's second book on his illness, followed the tremendous success of *To the Friend Who Did Not Save My Life* (*A l'ami qui ne m'a pas sauvé la vie*) a year earlier. Up to that point, Guibert had remained a little-known writer with a readership consisting mostly of gay men and whose fame barely exceeded Parisian circles. Now he had to face the thorny question of his relationship with a mainstream audience. Was a kind of community possible with them at all? How could his writing move away from the autobiographical and constitute instead an act of bearing witness? By placing the episode in the café early in a book he knows will meet a broad readership, Guibert may have provided us with an allegory of reading, enjoining us to handle him as the waiters did. Given the fact that dominant French culture considers both sexuality and illness private matters, one is expected to handle them with discretion. When reading Guibert's book we should use tact but also avoid the erasure that often results from French universalism. If tact represents a willing failure of language, a tactful mode of reading would be a way to share in the other's failure by foregrounding one's own—and one's own otherness, since otherness and failure are mutually defining as forms of alienation. In that sense, we may use tact as a basis for community—community *in* difference and community *as* difference.

A FART JOKE FROM PROUST

The character of Charlus, like Proust, who himself owes a lot to Balzac and Flaubert before him, can sometimes turn an unforgiving eye to the faults and lapses of other human beings—or literary creations. One day, for reasons having to do with his own unacknowledged shortcomings—desire, possessiveness, jealousy, and the like—Charlus becomes infuriated by the poor manners of his lover Morel's fiancée and, in the end, by Morel's own lack of class. This is all in bad faith, naturally, since class difference is at the root of Charlus's desire for the young violinist. And this may explain why the Baron explodes with such anger and piles up vulgarity upon vulgarity as he excoriates the musician, playing wittily with the various senses of tact and a rather unpoetic *dérèglement de tous les sens*:

> The tailor's niece having said one day to Morel: "That's all right
> then, come to-morrow and I'll stand you a tea," the Baron had quite
> justifiably considered this expression very vulgar on the lips of a
> person whom he regarded as almost a prospective daughter-in-law,
> but as he enjoyed being offensive and became carried away by his
> own anger, instead of simply saying to Morel that he begged him to
> give her a lesson in polite manners, the whole of their homeward
> walk was a succession of violent scenes. In the most insolent, the
> most arrogant tone: "So your 'touch' which, I can see, is not neces-
> sarily allied to 'tact,' has hindered the normal development of your
> sense of smell, since you could allow that fetid expression 'stand a
> tea'—at fifteen centimes, I suppose—to waft its stench of sewage
> to my regal nostrils? When you have come to the end of a violin
> solo, have you ever seen yourself in my house rewarded with a fart,
> instead of frenzied applause, or a silence more eloquent still, since
> it is due to exhaustion from the effort to restrain, not what your
> young woman lavishes upon you, but the sob that you have brought
> to my lips?"

In the original French version, the envoi of Charlus's tirade ("la peur de ne pouvoir retenir, non ce que votre fiancée nous prodigue, mais le sanglot que vous avez amené au bord des lèvres") is nothing short of outrageous. The play on the verb *retenir* explicitly invokes matters baser than emotions, and I'll let you figure out what the expression *avoir le cigare au bord des lèvres* refers to and why Charlus possibly alludes to it. (I haven't been able to find out when the expression made its lovely entry into French culture, but it sure smells like belle époque to me.) As for the eloquent silence that greets a violin solo, it indexes in the context of Charlus's earlier play on the archaic meaning of tact, what the audience's refined sense of aesthetic judgment owes to the repression of bodily function.

What better way, in fact, to demonstrate someone's hopeless lack of refinement than to liken their social artlessness to their alleged inability to rise above corporeality? Morel's musical talent that, along with serving as Charlus's lover, allowed him to climb up the social ladder is cruelly referred to as his "touch." Playing with semantic instability like a cat with a terrorized mouse wondering whether it shall live or die, the Baron means to remind Morel of his lover's precarious situation. Will the young musician and his "touch" fall back into lower-class bodily recesses whence they came or rise to aesthetic and social heights? Who's to know? Ambivalence also defines Charlus, since his desire for Morel's physical touch must, in high society, appear masked by an interest in his musical one.

TOUCH AND OTHER SENSES

In classical Western thought, touch is often presented as the most basic of all senses, the fertile humus, the original indifferentiation from which the others may grow and separate themselves from the rest. Touch stands as the opposite of sight that way. If the former remains firmly on the ground, the latter flies way, way up there alongside the stars. Touch is of the body, sight of the soul.

As I unearth tact's older meaning of touch—the meaning it had before sight became the dominant sense, the one above all others—I do not advocate a return to some sort of original plenitude, when all five senses were supposedly integrated and they provided a holistic apprehension of the world. I don't believe that such full incorporation ever existed anywhere at any time, only that people have conceptualized and experienced the interrelation of the senses in many different ways. I thus want to make it clear that tact, reembodied but still social, is inseparable from sight. I also try to restore tact's musical meaning and, with it, the aural dimension it possessed when the so-called lowest and most corporeal of all the senses stood in proximity to the so-called highest and most abstract of all the arts. And we know that it is etymologically related to taste. What matters is the play of the senses, not some illusory, and politically dubious, fusion of them.

IMMODESTY

Between June 1990 and March 1991, at the request of a television producer, Hervé Guibert filmed his daily life with a camcorder. The outcome was a film titled *Modesty or Immodesty* (*La pudeur ou l'impudeur*), one that, despite its author's best efforts, was broadcast only after his death. The film is at once moving and disturbing in many ways, as the title intimates. What are we to make of the blunt spectacle of a young man dying of AIDS? Was Guibert an exhibitionist, as so many of his detractors and quite a few of his fans have contended? The film does contain several scenes centered on his naked, wasted body, and they are tough to take. A shower scene, in particular, hides very little of the ravages of the illness and, like most images of people wasting away, these also show, in a sense, what is no longer there. Guibert's directness, it seemed, could incite either morbid fascination or utter rejection on the part of viewers.

In one very brief scene near the beginning of the movie, for instance, we catch a glimpse of Hervé defecating. He has left the door open, and we can see him sitting on the toilet in one of these small French WC's, naked, his head in his hands and his elbows on his knees—an odd variation on Rodin's *Thinker*. The artistic dimension of the image is emphasized by the way Hervé's body is framed. He has positioned the camera at such an angle that a funnel-like structure of white doors and hallways directs our gaze straight at him. There is basically nothing else to see, no way for us to deflect our gaze or pretend to do so.

Later on in the movie, we encounter an almost identical repetition of that scene. In the second one, Hervé has just gotten dressed and prepares to go out. Taken with a sudden bout of diarrhea, he "rushes" to the bathroom. (I use quotation marks here because he obviously found the time to position the camcorder and start the recording.) This time, however, he isn't naked and we hear the sound of his bowel movement, but the picture is framed exactly like the first one and Hervé sits in the same position, framed like a painting, posing like a sculpture—*The Shitter*.

As is the case with the three films about film, both scenes foreground the act of viewing, problematizing it in the way these movies do, but, thanks to its visual references to high art rather than trash, raising more direct questions about modern aesthetics. The open door hints at our possible voyeurism, of course, just as it does at Guibert's exhibitionism. But the funnel-like construction of the images amplifies and thus brings attention to the single-viewer perspective of post-Renaissance art. At the same time, foregrounding the frame emphasizes the fact that we are indeed looking at a carefully constructed picture and that we the viewers stand outside it. The image magnifies the supposedly unbridgeable distance between subject and object of the gaze and reveals its naturalness as an effect of representation itself. Indeed, right after the shower scene and with a similar doubling effect, Hervé's voice-over describes the daily act of looking at his own nakedness in the mirror, as we are watching him doing just that. The result is troubling. If we are both looking at him, he and I are essentially standing side by side, contiguous rather than at a safe objectifying distance.

Immediately following the second diarrhea scene with one of a routine hospital appointment, Guibert establishes a stark visual (and political) connection between aesthetics and medicine, as if to remind his audience that the two are endowed with the same power to objectify and expel. If he is to make contact with us, then, he must avoid amplifying the exclusionary outcome of these two modern forms of viewership. The question is "How?" Is it enough to exaggerate and denaturalize? Guibert cannot make contact all on his own. This can be achieved only with our assent. All he can do is make contact possible—leave doors open and open up potentialities. Where the three films opposed modern aesthetics by urging their audience to move away from what passes for beauty, Guibert's film, in a way, asks us to approach and touch what reason and our better judgment tell us to repel. What happens next is up to us, and it will depend largely on how we react to the discomfort we are bound to feel when a social boundary has been breached and we find ourselves confronted so directly with "objects" that our traditional notions of taste normally shun.

But even though French culture tends to see terminal illness and uncontrolled bodily functions as private matters, looking at them doesn't automatically entail transgression. In a medical movie, for example, or in a "tell-all" kind of documentary, both AIDS and diarrhea may be, if not pleasant, perfectly watchable, and their watchability results from the genres that frame the images for us. What exactly we would see, though, is a different matter. By embedding the act of looking in the structure of the image, Guibert makes it possible for us to question the way we watch and, by doing so, he asks us to see. We may lean toward Hervé and fulfill our end of the cont(r)act, or we may play it safe and move away. We still have that freedom. And if we opt for the latter, two options are offered us: radical disgust and disembodied aestheticization, which stand, each in their own way, as the (always failing) refusal of contiguity or nearness, that is to say, of contact.

That disgust, as I alluded to earlier, is a reflex of exclusion would seem to go without saying. But beyond the obvious, what defines this most emotional of emotions is also its fusion of all senses into some sort of impregnable fortress. Disgust isn't exclusionary only because it pertains to repulsion but also, and the two are corollaries, because more than any other affect, perhaps it turns its back on analysis and fuses the self into a perfect, nonrelational entity. Or rather the fiction thereof, which explains why disgust is the "ideal" fascist emotion.

As for disembodied aestheticization, it presupposes the division of the senses into discrete means of cognition. In other words, it relies on the faculty to discern and on the separation of subject and object. It is also concerned with the creation and enjoyment of forms. By contrast, not only does diarrhea evoke the formlessness and the undoing of the self, as do wasting illnesses such as AIDS, but because "form" also refers to acceptable or proper behavior, its absence characterizes immodesty as well. Hervé's body disrupts the power of "the body," especially the nude body, to symbolize (an ideal) and the social order that rests on this transcending operation. What Guibert's images show us, in the end, is a body that is neither form nor formlessness but transformation, and what opens up in the gap between artistic fulfillment and visceral revulsion is the creative possibility of contact itself. This possibility, of course, was always there. Disincorporated aesthetics cannot sever the link to the corporeal sensing of *aesthesis*. As for disgust, it is a reaction, and, as such, it always confirms what it repels. If abstract aesthetics and disgust always fail in the end, it is because they are forms of denial.

The point of contact, on the other hand, is difference embraced as alteration, an ongoing process in itself and for itself. Contact doesn't tend toward a goal to be achieved even if only as a theoretical *telos*. One can only be in contact if we understand it as a perpetually dynamic, relational ontology that all at once makes and unmakes the self. And we can make contact—again and again and again—only if we see this making as making do, a kind of bricolage that always lays itself bare as a process of transformation of what's at hand with no other purpose than to serve, modestly, the needs of the powerless.

REENTERING THE MOVIE THEATER'S RESTROOM

I know, I know, you've probably had your fill of such tasteless matters, but it'll only take a minute, I promise.

A scene in John Rechy's *Numbers* evokes the link between the old, musical meaning of *Takt* and the possibility of contact in the present opened up thanks to the return of the past. It gives the impression that the quest for contact had led to the rediscovery of ancient meanings, unearthed alive, active, productive into the present. Former hustler Johnny—you've met him before—makes his way into the theater following a somewhat disjointed, yet discernible, rhythm: "He knows all this is a matter of marking time, because: already he's walking up the stairs. But he stops suddenly . . . pauses . . . descends—starts hurriedly to walk toward the exit, decides not to leave, and goes down the stairs toward the head instead."

The past reemerges suddenly, reminding us that the archaic practice of impersonal sex finds its home in an obsolete setting and that contact between past and present is as simple a matter as leaving a door open:

> Quite probably this theater once housed elaborate productions—
> vaudeville, perhaps even opera. Its men's lounge has all the tattered
> elegance of such a house—carpets (large chunks missing; like an
> uncompleted jigsaw puzzle), stuffed chairs (lopsided lumps where
> the coils threaten to spring through), even a statue-lamp of a naked
> woman (she's so old-fashioned that she appears curiously clothed).
> Beyond—the door open—is the fluorescent-lighted restroom.

Johnny walks in, and what follows is the familiar dance of cruising and pretending with another patron:

> The man moves over to the urinal immediately next to him. Johnny
> can hear his own heart pumping—rather two hearts, one pumping
> in each ear. . . . He has stood like this before, in toilets of bars and
> bus stations, of Pershing Square—luring interested men by shaking
> his cock before the urinal long after he was through—but only to
> entice, only preparatory to leaving and expecting to be followed,
> propositioned, paid—never consummating the implied contact in
> the restroom, however. But that was three years ago.

The *Takt* Johnny's heart beats in his ears immediately recalls past occurrences and underlies the prelude to contact. Having, for all practical purposes, bypassed the modern phase of disembodiment, the old *Takt* implies, that is to say, contains the social as a pleasurable physical engagement with others. Seemingly obsolete, it still allows people sidelined by modernity to play together without having to rely on the policing operation of autonomous selfhood.

Imagine a woolly mammoth, once frozen and now thawed, prancing around as if nothing happened—a gay woolly mammoth.

TACT AND INTIMATION

When Guibert describes various physical interactions between patient and health care professionals, both in his film and in his books, he touches on the question of pleasure. I say "touches" because intimacy remains mostly intimated here. Tactile interactions provide Hervé with a degree of relief and well-being, and the erotic intimation brings an opportunity to critique the dominant notions of intimacy. Indeed, the concept of intimacy has long been used to produce the modern self as deep, enclosed, privatized, and, as such, the object of "intimate knowledge"—a form of policing. Nowhere is this more obvious than in the medical context. The intimation of pleasure, however, is outward bound and all exteriority. It thus allows Hervé to turn the doctor–patient interaction into something like a real relation by keeping it all on the surface. If intimacy is depth, intimation is nearness.

FOUND OBJECTS (I): TACT AND BEARING WITNESS AS FORMS OF BRICOLAGE

A quick Internet search of "tact" once yielded a curious list of other terms attached to it. I noticed that qualities thought to be directly contiguous with tact roughly fell into two categories. Some referred to deep, somewhat intangible qualities, such as wisdom, forethought, or charisma, that pertain to the tactful person's inner ability to evaluate the situation he or she is facing. The others had more to do with the outer actions or words that are to follow that initial understanding. These words were resourcefulness, ingenuity, imagination, or creativity. Granted, many entries that came up in my search were want ads and job descriptions, but still, taken together, they made up a valuable overview of the way tact functions in the cultural imagination, perhaps even social practices.

When it isn't practiced as part of a larger yet veiled policing project, tact can offer a way to deal with difficult situations by making do with what's handy for the immediate and mutual relief of all involved. Carmen's question to the dying Sylviane, for example, doesn't rest on the overall superiority of the former over the latter. After all, given what the friends were going through together in Auschwitz, the roles could just as well have been reversed. What is also striking in the passage is the fact that Carmen uses, on purpose, a perfectly hackneyed phrase in a context that seems shockingly incommensurate. But a platitude, in a sense, is something easily available to all. Its flat surface conceals no depth. It is simply there, one doesn't have to look for it or wonder who will be able to understand it because everybody will be. Those who have little may then seize on it and reinvest it with a new meaning.

Delbo also tells of the purposefully trivial—but tactful—last words that dying women would often utter so as to remove all momentousness to death and not discourage their friends.

> So you believed that only solemn words rise to the lips of the dying because solemn rhetoric flourishes naturally on deathbeds a bed is always dressed for funeral rites with the family assembled around it sincere pain and the appropriate demeanor.
>   Naked on the charnel house's pallets, almost all our comrades said, "I'm going to kick the bucket."
>   They were naked on a naked board.
>   They were dirty and the boards were soiled with pus and diarrhea.

This use of trivial words, as opposed to grander ones supported by institutions and rituals and designed to maintain societal continuity, also betrays the fact that master discourses had no more currency in Auschwitz, a place where inmates could envision no future beyond the end of the day. The extraordinary delicacy of the dying friends cannot be tied to a system of domination. In truth, it acts against one—Nazism—by tactically inhabiting another, the social conformity of the society they had left behind.

This form of tactful bricolage also characterizes witnessing practices in the face of events so disastrous that they have no transcendence, point to no grand purpose or scheme of things. I mentioned, in this book and elsewhere, how Delbo, in order to appeal to her readers for greater proximity with an experience that will always escape them, makes use of literary clichés, stock images, and shared cultural assumptions, thus establishing common ground while protecting herself (and us) from totalizing knowledge. And in case we miss her point, she makes it clear that the content of these words can no longer be believed and that she uses them only to make contact. These words are rubble, and bearing witness to traumatic events takes place on rubble. It makes use of the remnants of concepts and values no longer in use—at least not for what they were originally intended to do. This requires resourcefulness and ingenuity to make small meanings and sustain small actions in the here and now with discarded bits and pieces of broken ideology, art, culture, institutions, and the like.

If, as Goffman explains, the world becomes broken in the event of social embarrassment—he also calls this event a "false note" and a "dissonance"—we still have the freedom to resist the urge to fix it up and restore it to its old pristine state—to resolve the discordance. We may opt instead to remake the world in a different way. To see tact in its perpetual presentness, in its need to be reinvented each time, is to understand it as a way to make do and make contact within the narrow landscape of a given interaction. In that sense, tact does not give us a way to repair the world as a whole but, rather, to patch things up for a while just so we may live a little better, here, now, together. One could even go as far as saying that there is in fact no such thing as tact, only tactful gestures, and that the process of *sharing* never ends in the resolution of a *shared*. Tact, as a "thing," has no more existence than the emperor's new clothes.

The immediate exhaustion that characterizes tact, should one choose to use it this way, is what prevents its ethics from constituting a moral system, with rules of conduct that turn people into compliant subjects. The ethical question that tact poses may not be "What should I do" but "What should

I not do?" It is less about doing the right thing than not doing the wrong thing. Tact, then, could make up the (inevitably shaky) ground of a kind of negative ethics. This would account for the fact that tact, once reembodied, cannot produce ethical subjects, that is, individuals with depth and interiority whose tactful behavior is to be measured in relation to a norm and constructs them as normalized subjects (or subjugates them). It would be more helpful instead to think in terms of ethical acts, in relation to people, that can be determined only in specific situations that, like dysclosure, can never recur identically. If proper behavior toward others inevitably refers to a set of norms that keep the others at bay and constitutes them as others, to act is to be understood here as to act out, alongside each other, and to perform something like collective personhood. This may then serve the needs of people whose sense of self is momentarily shattered or suspended by situations that unveil their weakness. Tact, then, may figure a form of embodied ethics, to be actualized only in contexts of copresence, which is what makes it particularly useful for dealing with HIV. But instead of repairing the tactee's broken self in a normative fashion, tact as contact allows the tactor to agree to be broken as well—or rather breaking. If I expose my weaknesses, it isn't for all to see but for all to share.

TACTFULNESS TO THE DEAD

Describing a certain Taoist ritual in which the immortals go through a symbolic death and burial to avoid upsetting the world of the merely living, Barthes concludes: "Admirable concern for others, pure tact: to take on the appearance of being dead so as not to shock, hurt, disconcert those who die." This is what he calls "consideration" in both senses of the word.

FOUND OBJECTS (II): SOME BEAUTY

Hervé is on the bus one day, and he notices that the young woman sitting opposite him seems particularly agitated, unnerved by his presence. The telltale sign is that she carefully avoids looking at him, "as if she were asking herself about whether she really had the right to undertake the step she was about to make, about whether it would be interpreted as tact [délicatesse] or rudeness, she was trying to find suitable words, picking them carefully, polishing their expression, even if circumstances should prevent her from ever uttering them." Hervé gets up in preparation for getting off the bus; the woman does the same. Finally, she overcomes her hesitation and speaks out:

> With a subtle smile, full of graciousness and discretion, she said: "You remind me of a very well-known writer. . . ." I replied: "I'm not so sure about the well known. . . ." She: "I've made no mistake. I just wanted to tell you that I find you very handsome." At that moment, without another word, without turning round, she disappeared to the right, and I turned to the left, overwhelmed, grateful, on the brink of tears. Yes, it was necessary to find beauty in the sick, in the dying. Until then I had not accepted such a thing.

We notice once more the economy of language that characterizes the interaction ("without another word") as well as its indirectness. If Hervé is so moved by the encounter it is because he rightfully reads it as an understated gesture of solidarity and kindness. But in the context of a random encounter on a city bus, I was struck by the word "find"—the original French text reads: "je vous trouve très beau" and "il fallait trouver de la beauté aux malades, aux mourants."

Hervé had once been baffled, scandalized even, when his lover and best friend Jules told him he found beautiful an extremely frail Robert Mapplethorpe, so young but looking so old, in the photo that a newspaper had published on its front page after the photographer's death from AIDS. Hervé had erred by remaining within the dominant social viewpoint that equates youth with beauty and beauty with health. The encounter with the young woman on the bus allows him to reconsider this initial reaction and rethink the connection among the three. But how is beauty redefined in a way that Hervé may now embrace? To find beauty, in this passage, doesn't suggest a discovery, as if beauty had always been there, immutable and ready to be revealed as an inescapable truth—quite the contrary. The partitive—

de la beauté, as opposed to *la beauté*—reinforces the smallness, incompleteness, and contingency of beauty here. Some beauty, or some kind of beauty, results from the contact between an "I" and a "you," as the speech act the woman uses—"I just wanted to tell you"—emphasizes. I find you by accident and I find you beautiful; this is the way such things happen in big cities, but the act of telling transforms the encounter into a contact.

Sight hardly seems involved at all here. Hervé's beauty is of the dynamic, not the formal, kind. Like Mapplethorpe in that picture, he is near death and both he and his beauty are passing. His body is not the earthly vessel of an ideal that, as such, must remain inaccessible, but the locus of social relations enacted by means of touch (or in this case something like touch: contact), and Hervé is touched by it. The fact that the participants in the encounter each go their separate ways in the end and will in all likelihood never meet again—they meet on a bus and were going somewhere else—emphasizes that transitoriness is what it's all about. What makes the woman's reaction tactful in a way that doesn't police and exclude Hervé is that her gesture doesn't seek to restore any kind of social order or aesthetic harmony—the visible form as an expression of an ideal—but rather to maintain incongruity, that of a young man near death on a bus and the unexpected encounter between an author and a reader, as an effect of context and relationality. (Given the fact that the scene wasn't witnessed by a third party, it is true that there was little incentive for the woman to exclude Hervé for the purpose of class-based bonding. I believe, however, that the third party need not be actually present and that he or she may be simply imagined—or postponed, if one were later to tell the story of "how I behaved with tact.") Interestingly enough, the woman's simple words, "I just wanted to tell you," echo the ones that often precede a disclosure. It is as if she sought to mirror the very act that had suddenly made Guibert "a very well-known writer," as if, in addition to praising his success and beauty, she took on some of the social marginalization that disclosures always presuppose. This, in essence, is what I meant earlier by the phrase "compatible discordance." Beyond HIV, tact may serve as a general model for a poetic form of reading the social and dealing with others—a form of contact with people one fails fully to comprehend. We may go down different streets in the end, but that doesn't mean we can't touch each other. That's why we have streets. And metro stations, where those who have fallen on hard times may play music to make a small living.

Contact

LEAVING THE DOOR OPEN

On Wednesday, May 24, 2006, at three o'clock in the afternoon, my life unexpectedly became a huge and shocking mess. Since then, it has gradually transformed into a small, slow-burning chaos. "You should write about this," my friend Testuya suggested the day I told him. I laughed. "What's there to write? I'm HIV positive. It sucks. Then what?" Thinking about a chronic disease, I now feel I have written a text that is itself ill, like a mad book about confusion, and I'm tired. I imagined that with my life in shambles I'd fit at last into a chaotic world or, if this too failed, that there might be a chance at hand for me to move closer and about, without the fear of falling right into the gaps I'd been trying to bridge. But shreds and shards make for an odd sort of normalcy. Not a big surprise there, I guess, and I didn't start this book in the hope that it would help me recapture some illusory cohesion or paradise lost I never possessed to begin with. What, I wondered, does it feel like to be HIV positive in a world at war? Uneventful is the answer. I have HIV and that's that. Like the tiny tinny sound seeping from someone's earphones as they listen to MP3s, with the voices screaming in one person's ears all but inaudible to other people standing right next to them, I blend into the surrounding noise, not undetectable so much as undetected. So I'll just turn in now, throw in the towel. I'll leave the door open, though. Just because I prefer to stay at a distance doesn't mean I'm out of sight or out of touch, quite the contrary. I won't come out, but by all means let yourself in. Or, if you prefer, we can slow dance at the doorstep, sway with the sensuous rhythm and draw little circles as our bodies mingle and tangle ever more tightly to the music we make, cruising on a slow boat to China.

THE UNEXPECTED CODA: MAY 24, 2011

Osama bin Laden is still dead and I'm still HIV positive. Lucky me. As I'm completing the first draft of my manuscript, I'm looking back on five years. I, America, and many people around the world are heading toward the tenth anniversary of 9/11 and of the invasion of Afghanistan.

A couple of weeks ago I was back in my doctor's office. Although the nurse didn't take me to the same exact room as five years earlier and the purpose of my visit was far more benign, it was the same doctor. I hadn't seen him in a while. I have, after all, been cheating on him with the guy at infectious diseases. So he asked me how I was doing, meaning AIDSwise of course. I told him I had just completed this book and that he was the hero of the opening section. And before we knew it we found ourselves talking about that day five years earlier, a day, as it turned out, he remembers as clearly as I do. ("You were supposed to go to Canada.") His attention had focused on different details—the friend who had given me a ride was sitting in the waiting room looking "like a deer in the headlights"; and he remembers walking toward the examination room as vividly as I remember the car ride to his practice—as a short trip we both had taken on many occasions before but that was this time saturated with sadness and anxiety.

In the end, our brief five-year anniversary conversation wasn't especially complex or meaningful—at least, not on the surface of it, not in the transparent sense of the words we exchanged, but like the nicest anniversaries it was sweet and resolutely unshowy. It all felt very restrained, a bit hesitant and a bit awkward, with a touch perhaps of the sort of shyness that isn't quite shyness but, with eyes averting other eyes, looks like it when it must give palpable form to the fear, inexpressible by nature, of upsetting a delicate balance. My doctor's lament about how difficult it is to give bad news to patients did not come out as tactless at all, like the erasure of my own pain. What makes this task so difficult is the fact that, as was the case with me, patients who are called in urgently to discuss their test results already know what the news is and that it isn't good. The doctor finds himself or herself in the position, obvious to all present, of mimicking the giving of the news already received while well aware that, as a result, much more than news must be conveyed, and with far greater delicacy, by the silent edges that surround these brutal words. Similarly, beyond the words of our recent conversation, or perhaps beside them, near them, lay an unspoken, delicate reality: he hadn't given me some bad news five years earlier; in his own way he had shared it. And violent as this initial contact may have been to both of us, its ripples caress us softly now.

(To the unusual suspect
I hope that you are well)

NAMES

In many ways unplanned (I unexpectedly found myself forced to envisage a new life when I wasn't done messing up the old one yet), this book makes do with what's at hand, what's near and free for the taking. So yes, I talk about myself a lot, it's true, and I understand that some academics find this distasteful in our line of work, but how else, I wonder, may one reflect meaningfully on tact if not at the risk of tactlessness? Furthermore, mine is a self like all selves, really, caught in external forces that shape it in relation to other selves. All the things I wrote on in these pages—9/11, war, torture, yellow stars on lapels, clandestine abortions, the forced unveiling of Muslim women, the incessant brutality of the police, the perils and joys of public sex—are not interchangeable with HIV, the book's impetus and a virus that more and more people are now lucky to be living with instead of dying of; but they are its neighbors. One isn't HIV positive in a vacuum but in the world, near the bodies, actions, and feelings of the people with whom we share this world.

To the extent that being HIV positive—under a successful treatment and without crippling side effects—does actually feel like anything at all, it is only in the way you relate to the world around you and the world relates to you. Millions of people are living with HIV, and more and more have access to life-prolonging treatments, while other people continue to become infected. In other words, more and more of us will be sharing that experience. But as I soon came to realize, one doesn't share HIV only with people who have it. Living with HIV means living alongside people without HIV in a world where the virus is saturated with meaning. It is inevitable that a book about the fear of contact should largely be about them, about that world and about saturation. The life of the mind takes place in the world, after all. And one inhabits the world with one's body—well, maybe not only with one's body, but to do it that way often brings life a unique texture. Queers like me, and presumably all groups of people pushed aside for their irreducible corporeality, find themselves singularly well positioned as a result to propose and, more important, practice the reembodiment of taste, tact, and thought that this book advocates.

Living in such promiscuity often requires what in French is called *faire avec*, a kind of improvisational making-do that bespeaks the handyperson rather than the professional. It also requires on the part of all involved that they draw on the fragile resources of tact. The ultimate point of this essay is that the two—making do and tactfulness—not only have a lot in common but also a lot to tell us about how to live with HIV. Making do may feel constraining, evidently, but may also turn out to be a source of pleasure, of the modest sort one sometimes derives from ingenuity and dexterity and from the short-lived satisfaction found in small victories. Such is the spirit in which these pages were written. Treading water and gasping for air, I didn't embark on a quest; I flailed and groped and took hold of whatever I could reach. Making contact is what it's been all about. What comes after that is of little concern right now; what came before is a different story told here only in bits and pieces. Like Blanche DuBois, this book's tutelary goddess, I have always depended on the kindness of strangers and I do now more than ever.

Luckily, I received a lot of kindness from strangers along the way, as well as incredible support from my friends. To attempt to thank everyone by name, real or made up, would expose me to the risk of tactless oversights—a risk I'd be wise not to take. I won't even try to be exhaustive, then, and will limit myself to those whose fingerprints are all over these pages.

Ross Chambers, Juli Highfill, Nicolas Dupeyron, Bruno Boniface, David Halperin, and Matthieu Dupas have been tireless interlocutors from the start. This book simply would not have been the same without them. David Carroll and Marie-Hélène Huet graciously agreed to write letters in support of my project, and I hope that the final result won't disappoint them. Kane Race, of course, is special.

I presented many parts of this book at conferences and lectures over the past few years, and I have been overwhelmed by the support and incredibly insightful input that people provided. Many thanks to everyone.

I am tremendously grateful to my editor, Richard Morrison, whose support and personal involvement have touched me. Warm thanks also go to three anonymous readers whose reports were so unusually engaged and thoughtful that their suggestions helped me make this book much, much better.

My gratitude to my doctor and his team is, literally, undying.

I owe many thanks to the University of Michigan, in particular the Department of Romance Languages and Literatures, for its very generous support. I was fortunate and greatly honored to have been the recipient of a John Simon Guggenheim Memorial Foundation Fellowship that allowed me to complete the book's first draft.

As for the others, those who helped me get through far more than just the writing of the book, you know who you are, and if you don't, that's probably because you live halfway around the world. I may one day forget some of your names, but the feel of your skin will stay with me forever. I love you all. A book called *The Nearness of Others* belongs to you, and I dedicate it to everyone this stupid pandemic has hurt.

NOTES

Footnotes

6   This quotation is from Adam Mars-Jones's introduction to his volume of short stories about AIDS titled *Monopolies of Loss*, 2.

RB on TB

7   The photograph and caption appear in *Roland Barthes by Roland Barthes*, 30.

Depressed Thinking

18   On melancholia as social phenomenon and a kind of thought in its own right, see Lepenies, *Melancholy and Society*; Kristeva, *Soleil noir*; and Chambers, *Mélancolie et opposition*.

Making Sense

19   All quotations are from Feinberg, *Eighty-Sixed*, 183.

How Can Plain Curiosity Be Unkind?

29   Kureishi, *My Ear at His Heart*, 94.

Speaking of HIV

36   The long quotation is from the beginning of Hervé Guibert's first book dealing with his illness, *To the Friend Who Did Not Save My Life*, 6.

Tough as Nail Polish

40   For a typical example of how early AIDS activists and critics advocated an embrace, rather than rejection, of gay collective values, see Douglas Crimp, "How to Have Promiscuity in an Epidemic." For a more recent argument about the positive uses of camp in the face of the epidemic, see chapter 5 of Kane Race's book *Pleasure Consuming Medicine*.

From Hervé Guibert's Hospital Diary (I)

43   All these quotations are from Guibert, *Cytomégalovirus*, and the translations are mine. "I will ask": 14; "Hospital is hell": 20; "You have to demand respect": 29; "Allow me, Madam": 41–42; "To turn psychological torture": 54; "This morning": 57; "You will have to wait": 58; "I was martyred for peanuts": 63.

Hospital Visits

46   The book I envy was written by Mark Cichocki, and it's called *Living with HIV*. While I'm at it, I should thank Mark for being such a great nurse.

From Hervé Guibert's Hospital Diary (II)

47   Again, from Guibert, *Cytomégalovirus*, 68.

Nearness and Neighborliness

61   Delbo's epigraph is from *Auschwitz and After*, 1.

62   I discuss neighborhoods in my book *My Father and I*.

Beckoning and Appealing

64   Barthes's discussion of the photography is in *Camera Lucida*.

Incomplete Strangers

67   My thinking about the intimation and intimacy, here and later in the book, is indebted to long discussions with Juli Highfill, usually over dinner and drinks. Many thanks.

Ground Zero

68   The quotation is from the Plume edition, 22.

Naked Arab Bodies

72   The quotation by Jean-Luc Nancy comes from *La pensée dérobée*, 13 (my translation).

73   Puar, *Terrorist Assemblages*, 110–11.

73   *Riz noir*, by Anna Moï, is quoted from the Folio edition of the book, 27.

Truth and Torture

78   Scarry, *Body in Pain*, 29.

79   I translated the excerpt from Bizot's book, *Le silence du bourreau*, 46. For stylistic reasons, I decided to keep the masculine pronouns of the original French.

Dining with French People

80 See Scott, *Politics of the Veil*, and Bowen, *Why the French Don't Like Headscarves*.

82 Rancière's discussion of the police vs. equality appears in *The Shores of Politics*.

83 The discussion of visibility and its problems draws on Foucault's *History of Sexuality*, vol. 1.

85 "Muslims are now in a similar position": Scott, *Politics of the Veil*, 117.

86 Diprose, *Corporeal Generosity*, 61.

Encountering the Strange

87 See Davidson, *Only Muslim*.

Times Square Lost

90 Kureishi's remark comes from his novel *Something to Tell You*, 99.

From Public Schools to Public Pools

93 For this tidbit about Denmark, I thank Peter Edelberg.

Particular Bodies

94–95 Jullien, *Impossible Nude*. The ideas I discuss here are found throughout Jullien's essay, but the passages I quote are on page 111.

One Drop of Blood

103 About the oil spill story, see Saulny, "Cajuns on Gulf Worry They May Need to Move On Once Again."

104 See Wiltse, *Contested Waters*.

105 On the question of risk and how it differs from danger, see in particular Deborah Lupton's *Risk* and, in the specific context of HIV and AIDS, Halperin's *What Do Gay Men Want?*

106 For the Louganis quotation, *Breaking the Surface*, xiii.

Shame and Experience

109 Bersani and Phillips, *Intimacies*, 33.

The Doorstep of Shame

110 Ernaux, *Shame*: "I rushed into the store": 93.

Forget Your Health

111, 113 Diprose, *Corporeal Generosity*: "But memory and forgetting": 157; "generosity is the passivity of exposure" and "Before the rational community": 168.

Obama's Disclosures, Forever Deferred

115   "When he says he's a Christian": Senate minority leader Mitch McConnell and Speaker of the House John Boehner have both said that, and many others have made similar comments.

Adventures in Online Cruising

119   "The obligation to confess": *The History of Sexuality*, 1:60.

120   Heartfelt thanks to Trevor Hoppe for sharing his work and unsurpassable expertise on HIV criminalization. His data on nondisclosure and sex offender registries have been especially helpful to me here.

120   J. J. Prescott made his comment at the University of Michigan on January 16, 2012, during "A Panel Discussion of the Michigan Sex Offender Registry" organized by the Prison Creative Arts Project. While HIV nondisclosure is a crime in Michigan, the state does not mandate placement on the sex offender registry for people convicted under that law.

120   Patterson, *Slavery and Social Death*, 41.

121   On the modalities of gay online cruising in relation to HIV disclosure, see Race, "Click Here for HIV Status."

124   My point on the tension between symbolism and thought is indebted to the work of Victor Turner, as discussed by Patterson in *Slavery and Social Death*, 35–36.

125   On the 1973 Acanfora case in Maryland, see Sedgwick, *Epistemology*, 69–70.

125   On French responses to the epidemic, see my *AIDS in French Culture*.

125   Chambers, *Untimely Interventions*. "Flaunting is, par excellence": 239; "They have to get themselves read": 289.

On the Question of Barebacking, Very Briefly

128   For further reading, I send the readers to the authors and texts I referenced: Halperin, *What Do Gay Men Want?*; Dean, *Unlimited Intimacy*; Bersani and Phillips, *Intimacies*; and Tomso, "Bug Chasing, Barebacking, and the Risks of Care" and "Viral Sex and the Politics of Life."

Reasons to Exclude

132   On the death of the author in AIDS writing, see Chambers, *Facing It*.

The Stories of AIDS

133   The theory of genres as organizers of social relations is Anne Freadman's.

A Brief History of HIV/AIDS Disclosure

137   Christophe Broqua's study of ACT UP–Paris and ACT UP's own book provided me with good sources of information for this discussion. Here, too, Freadman's work informs my thinking about genre. I also found Asha Persson and Wendy Richards's work on HIV disclosure among heterosexuals very useful.

Founding Mothers

141   Moore, *PWA*, xxix.

141–42   Weir, *What I Did Wrong*, 60.

Uttering AIDS

144   The study of disclosure is *Mortal Secrets*, and it is much more interesting than its tasteless title may suggest. The quotation is on page 1.

144–45   In addition to this book, I found Green et al.'s *Privacy and Disclosure of HIV* a useful resource.

146   Mark Trautwein's comment is from his op-ed piece in the *New York Times*.

147   On the problematic reliance of closet and coming-out metaphors among heterosexuals with HIV, see the essay by Persson and Richards, "From Closet to Heterotopia."

What I Said and How I Said It

150–51   On the coded ways in which HIV positive gay men disclose their status to peers, see Halperin, *What Do Gay Men Want?*

154   Johnson, *Geography of the Heart*: "There's something you ought to know": 30; "He spoke the terrible facts aloud": 30–31.

155   The book of gay etiquette is *The Essential Book of Gay Manners and Etiquette*, by Steven Petrow.

So Am I

159   Butler, "Imitation and Gender Insubordination," 15.

160   Paul Reed's novel is titled *Facing It*. It isn't a great novel but, given that it appeared so early in the epidemic, it constitutes a fascinating document (109).

Compatible Discordance

164   The works of Emile Benveniste and J. L. Austin are obvious references in this discussion of the pragmatics of utterance as it pertains to disclosure.

166   Brodkey, *This Wild Darkness*: "the overwhelming majority of middle-

class AIDS patients": 86; "The overwhelmingly powerful thrust of bourgeois life": 114.

The Battlefield of the Body

171–79   Ernaux, *Happening* (some translations have been modified): "I kept picturing the same blurred scene": 10; "I got off at Barbès métro station": 7; "I realized that I had lived through events": 11; "His face instantly took on an intrigued, thrilled expression": 26; "I didn't think that Jean T had shown contempt for me": 27–28; "I knew she was greedy for secrets": 47; "The same situation will probably occur": 78; "I realize this": 47 [62 in the French text]; "compared to such people": 42 [55]; "women in Surrealist writing": 37; "Somehow I felt there existed a connection": 24–26; "Connecting different spheres of knowledge": 38; "Clearly, money was a strong motive": 60 [80]; "She attended to her business": 59 [79]; "Although abortion was mentioned": 30; "I don't believe there is a single museum": 67; "I realize this account may exasperate or repel readers": 44 [58]; "I'm no fucking plumber": 79; "In my mind": 80 [108]; "As I am writing this": 68 [92].

176   Brodkey, *This Wild Darkness*: "logic and intelligence depend on a future": 145.

176   Huffer, *Mad for Foucault*, 18.

176   I thank Matthieu Dupas for sharing the idea of the witch as the dark side of science.

Dysclosure

181   Delbo, *Auschwitz and After*.

181   Améry, *At the Mind's Limits*.

181   Brison, *Aftermath*.

182   Feinberg, *Spontaneous Combustion*, 191–92.

184   Scarry, *Body in Pain*, 27.

Towel Stories (III)

187   The song "On a Slow Boat to China" is by Frank Loesser.

Intimacy in Public

191   Schulman, *People in Trouble*, 78.

191–92   This entire passage is from Weir, *What I Did Wrong*, 58.

Accounting for Taste

193–96   A great deal of this section is indebted to Juli Highfill, *Modernism and Its Merchandise*. See also Kolb, *Ambiguity of Taste*.

194   Wald, *Contagious*, 12.

Reembodiment and Discomfort

198 Butler, "Critically Queer," 18.

Reentering the Movie Theater

201 Tsai tells the story of the making of the movie and of his attempts to save the place in an interview with Michael Berry published in *Speaking in Images*; see page 388 in particular.

203 Williams, "Mysteries of the Joy Rio": "He did not go far": 101. The italics, here and in all the other quotations from Williams, are mine.

204 Chambers, *Story and Situation*: "'narratorial' (versus 'narrative') authority": 51; "promoting a *relational*, not informational, concept of discourse": 53.

205 Foucault, *History of Sexuality*, vol. 1: "modern society": 47.

207 Williams, "Hard Candy": "For the Joy Rio is by no means an ordinary theater": 341.

207–8 Rechy, *Numbers*, 95.

Moving in Queer Circles

209–10 Dean, *Unlimited Intimacy*, 187.

210 From Bruce Benderson's essay "Sex and Isolation" in the eponymous book, 26.

212–13 Guy Hocquenghem's *Le gay voyage* has not been translated into English, so I tried my best, with a little help from my friends, to approximate its lyricism. "Hands jerk to the beat of ancient oars": 135; "This is Arab-style cinema": 136; "The neighborhood queens": 135.

213 Leavitt, *Lost Language of Cranes*: "The place he is going has no beginning or end": 79; "The hand strokes Philip's thigh": 81.

Spaces, People, and Actions (I)

216–17 In *Melancholy Drift*, Jean Ma proposes a more systematic reading of Tsai's film in light of Barthes's essay than I attempt to do here. See pages 108–11 in particular.

Spaces, People, and Actions (II)

220 Williams, "Mysteries of the Joy Rio": "The angel of such a place": 103–4.

221 Reechy, *Numbers*, 39–40, 41, 94.

223–24 Howie, *Claustrophilia*: "To touch is to experience a limit": 7; "such an ontology": 7–8.

Again, Where Are the Police?

226–27 I am grateful to Marta Marín-Dòmine for sharing this insight about women as disposable caregivers.

227   Holleran, *Beauty of Men*, 182.

227–28   Coe, *Such Times*, 94.

228   Williams, "Mysteries of the Joy Rio": "According to Emil Kroger": 103.

228   Taussig, *Defacement*, 4. In this passage, Taussig is referencing Freud.

230   On circularity and homosexuality, see Hocquenghem, *Homosexual Desire*.

231   Howie, *Claustrophilia*: "the fundamentally erotic approximations of anachronism": 7.

231   Ricco, *Logic of the Lure*, 10.

Hostile Bodies (and the People Who Love Them)

239   Moore, *PWA*, xxv.

Sharing: From Disclosure to Tact

242–43   Shurin, *Unbound*: "We have conversations in various forms" and "His news precedes him": 17; "Sometimes we know things about each other": 17–18; "Eric was my good friend T's sometime lover": 19; "His desire to charm outpointed his powerful adversary," "it was for *him* I did it," "I was nervous," "Almost immediately, he showed me": 20.

Tactful Encounters

247   Guibert's reference to the Nazi doctor is in *The Compassion Protocol*.

247   I proposed detailed readings of Dreuilhe's *Mortal Embrace* in *My Father and I* and "AIDS/Holocaust: Metaphor and French Universalism."

248   See Crimp, "Portrait of People with AIDS."

250   See Chambers, "Long Howl."

Tact and Delicacy (II)

253–55   Barthes, *Neutral*: "Tied to language, founded by it, tact": 34–35; *prendre la tangente* vs. dodging: 167 (French text), 127 (English text); "Sade's very utterance": 29–30 [58–59].

255   Sade's words, "the most singular and bizarre of them," are quoted in Barthes, *Sade, Fourier, Loyola*, 190 [174].

255   The quotation "vous savez que personne n'analyse les choses comme moi" appears, with the rest of the letter, in volume 12 of Sade's *Oeuvres complètes*, 412.

Tact and Delicacy (III)

257   Jung, "Psychological Aspects of the Mother Archetype," vol. 9, pt. 1 of *The Collected Works of C. G. Jung*, 86–87.

257–58   Quoted in Lohser and Newton, *Unorthodox Freud*: "The 'Recommendations on Technique' I wrote long ago": 15; "All those who have no tact": 16.

258   For an in-depth discussion of homosexuality's association with archaism, see my book *My Father and I*.

Tact, Power, and the Police (I)

259   Some basic characteristics of tact are fairly well explained in van Manen's *Tact of Teaching*.

260   Foucault, *History of Sexuality*, 1:17–18.

261   Adorno, *Minima Moralia*: "For tact, we now know, has its precise historical hour": 36; "when emancipated, [tact] confronts the individual as an absolute": 37. I thank George Hoffmann for bringing this essay to my attention.

261–62   Sartre, *Anti-Semite and Jew*, 124.

264   Jean-Luc Nancy's idea of fascism as the community of fusion is developed in *The Inoperative Community*.

264   Racine's line and Maurras's assertion that the Jews are unable to understand it is quoted in *Anti-Semite and Jew*, 24, where Sartre also uses the metaphor of fusion to describe anti-Semitic affect.

Tact, Power, and the Police (II)

266, 268, 270   Goffman, *Interaction Ritual*: "to appear flustered": 101–2; "During interaction": 105–6; "sharing this sentiment," "By the standards of the wider society," "But of course the trouble does not stop with the guilty pair": 106.

266   Scarry, *Body in Pain*, 27.

267   Giddens, *Social Theory*, 113.

269   Rancière, *On the Shores of Politics*, 82.

270   Barthes, *Sade, Fourier, Loyola*, 170–71 (translation modified).

Tact and Contamination

271, 272, 273   Littell, *Kindly Ones*: "I found it": 664; "insisted that, yes": 665; "but perhaps it was also": 665; "for that there could only have been one reason": 666 [952].

271   There is a detailed discussion of the euphemisms used by the Nazis in relation to the Holocaust in Arendt's *Eichmann in Jerusalem*.

272   I found this translation of Himmler's speech on www.holocaust-history.org. I modified it a little.

Tact and Silence

274   Barthes, *Neutral*: "*tacere*": 22; "In such a 'semiology,'" "in fact, in every 'totalitarian' or 'totalizing' society," "'imprisoned by reason of implicitness'": 24 [52].

275–76   Zerubavel, *Elephant in the Room*: "between the private act of noticing and the public act of acknowledging": 2; "And the difference between what we actually notice": 31; "examine institutionalized prohibitions": 15; "In other words, the very act of avoiding the elephant is itself an elephant!": 53.

277   Rancière, *Shores of Politics*, 69–70.

Tact and Failure

278   Delbo, *Mesure de nos jours*, 144–45; "The tenderness in Carmen's voice was true": 145 (my translation).

The Kindness of Strangers

281   Williams, *Streetcar Named Desire*: "There was something different about the boy": 182–83; "and all I knew was that I'd failed him," "Then I found out," "Afterwards we pretended": 183; "I saw! I know! You disgust me": 184.

Sunday in the Park with . . . ?

283–84   Holleran, *Ground Zero*, 78–79; "thinking, *There is no need to stay*," "I left O.'s block," "the sites of those strolls," "I looked back, and we began to circle": 79; "his friends were dying": 47; "we said nothing": 80.

283   Delbo, *Mesure de nos jours*, 313 [145].

283–84   Davis, *Valley of the Shadow*, 145.

284   Barthes, *Journal de deuil*, 212.

The Yellow Star

285–88   "I was very courageous": 54 [57–58]; "I got to the main courtyard of the Sorbonne": 55–56 [59–60]; "We talked about the exam" 56 [60]; "My confidence got a boost": 57–58 [61–62]; "Yesterday at the Sorbonne": 165–66 [178–79]; "How to escape this dilemma," "Souls like that": 166; [179] (my emphasis).

289   Sartre, *Anti-Semite and Jew*, 77.

290   For Derrida on the gift, go to *Glas*, *Mémoires: For Paul de Man*, and *Ulysse Gramophone: Deux mots pour Joyce*.

Tact as Social Music Making

291–93, 295   Guibert, *Compassion Protocol*: "Not a single word was uttered": 4 [12] (translation modified, my emphases); "I understand": 22; "who never utters one word more or less than is necessary": [29] (my translation); "I'm so knocked out": 5; "That was the contract we embarked upon": 6 [14] (my emphasis); "The alveolar lavage": 62 [75] (translation modified).

293　On *Takt*, see van Manen, *Tact of Teaching*.

293, 294　The episode of the concert in Venice is recounted by Goethe in his *Travels in Italy*, 129 (translation modified); that of the concert in Naples is found in Berlioz's *Mémoires*, 1:260. I thank Ross Chambers for passing these excerpts on to me.

A Fart Joke from Proust

297　Need I express how grateful I am to Katherine Ibbett for having reminded me of this lovely passage? It is found in *The Captive*, page 482, of the Wordsworth two-volume edition and, for the French, in *La prisonnière*, volume 11 of the fifteen-volume Gallimard edition of 1946–47.

Touch and Other Senses

299　On touch as the most basic of all senses, see Donald A. Landes's reading of Nancy and Derrida, in "*Le toucher* and the *Corpus* of Tact."

Reentering the Movie Theater's Restroom

303　Rechy, *Numbers*: "he knows all this is a matter of marking time": 40; "Quite probably this theater": 40–41; "The man moves over": 42.

Found Objects (I): Tact and Bearing Witness as Forms of Bricolage

306　Delbo, *Auschwitz and After*, 108.

307　Goffman, *Interaction Ritual*, 99.

Tactfulness to the Dead

309　Barthes, *Neutral*, 33–34.

Found Objects (II): Some Beauty

310　Guibert, *Compassion Protocol*: "as if she were asking herself": 97 [114] (translation modified); "With a subtle smile": 98 [115] (translation modified).

BIBLIOGRAPHY

ACT UP–Paris. *La sida: Combien de divisions?* Paris: Dagorno, 1994.

Adorno, Theodor. *Minima Moralia: Reflections from Damaged Life.* Trans. by E. F. N. Jephcott. New York: Verso, 1978. Trans. of *Minima Moralia.* Frankfurt am Main: Suhrkamp Verlag, 1951.

Althusser, Louis. "Ideology and State Ideological Apparatuses." *Lenin and Philosophy and Other Essays.* London: New Left Books, 1971.

Améry, Jean. *At the Mind's Limits: Contemplations by a Survivor on Auschwitz and Its Realities.* Trans. by Sidney Rosenfeld and Stella P. Rosenfeld. Bloomington: Indiana University Press, 1980. Trans. of *Jenseits von Schuld und Sühne: Bewälti-gungsversuche eines Überwältigen.* Munich: Szczesny, 1966.

Arendt, Hannah. *Eichmann in Jerusalem: A Report on the Banality of Evil.* New York: Viking, 1963.

Austin, John Langshaw. *How to Do Things with Words.* Cambridge, Mass.: Harvard University Press, 1962.

Barthes, Roland. *Camera Lucida: Reflections on Photography.* Trans. by Richard How-ard. New York: Hill and Wang, 1981. Trans. of *La chambre claire: Note sur la pho-tographie.* Paris: Gallimard/Seuil, 1980.

———. "The Death of the Author." In *The Rustle of Language.* Trans. by Richard How-ard. Berkeley: University of California Press, 1989. Trans. of *Le bruissement de la langue.* Paris: Seuil, 1984.

———. *Journal de deuil.* Paris: Seuil/Imec, 2009.

———. "Leaving the Movie Theater." In *The Rustle of Language.* Trans. by Richard Howard. Berkeley: University of California Press, 1989: 345–49. Trans. of *Le bruissement de la langue.* Paris: Seuil, 1984.

———. *Littérature et réalité.* Paris: Seuil, 1982.

———. *The Neutral.* Trans. by Rosalind E. Kraus and Denis Hollier. New York: Co-lumbia University Press, 2005. Trans. of *Le neuter.* Paris: Seuil, 2002.

———. *Roland Barthes by Roland Barthes.* Trans. by Richard Howard. Berkeley: Uni-versity of California Press, 1994. Trans. of *Roland Barthes par Roland Barthes.* Paris: Seuil, 1975.

———. *Sade, Fourier, Loyola.* Trans. by Richard Miller. New York: Hill and Wang, 1976. Trans. of *Sade, Fourier, Loyola.* Paris: Seuil, 1971.

The Basketball Diaries. Dir. Scott Calvert. New Line Cinema, 1995.

Benderson, Bruce. *Sex and Isolation and Other Essays.* Madison: University of Wisconsin Press, 2007.

Benveniste, Emile. *Problèmes de linguistique générale.* 2 vols. Paris: Gallimard, 1966, 1974.

Berlioz, Hector. *Mémoires.* Vol. 1. Paris: Garnier-Flammarion, 1969.

Berr, Hélène. *The Journal of Hélène Berr.* Trans. by David Bellos. New York: Weinstein Books, 2008. Trans. of *Journal.* Paris: Tallandier, 2008.

Berry, Michael. *Speaking in Images: Interviews with Contemporary Chinese Filmmakers.* New York: Columbia University Press, 2005.

Bersani, Leo, and Adam Phillips. *Intimacies.* Chicago: University of Chicago Press, 2008.

Bizot, François. *Le silence du bourreau.* Paris: Flammarion, 2011.

Bourdieu, Pierre. *Distinction: A Social Critique of the Judgment of Taste.* Trans. by Richard Nice. Cambridge, Mass.: Harvard University Press, 1984. Trans. of *La distinction: Critique sociale du jugement.* Paris: Minuit, 1979.

Bowen, John R. *Why the French Don't Like Headscarves: Islam, the State, and Public Space.* Princeton, N.J.: Princeton University Press, 2007.

Breaking the Surface: The Greg Louganis Story. Dir. Steven Hillard Stern. Green/Epstein Productions, 1997.

Brison, Susan. *Aftermath: Violence and the Remaking of a Self.* Princeton, N.J.: Princeton University Press, 2002.

Brodkey, Harold. *This Wild Darkness: The Story of My Death.* New York: Metropolitan Books, 1996.

Broqua, Christophe. *Agir pour ne pas mourir: Act Up, les homosexuels et le sida.* Paris: Presses de la fondation nationale des sciences politiques, 2005.

Butler, Judith. "Critically Queer." *GLQ* 1.1 (1993): 17–32.

———. "Imitation and Gender Insubordination." In *Inside/Out: Lesbian Theories, Gay Theories,* ed. by Diana Fuss. New York: Routledge, 1991: 13–31.

Caron, David. "AIDS/Holocaust: Metaphor and French Universalism." *L'esprit créateur* 45.3 (2006): 63–73.

———. *AIDS in French Culture: Social Ills, Literary Cures.* Madison: University of Wisconsin Press, 2001.

———. *My Father and I: The Marais and the Queerness of Community.* Ithaca, N.Y.: Cornell University Press, 2009.

———. "Shame on Me, or the Naked Truth about Me and Marlene Dietrich." In *Gay Shame,* ed. by David M. Halperin and Valerie Traub. Chicago: University of Chicago Press, 2009: 117–31.

Certeau, Michel de. *The Practice of Everyday Life.* Trans. by Steven Rendall. Minneapolis: University of Minnesota Press, 1998. Trans. of *L'invention du quotidien.* Paris: Gallimard, 1980.

Chambers, Ross. *Facing It: AIDS Diaries and the Death of the Author*. Ann Arbor: University of Michigan Press, 1998.

———. "The Long Howl: Serial Torture." *Yale French Studies* 118–19 (2010): 39–51.

———. *Mélancolie et opposition: Les débuts du modernisme en France*. Paris: Corti, 1987.

———. *Story and Situation: Narrative Seduction and the Power of Fiction*. Minneapolis: University of Minnesota Press, 1984.

———. *Untimely Interventions: AIDS Writing, Testimonial, and the Rhetoric of Haunting*. Ann Arbor: University of Michigan Press, 2004.

Cichocki, Mark. *Living with HIV: A Patient's Guide*. Jefferson, N.C.: McFarland, 2009.

Coe, Christopher. *Such Times*. New York: Harcourt Brace, 1993.

Cole, Joshua. "Intimate Acts and Unspeakable Relations: Remembering Torture and the War for Algerian Independence." In *Memory, Empire, and Postcolonialism: Legacies of French Colonialism*, ed. by Alec G. Hargreaves. Lanham, Md.: Lexington Books, 2005: 125–41.

Crimp, Douglas, ed. *AIDS: Cultural Analysis, Cultural Activism*. Cambridge, Mass.: MIT Press, 1988.

———. "How to Have Promiscuity in an Epidemic." In Crimp, *AIDS*: 237–71.

———. "Portrait of People with AIDS." In *Cultural Studies*, ed. by Lawrence Grossberg, Cary Nelson, and Paula Treichler. New York: Routledge, 1991: 117–30.

Davidson, Naomi. *Only Muslim: Embodying Islam in Twentieth-Century France*. Ithaca, N.Y.: Cornell University Press, 2012.

Davis, Christopher. *Valley of the Shadow*. New York: Stonewall Inn, 1988.

Dean, Tim. *Unlimited Intimacy: Reflections on the Subculture of Barebacking*. Chicago: University of Chicago Press, 2009.

Delany, Samuel R. *Tines Square Red, Times Square Blue*. New York: New York University Press, 1999.

Delbo, Charlotte. *Aucun de nous ne reviendra*. Paris: Minuit, 1970.

———. *Auschwitz and After*. Trans. by Rosette C. Lamont. New Haven, Conn.: Yale University Press, 1995.

———. *Une connaissance inutile*. Paris: Minuit, 1970.

———. *Mesure de nos jours*. Paris: Minuit, 1971.

DeLillo, Don. *Falling Man*. New York: Picador, 2007.

Derrida, Jacques. *Glas*. Trans. by John P. Leavy and Richard Rand. Lincoln: University of Nebraska Press, 1986. Trans. of *Glas*. Paris: Galilée, 1974.

———. *Mémoires: For Paul de Man*. Trans. by Cecile Lindsay, Jonathan Culler, and Eduardo Cadava. New York: Columbia University Press, 1986. Trans. of *Mémoires, pour Paul de Man*. Paris: 1988.

———. *Ulysse Gramophone: Deux mots pour Joyce*. Paris: Galilée, 1987.

Diprose, Rosalyn. *Corporeal Generosity: On Giving with Nietzsche, Merleau-Ponty, and Levinas*. Albany: State University of New York Press, 2002.

Dolnick, Sam. "A Long Jump to Manhood in the Bronx." *New York Times*, July 18, 2010.

Douthat, Ross. "Islam and the Two Americas." www.nytimes.com/2010/08/16
/opinion/ (accessed December 6, 2010).

Dragon Gate Inn (*Long men ke zhen*). Dir. King Hu. Union Film Company, 1967.

Dreuilhe, Alain Emmanuel. *Mortal Embrace: Living with AIDS.* Trans. by Linda Coverdale. New York: Hill and Wang, 1988. Trans. of *Corps à corps: Journal de sida.*
Paris: Gallimard, 1987.

Ernaux, Annie. *Happening.* Trans. by Tanya Leslie. New York: Seven Stories, 2001.
Trans. of *L'événement.* Paris: Gallimard, 2000.

———. *Shame.* Trans. by Tanya Leslie. New York: Seven Stories, 1998. Trans. of *La
honte.* Paris: Gallimard, 1997.

Feinberg, David B. *Eighty-Sixed.* New York: Viking, 1989.

———. *Spontaneous Combustion.* New York: Viking, 1991.

Ferenczi, Sándor. "The Elasticity of Psycho-Analytic Technique." In *Final Contributions
to the Problems and Methods of Psychoanalysis,.* Ed. by Michael Balint, trans. by Eric
Mosbacher and others. London: Hogarth, 1955.

Foucault, Michel. *The Archeology of Knowledge.* Trans. by A. M. Sheridan Smith. New
York: Pantheon, 1972. Trans. of *L'archéologie du savoir.* Paris: Gallimard, 1969.

———. *The History of Sexuality.* Trans. by Robert Hurley. New York: Pantheon, 1978.
Trans. of *Histoire de la sexualité.* Paris: Gallimard, 1976.

Freadman, Anne, and Amanda Macdonald. *What Is This Thing Called Genre? Four Essays in the Semiotics of Genre.* Mount Nebo, Queensland: Boombana Publications,
1992.

Freud, Sigmund. "'Wild' Psycho-Analysis." *Standard Edition,* vol. 11. Trans. and ed. by
James Strachey. London: Hogarth, 1957: 221–27.

Giddens, Anthony. *Social Theory and Modern Sociology.* Cambridge: Polity, 1987.

Goethe, J. W. von. *Letters from Switzerland and Travels in Italy.* Ed. by Frederic Henry
Hedge and L. Noa. Trans. by Alexander James William Morrison. Boston: S. E.
Cassino, 1884. Trans. of *Italienische Reise,* 1816–17.

Goffman, Erving. *Interaction Ritual: Essays on Face-to-Face Behavior.* New York: Pantheon, 1967.

———. *Stigma: Notes on the Management of Spoiled Identity.* New York: Simon and
Schuster, 1963.

Goodbye, Dragon Inn (*Bu san*). Dir. Tsai Ming-Liang. Homegreen Films, 2003.

Green, Kathryn, Valerian J. Derlega, Gust A. Yep, and Sandra Petronio. *Privacy and
Disclosure of HIV in Interpersonal Relationships: A Sourcebook for Researchers and
Practitioners.* Mahwah, N.J.: Lawrence Erlbaum Associates, 2003.

Guibert, Hervé. *The Compassion Protocol.* Trans. by James Kirkup. New York: Braziller,
1994. Trans. of *Le Protocole compassionnel.* Paris: Gallimard, 1991.

———. *Cytomégalovirus.* Paris: Seuil, 1992.

———. *To the Friend Who Did Not Save My Life.* Trans. by Linda Coverdale. New
York: High Risk Books, 1994. Trans. of *A l'ami qui ne m'a pas sauvé la vie.* Paris:
Gallimard, 1990.

Halperin, David M. *What Do Gay Men Want? Essays on Sex, Risk, and Subjectivity.* Ann Arbor: University of Michigan Press, 2007.

Highfill, Juli. *Modernism and Its Merchandise: The Spanish Avant-Garde and Material Culture.* University Park: Pennsylvania State University Press, 2014.

Himmler, Heinrich. Address, October 4, 1943, Posen, Poland. www.holocaust-history org/himmler-poznan/speech-text.shtml (accessed May 27, 2011).

Hocquenghem, Guy. *Le gay voyage: Guide et regard homosexuels sur les grandes métropoles.* Paris: Albin Michel, 1980.

———. *Homosexual Desire.* Trans. by Daniella Dangoor. London: Allison and Busby, 1978. Trans. of *Le désir homosexuel.* Paris: Editions universitaires, 1972.

Hofmann, Regan. "Sweet Home Alabama." *Poz*, April 2008, 22–25.

Holleran, Andrew. *The Beauty of Men.* New York: Morrow, 1996.

———. *Ground Zero.* New York: Morrow, 1988.

Howie, Cary. *Claustrophilia: The Erotics of Enclosure in Medieval Literature.* New York: Palgrave, 2007.

Huffer, Lynne. *Mad for Foucault: Rethinking the Foundations of Queer Theory.* New York: Columbia University Press, 2010.

Johnson, Fenton. *Geography of the Heart.* New York: Scribner, 1996.

Jullien, François. *The Impossible Nude: Chinese Art and Western Aesthetics.* Trans. by Maev de la Guardia. Chicago: Chicago University Press, 2007. Trans. of *Le nu impossible.* Paris: Seuil, 2000.

Jung, Carl Gustav. *The Archetypes and the Collective Unconscious.* Vol. 9, part 1 of *The Collected Works of C. G. Jung.* Ed. by Sir Herbert Read, Michael Fordham, and Gerhard Adler. Trans. by R. F. C. Hull. New York: Pantheon Books, 1959.

Klitzman, Robert, and Ronald Beyer. *Mortal Secrets: Truth and Lies in the Age of AIDS.* Baltimore, Md.: Johns Hopkins University Press, 2003.

Kolb, Jocelyne. *The Ambiguity of Taste: Freedom and Food in European Romanticism.* Ann Arbor: University of Michigan Press, 1995.

Kristeva, Julia. *Soleil noir: Dépression et mélancolie.* Paris: Gallimard, 1987.

Kureishi, Hanif. *My Ear at His Heart: Reading My Father.* London: Faber and Faber, 2004.

———. *Something to Tell You.* New York: Scribner, 2008.

Landes, Donald A. "*Le toucher* and the *Corpus* of Tact: Exploring Touch and Technicity with Jacques Derrida and Jean-Luc Nancy." *L'Esprit Créateur* 47.3 (2007): 80–92.

Laqueur, Thomas. *Making Sex: Body and Gender from the Greeks to Freud.* Cambridge, Mass.: Harvard University Press, 1990.

Leavitt, David. *The Lost Language of Cranes.* New York: Knopf, 1986.

———. "Saturn Street." In *Arkansas: Three Novellas.* Boston: Houghton Mifflin, 1997.

Lepenies, Wolf. *Melancholy and Society.* Trans. by Jeremy Gaines and Doris Jones. Cambridge, Mass.: Harvard University Press, 1992. Trans. of *Melancholie und Gesellschaft.* Frankfurt: Suhrkamp, 1969.

Lingis, Alphonso. *The Community of Those Who Have Nothing in Common*. Blooming-ton: Indiana University Press, 1994.

Littell, Jonathan. *The Kindly Ones*. Trans. by Charlotte Mandell. New York: Harper, 2009. Trans. of *Les bienveillantes*. Paris: Gallimard, 2006.

Lohser, Beate, and Peter M. Newton. *Unorthodox Freud: The View from the Couch*. New York: Guilford, 1996.

Louganis, Greg, with Eric Marcus. *Breaking the Surface*. New York: Random House, 1995.

Lupton, Deborah. *Risk*. London: Routledge, 1999.

Ma, Jean. *Melancholy Drift: Marking Time in Chinese Cinema*. Hong Kong: Hong Kong University Press, 2010.

Manen, Max van. *The Tact of Teaching: The Meaning of Pedagogical Thoughtfulness*. Al-bany: State University of New York Press, 1991.

Mars-Jones, Adam. *Monopolies of Loss*. New York: Knopf, 1993.

Moï, Anna. *Riz noir*. Paris: Gallimard, 2004.

Montaigne, Michel de. "De la conscience." In *Les Essais*. Vol. 2. Paris: PUF/Quaridge, 1988: 366–69.

Moore, Oscar. *PWA: Looking AIDS in the Face*. London: Picador, 1996.

Nancy, Jean-Luc. *The Inoperative Community*. Trans. by Peter Conner, Lisa Garbus, Michael Holland, and Simona Sawhney. Minneapolis: University of Minnesota Press, 1991. Trans. of *La communauté désoeuvrée*. Paris: Christian Bourgois, 1986.

———. *La pensée dérobée*. Paris: Galilée, 2001.

Olympia. Dir. Leni Riefenstahl. International Olympic Committee, 1938.

Patterson, Orlando. *Slavery and Social Death: A Comparative Study*. Cambridge, Mass.: Harvard University Press, 1982.

Persson, Asha, and Wendy Richards. "From Closet to Heterotopia: A Conceptual Exploration of Disclosure and 'Passing' among Heterosexuals Living with HIV." *Culture, Health, and Sexuality* 10.1 (2008): 73–86.

Petrow, Steven, with Nick Steele. *The Essential Book of Gay Manners and Etiquette*. New York: Harper, 1995.

Poison. Dir. Todd Haynes. Bronze Eye Productions, 1991.

Porn Theater (*La chatte à deux têtes*). Dir. Jacques Nolot. Elia Films, 2002.

Proust, Marcel. *Remembrance of Things Past*. Trans. by C. K. Scott Moncrief and Ste-phen Hudson. London: Wordsworth, 2006. Trans. of *A la recherche du temps per-du*. Paris: Gallimard, 1946–47.

Puar, Jasbir K. *Terrorist Assemblages: Homonationalism in Queer Times*. Durham, N.C.: Duke University Press, 2007.

La pudeur ou l'impudeur. Dir. Hervé Guibert. TF1: 1992.

Race, Kane. "Click Here for HIV Status: Shifting Templates of Sexual Negotiation." *Emotion, Space, and Society* (2010), doi: 10.10.16/j.emospa.2010.01.003.

————. *Pleasure Consuming Medicine: The Queer Politics of Drugs.* Durham, N.C.: Duke University Press, 2009.

Rancière, Jacques. *The Shores of Politics.* Trans. by Liz Heron. London: Verso, 1995. Trans. of *Aux bords du politique.* Paris: Osiris, 1992.

Rechy, John. *Numbers.* New York: Grove, 1967.

Reed, Paul. *Facing It: A Novel of AIDS.* San Francisco: Gay Sunshine, 1984.

Renan, Ernest. *Qu'est-ce qu'une nation?* Paris: Mille et une nuits, 1997.

Ricco, John Paul. *The Logic of the Lure.* Chicago: University of Chicago Press, 2002.

"The Rise of Muslim Europe: What It Means for the Jews and Israel." *Jewish Journal of Greater Los Angeles* 24.2 (2009): 10–12.

Ross, Andrew. *The Celebration Chronicles: Life, Liberty, and the Pursuit of Property Value in Disney's New Town.* New York: Ballantine Books, 2000.

Ross, Kristin. *May '68 and Its Afterlives.* Chicago: University of Chicago Press, 2002.

Sade, Donatien Alphonse François de. *Oeuvres complètes.* Vol. 12. Ed. by Gilbert Lely. Paris: Cercle du livre précieux, 1966.

Said, Edward. *Orientalism.* New York: Pantheon, 1978.

Sartre, Jean-Paul. *Anti-Semite and Jew.* Trans. by George J. Becker. New York: Schocken Books, 1948. Trans. of *Réflexions sur la question juive.* Paris: Gallimard, 1954.

Saulny, Susan. "Cajuns on Gulf Worry They May Need to Move On Once Again." *New York Times,* July 19, 2010.

Scarry, Elaine. *The Body in Pain: The Making and Unmaking of the World.* New York: Oxford University Press, 1985.

Schulman, Sarah. *People in Trouble.* New York: Dutton, 1990.

Scott, Joan Wallach. *The Politics of the Veil.* Princeton, N.J.: Princeton University Press, 2007.

Sedgwick, Eve Kosofsky. *Epistemology of the Closet.* Berkeley: University of California Press, 1990.

Serbis. Dir. Brillante Ma Mendoza. Centerstage Productions, 2008.

Shoah. Dir. Claude Lanzmann. Les Films Aleph and Historia Films, 1985.

Shurin, Aaron. *Unbound: A Book of AIDS.* Los Angeles: Sun and Moon, 1997.

Stolen Kisses (Baisers Volés). Dir. François Truffaut. Les films du carosse, 1969.

Taussig, Michael. *Defacement: Public Secrecy and the Labor of the Negative.* Stanford, Calif.: Stanford University Press, 1999.

Taxi to the Dark Side. Dir. Alex Gibney. Jigsaw Productions, 2007.

The Thorn Birds. David Wolper-Stan Margulies Productions, 1983.

Tomso, Gregory. "Bug Chasing, Barebacking, and the Risks of Care." *Literature and Medicine* 23.1 (2004): 88–111.

————. "Viral Sex and the Politics of Life." *South Atlantic Quarterly* 107.2 (2008): 265–85.

Trautwein, Mark. "The Death Sentence That Defined My Life." *New York Times,* June 5, 2011.

Trop de Bonheur. Dir. Cédric Kahn. IMA Productions, 1994.

Turner, Victor. *The Forest of Symbols.* Ithaca, N.Y.: Cornell University Press, 1967.

The Umbrellas of Cherbourg (Les parapluies de Cherbourg). Dir. Jacques Demy. Parc Film, 1964.

Wald, Priscilla. *Contagious: Cultures, Carriers, and the Outbreak Narrative.* Durham, N.C.: Duke University Press, 2008.

Weir, John. *What I Did Wrong.* New York: Viking, 2006.

Wild Reeds (Les roseaux sauvages). Dir. André Téchiné. IMA Fils/Les films Alain Sarde, 1994.

Williams, Tennessee. "The Mysteries of the Joy Rio" and "Hard Candy." In *Collected Stories.* New York: New Directions, 1985.

———. *A Streetcar Named Desire.* New York: Penguin, 1980.

Wiltse, Jess. *Contested Waters: A Social History of Swimming Pools in America.* Chapel Hill: University of North Carolina Press, 2007.

Yaeger, Patricia. "Testimony without Intimacy." *Poetics Today* 27.2 (2006): 399–423.

Zerubavel, Eviatar. *The Elephant in the Room: Silence and Denial in Everyday Life.* Oxford: Oxford University Press, 2006.

DAVID CARON is professor of French and women's studies at the University of Michigan. He is the author of *AIDS in French Culture: Social Ills, Literary Cures* and *My Father and I: The Marais and the Queerness of Community*. He is coeditor of *Les revenantes: Charlotte Delbo, la voix d'une communauté à jamais déportée*. He has written on HIV/AIDS, the Holocaust, and French and gay literature and culture, and has been the recipient of fellowships from the National Endowment for the Humanities and the John Simon Guggenheim Memorial Foundation.